Drinking
Water
and
Health

Volume 2

SAFE DRINKING WATER COMMITTEE

Board on Toxicology and
   Environmental Health Hazards
Assembly of Life Sciences
National Research Council

NATIONAL ACADEMY PRESS
Washington, D.C. 1980

ALL377

The National Research Council was established by the National Academy of Sciences in 1916 to associate the broad community of science and technology with the Academy's purposes of furthering knowledge and of advising the federal government. The Council operates in accordance with general policies determined by the Academy under the authority of its Congressional charter of 1863, which establishes the Academy as a private, non-profit, self-governing membership corporation. The Council has become the principal operating agency of both the Academy of Sciences and the National Academy of Engineering in the conduct of their services to the government, the public, and the scientific and engineering communities. It is administered jointly by both Academies and the Institute of Medicine. The Academy of Engineering and the Institute of Medicine were established in 1964 and 1970, respectively, under the charter of the Academy of Sciences.

NOTICE: The project that is the subject of this report was approved by the Governing Board of the National Research Council, whose members are drawn from the Councils of the National Academy of Sciences, the National Academy of Engineering, and the Institute of Medicine. The members of the Committee responsible for the report were chosen for their competences and with regard for appropriate balance.

This report has been reviewed by a group other than the authors according to procedures approved by a Report Review Committee consisting of members of the National Academy of Sciences, the National Academy of Engineering, and the Institute of Medicine.

At the request of and funded by the
U.S. Environmental Protection Agency
Contract No. 68-01-3169

Library of Congress Catalog Card Number: 77-89284

International Standard Book Number 0-309-02931-7

Available from

NATIONAL ACADEMY PRESS
2101 Constitution Avenue, N.W.
Washington, D.C. 20418

Printed in the United States of America

List of Participants

SAFE DRINKING WATER COMMITTEE

JOHN DOULL, University of Kansas Medical Center, Kansas City, *Chairman*

J. CARRELL MORRIS, Harvard University, Cambridge, Massachusetts, *Vice Chairman*

JOSEPH F. BORZELLECA, Medical College of Virginia, Richmond

RICHARD S. ENGELBRECHT, University of Illinois, Urbana

DAVID G. HOEL, National Institute of Environmental Health Sciences, Research Triangle Park, North Carolina

CORNELIUS W. KRUSÉ, Johns Hopkins University, Baltimore

EDWIN H. LENNETTE, California Department of Health, Berkeley

SHELDON D. MURPHY, University of Texas Medical School of Houston

PAUL M. NEWBERNE, Massachusetts Institute of Technology, Cambridge

MALCOLM C. PIKE, University of Southern California, Los Angeles

MARVIN A. SCHNEIDERMAN, National Cancer Institute, Bethesda, Maryland

RONALD C. SHANK, University of California, Irvine

IRWIN H. SUFFET, Drexel University, Philadelphia

SHELDON WOLFF, University of California, San Francisco

NAS–NRC Staff

RILEY D. HOUSEWRIGHT, *Project Director*
ROBERT J. GOLDEN, *Assistant Project Director*
ROY WIDDUS, *Staff Officer*
FRANCES M. PETER, *Editor*

Subcommittee on Adsorption

IRWIN H. SUFFET, Drexel University, Philadelphia, *Chairman*
MARTIN ALEXANDER, Cornell University, Ithaca, New York
JOHN T. COOKSON, JR., JTC Environmental Consultants, Inc., Bethesda, Maryland
FRANCIS DIGIANO, University of Massachusetts, Amherst
ROBERT KUNIN, Yardley, Pennsylvania
JOSEPH SHANDS, University of Florida, Gainesville
VERNON L. SNOEYINK, University of Illinois, Urbana

Subcommittee on Chemistry of Disinfectants and Products

J. CARRELL MORRIS, Harvard University, Cambridge, Massachusetts, *Chairman*
RUSSELL F. CHRISTMAN, University of North Carolina, Chapel Hill, *Vice Chairman*
WILLIAM H. GLAZE, North Texas State University, Denton
ROBERT C. HOEHN, Virginia Polytechnic Institute and State University, Blacksburg
ROBERT L. JOLLEY, Oak Ridge National Laboratory, Tennessee

Subcommittee on Efficacy of Disinfection

RICHARD S. ENGELBRECHT, University of Illinois, Urbana, *Chairman*
MARTIN FAVERO, Center for Disease Control, Phoenix, Arizona
ARNOLD GREENBERG, California Department of Health, Berkeley
J. DONALD JOHNSON, University of North Carolina, Chapel Hill
CORNELIUS W. KRUSÉ, Johns Hopkins University, Baltimore
EDWIN H. LENNETTE, California Department of Health, Berkeley
WALTER L. NEWTON, Fairfax, Virginia
VINCENT P. OLIVIERI, Johns Hopkins University, Baltimore
PASQUALE V. SCARPINO, University of Cincinnati
OTIS J. SPROUL, Ohio State University, Columbus

Consultant

MICHAEL J. McGUIRE, Metropolitan Water District of Southern California, Los Angeles

EPA Project Officer

JOSEPH COTRUVO, Office of Water Supply, U.S. Environmental Protection Agency, Washington, D.C.

EPA Liaison Representative

WILLIAM MARCUS, Office of Water Supply, U.S. Environmental Protection Agency, Washington, D.C.

Contents

Preface

In 1975 the National Academy of Sciences–National Research Council initiated a series of studies to meet the congressional mandate of the Safe Drinking Water Act (PL 93-523). Results of these studies were published in *Drinking Water and Health* (National Academy of Sciences, 1977). Amendments to the act in 1977 called for revisions of the studies "reflecting new information which has become available since the most recent previous report [and which] shall be reported to the Congress each two years thereafter" (see Appendix).

Results of studies completed by the Safe Drinking Water Committee since 1977 are contained in this book and a companion volume, *Drinking Water and Health,* Volume 3. This book contains an assessment of processes and chemicals for the disinfection of drinking water, identification of the by-products resulting from their use, and an evaluation of granular activated carbon for removal of organic and other contaminants from drinking water. Volume 3 contains evaluations of several epidemiological studies relating to drinking water and a chapter elaborating on the previous study of risk estimation (National Academy of Sciences, 1977). Another part is a toxicological evaluation of drinking water contaminants selected because they are by-products of disinfection or because of their potential involvement in spills. The final chapter examines the contribution of drinking water to mineral nutrition in humans. Particular attention is paid to differences between the amounts required for proper nutrition and the amount that results in toxic symptoms.

The general aproach to the study, and considerations that enter into evaluation of health effects and the reasons for selection of subjects, are discussed in the following paragraphs. The findings of the study are summarized at the end of each chapter and briefly in the Executive Summary.

Economic considerations are not a part of this study.

The goal of disinfecting water supplies is the elimination of the pathogens that are responsible for waterborne diseases. Chlorination is the most widely used method for disinfecting water supplies in the United States. It has been so successful that freedom from epidemics of waterborne diseases is now virtually taken for granted.

However, the discovery that chlorination can result in the formation of trihalomethanes (THM's) and other halogenated hydrocarbons has prompted a reexamination of available disinfection methodology to determine alternate agents or procedures.

Methods of disinfection are examined individually and their major characteristics and biocidal efficacy are compared by means of summary tables and the c · t (concentration, mg/liter, times contact time, min) values required for similar inactivations under identical conditions. The conclusions of the study are made on the basis of this evidence.

A major objective of the review of disinfectant chemistry is the identification of likely by-products that might be formed through the use of specific disinfectants. The prediction of possible products is intended to be a guide to those contaminants that might require removal or toxicological evaluation. The benefits of removing chemicals such as cyanides, phenols, and possibly other compounds by disinfectants and the use of combinations of disinfectants sequentially were not examined.

The chapter on granular activated carbon (GAC) identifies the compounds that may be removed or added to drinking water by the adsorption process with its attendant chemical and microbial processes. Some attention is given to an examination of potential health effects related to the use of adsorbants, but detailed toxicological and epidemiological implications resulting from the presence in drinking water of organic compounds are considered in separate chapters of this volume and Volume 3. The development of standards for GAC and the economic aspects of its use were not a part of this study.

It is a pleasure to express, on behalf of the committee and the subcommittees, a special note of thanks to the staff: Dr. Riley D. Housewright, Dr. Robert Golden, Dr. Roy Widdus, and Ms. Frances M. Peter whose informed and tireless efforts aided the committee in planning, conducting, and editing the study. We are grateful to Mr.

David Goff, Ms. Virginia White, and Ms. Edna Paulson who assisted in an extensive search of the scientific literature.

We also acknowledge the assistance of members of the staff of the Environmental Protection Agency, especially Dr. Joseph Cotruvo and Dr. William Marcus.

Organization of the meetings and preparation of the manuscripts were made easier by the dedicated secretarial services of Mrs. Delores Banks, Ms. Helen Harvin, and Ms. Merle Morgan.

JOHN DOULL, *Chairman*
Safe Drinking Water Committee

REFERENCE

National Academy of Sciences. 1977. Drinking Water and Health. Safe Drinking Water Committee, National Academy of Sciences, Washington, D.C. 939 pp.

I

Executive Summary

DISINFECTION

Chlorination is the most widely used method for disinfecting water supplies in the United States. It is convenient to use, effective against most waterborne pathogens, and continues disinfectant activity within the distribution system. Chlorination is the standard disinfectant against which others are compared.

However, chlorination can result in the formation of trihalomethanes (THM's) and other halogenated hydrocarbons. The discovery that some of these products are carcinogenic for experimental animals has prompted a reexamination of alternate disinfectants and procedures.

The comparative effectiveness of 12 disinfectants or processes for inactivating microorganisms (bacteria, viruses, protozoa) were evaluated. Chlorination, ozonization, and the use of chlorine dioxide come closest to meeting the criteria established for a drinking water disinfectant.

The ultimate choice among methods will require weighing the disinfectant efficacy, detailed in this evaluation, against the toxicity of the products produced by the use of a particular method of disinfection.

CHEMISTRY

The major objective of the review of disinfectant chemistry is the identification of products that are likely to be formed by the use of

1

specific disinfectants. The identification of known and theoretical products of disinfection, which is attempted herein, is intended to be a guide to those contaminants that might require removal or toxicological evaluation.

There is a large and rapidly growing body of scientific literature on the products of chlorination in drinking water. Comparable information for other disinfectants is scarce. This lack of data on alternative disinfectants should not lead to the conclusion that they are free of the difficulties encountered with chlorine. Quite apart from the question of their efficacy as alternative disinfectants, there remains the question, "Will the substitution of a disinfectant for chlorine in water treatment merely produce a different set of by-products whose effects on human health may be as significant, or more so, than those products known to be produced from chlorine?"

Clearly, each disinfectant chemical that was examined in this survey produces by-products that may occur in actual water treatment applications. Of particular concern are the following substances that are either known to or could result from the use of the various disinfectants.

From chlorine: the trihalomethanes (THM's), trichloroacetone (CCl_3COCH_3), and other largely uncharacterized chlorinated and oxidized intermediates that are formed from the complex set of precursors in natural waters; chloramines; chlorophenols; and the largely unknown products of dechlorination.

From ozone: epoxides, which theoretically result from unsaturated substrates such as oleic acid, although none have yet been found in drinking water; peroxides; and other highly oxidized intermediates such as glyoxal ($OHCCHO$) and methylglyoxal (CH_3COCHO) from aromatic precursors.

From bromine and iodine: THM's and other bromine and iodine analogs of chlorinated species; bromophenols; bromoindoles; bromoanisoles; plus the halogens themselves, which may remain in drinking water as residual.

From chlorine dioxide: chlorinated aromatic compounds; chlorate (ClO_3^-) and chlorite (ClO_2^-), which are often present as by-products or unreacted starting material from production of chloride dioxide; and chlorine dioxide itself.

This list, incomplete as it is, is compelling in that it shows that the use of each disinfectant could result in products that should be examined in more detail.

GRANULAR ACTIVATED CARBON

Raw water and disinfected water supplies may contain organic compounds that have been demonstrated to be carcinogenic or otherwise toxic in experimental animals or in epidemiological studies.

Properly operated granular activated carbon (GAC) systems can remove or effectively reduce the concentration of many of these harmful compounds. Less is known about synthetic resins than about GAC, but it is known that they can be applied to remove certain types of organic contaminants. This study of GAC provides data on adsorption isotherms, percent removal, and competitive equilibria of a wide variety of organic compounds.

The information available as of this date on the treatment of water with GAC provides no evidence that harmful health effects are produced by the process under proper operating conditions. However, there are incomplete studies on the possible production of such effects with virgin or regenerated carbon through

- reactions that may be catalyzed by the GAC surface;
- reactions of disinfectants with GAC or compounds adsorbed on it;
- reactions mediated by microorganisms that are part of the process;

or
- by the growth of undesirable microorganisms on GAC.

Studies are also needed on the properties of regenerated activated carbons and on the adsorption of additional contaminants with potential health effects.

The data regarding microorganisms on GAC beds and their metabolic products, including endotoxin production, are quite limited. The efficacy of biodegradation is believed to be less than adsorption, although microbial activity has been shown to remove organic compounds as measured by group parameters such as total organic carbon, potassium permanganate demand, chemical oxygen demand, and UV absorbance. No evidence was found for removal of specific organic compounds of potential harm to health by microbial activity. The evidence for and against prechlorination and preozonization enhancing biodegredation of organic compounds is presented.

GAC serves as a catalyst for some reactions in water systems, e.g., oxidation, reduction, and polymerization. These reactions can produce organic and inorganic species that were not present originally. However, little can be said concerning the degree of their occurrence during water treatment and their possible impact on public health.

Regeneration procedures influence the chemical properties of GAC. This, in turn, influences adsorption, catalytic properties, and leachable chemicals. The frequency of GAC regeneration is determined by the organic compounds in the water and their competitive interactions. The types and concentrations of organic compounds may vary widely in different locations and seasons of the year. Competitive interactions are complex and presently cannot be predicted without data from laboratory and/or pilot scale tests on the water to be treated.

While there is ample evidence for the effectiveness of GAC in removing many organics of health concern, more data are needed in the quantification of any harmful health effects related to the use of GAC. This need, however, should not prevent the present use of GAC at locations where analysis of the water supply clearly indicates the existence of a potential health hazard greater than that which would result from the use of GAC.

Clarification processes (coagulation, sedimentation, filtration) remove significant amounts of some organics, especially some types of THM precursors and relatively insoluble compounds that may be associated with particulates. In some cases, the removal of THM precursors by clarification may be sufficient to eliminate the need for an adsorption process.

II

The Disinfection of Drinking Water

The goal of disinfection of public water supplies is the elimination of the pathogens that are responsible for waterborne diseases. The transmission of diseases such as typhoid and paratyphoid fevers, cholera, salmonellosis, and shigellosis can be controlled with treatments that substantially reduce the total number of viable microorganisms in the water.

While the concentration of organisms in drinking water after effective disinfection may be exceedingly small, sterilization (i.e., killing *all* the microbes present) is not attempted. Sterilization is not only impractical, it cannot be maintained in the distribution system. Assessment of the reduction in microbes that is sufficient to protect against the transmission of pathogens in water is discussed below.

Chlorination is the most widely used method for disinfecting water supplies in the United States. The near universal adoption of this method can be attributed to its convenience and to its highly satisfactory performance as a disinfectant, which has been established by decades of use. It has been so successful that freedom from epidemics of waterborne diseases is now virtually taken for granted. As stated in *Drinking Water and Health* (National Academy of Sciences, 1977), "chlorination is the standard of disinfection against which others are compared."

However, the discovery that chlorination can result in the formation of trihalomethanes (THM's) and other halogenated hydrocarbons has prompted the reexamination of available disinfection methodology to determine alternative agents or procedures (Morris, 1975).

5

The method of choice for disinfecting water for human consumption depends on a variety of factors (Symons *et al.*, 1977). These include:

- its efficacy against waterborne pathogens (bacteria, viruses, protozoa, and helminths);
- the accuracy with which the process can be monitored and controlled;
- its ability to produce a residual that provides an added measure of protection against possible posttreatment contamination resulting from faults in the distribution system;
- the aesthetic quality of the treated water; and
- the availability of the technology for the adoption of the method on the scale that is required for public water supplies.

Economic factors will also play a part in the final decision; however, this study is confined to a discussion of the five factors listed above as they apply to various disinfectants.

The propensity of various disinfection methods to produce by-products having effects on health (other than those relating to the control of infectious diseases) and the possibility of eliminating or avoiding these undesirable by-products are also important factors to be weighed when making the final decisions about overall suitability of methods to disinfect drinking water. The subcommittee has not attempted to deal with these problems since the chemistry of disinfectants in water and the toxicology of expected by-products have been studied by other subcommittees of the Safe Drinking Water Committee, whose reports appear in Chapter III of this volume (Chemistry) and Chapter IV (Toxicity) of *Drinking Water and Health*, Vol. 3.

ORGANIZATION OF THE STUDY

The general considerations noted in the immediately following material should be borne in mind when considering each method of disinfection. Available information on the obvious major candidates for drinking water disinfection—chlorine, ozone, chlorine dioxide, iodine, and bromine—is then evaluated for each method individually in the following sections. Other less obvious possibilities are also examined to see if they have been overlooked unjustly in previous studies or if it might be profitable to conduct further experimentation on them. Disinfection by chloramines is dealt with in parallel with that effected by chlorine because of the close relationship the former has to chlorine disinfection under conditions that might normally be encountered in drinking water treatment.

The evaluations in this report are not exhaustive literature reviews but, rather, are selections of the studies that, in the judgment of the committee, provide the most accurate and relevant information on the biocidal activities of each method of disinfection. The analytical methods that are described in this report are those that are most likely to be used by persons involved in disinfection research or water treatment. A review of all existing analytical methods, some of which may be more sophisticated than those described below, would be impractical within the constraints of time and space available and is not within the scope of this document.

After the methods of disinfection are examined individually, their major characteristics and biocidal efficacy are compared by means of summary tables and c · t (concentration, in milligrams per liter, times contact time, in minutes) values required for similar inactivations under identical conditions. The conclusions of the study are then recorded on the basis of this evidence.

GENERAL ASPECTS OF DISINFECTION

In any comparison of disinfection methods, certain considerations should be discussed at the outset since they are relevant to most, if not all, methods. The quality of the raw water (i.e., its content of solids and material that will react with the disinfectant), treatment of the water prior to disinfection, and the manner in which the disinfectant is applied to the water will directly affect the efficacy of all disinfectants. Equally applicable to all methods are appropriate standards for verifying the adequacy of disinfection, differences in response to disinfectants between organisms that were obtained directly from the field and those that have been acclimated to laboratory culture, and the maintenance of potability from treatment plant to the consumer's tap. The use of chlorination as presented in examples in the following pages does not imply that it is necessarily the method of choice. Rather, this method has been studied more thoroughly than other methods.

Raw Water Quality

In addition to potential pathogens, raw water may contain contaminants that may interfere with the disinfection process or may be undesirable in the finished product. These contaminants include inorganic and organic molecules, particulates, and other organisms, e.g., invertebrates. Variations among these contaminants arise from differences in regional geochemistry and between ground- and surface-water sources.

DISINFECTANT DEMAND

Many inorganic and organic molecules that occur in raw water exert a "demand," i.e., a capacity to react with and consume the disinfectant. Therefore, higher "demand" waters require a greater dose to achieve a specific concentration of the active species of disinfectant. This demand must be satisfied to ensure adequate biocidal treatment.

Ferrous ions, nitrites, hydrogen sulfide, and various organic molecules exert a demand for oxidizing disinfectants such as chlorine. The bulk of the nonparticulate organic material in raw water occurs as naturally derived humic substances, i.e., humic, fulvic, and hymatomelanic acids, which contribute to color in water. The structure of these molecules is not yet fully understood. However, they are known to be polymeric and to contain aromatic rings and carboxyl, phenolic, alcoholic hydroxyl, and methoxyl functional groups. Humic substances, when reacting with and consuming applied chlorine, produce chloroform ($CHCl_3$) and other THM's. Water, particularly surface waters, may also contain synthetic organic molecules whose demand for disinfectant will be determined by their structure. Ammonia and amines in raw water will react with chlorine to yield chloramines that do have some biocidal activity, unlike most products of these side reactions. If chlorination progresses to the breakpoint, i.e., to a free-chlorine residual, these chloramines will be oxidized causing more added chlorine to be consumed before a specific free-chlorine level is achieved. This phenomenon is discussed more fully below.

The nature of the demand reactions varies with the composition of the water and the disinfectant. Removal of the demand substances leaves a water with a lower requirement for a disinfectant to achieve an equivalent degree of protection against transmission of a waterborne disease.

PHYSICAL AND CHEMICAL TREATMENTS

Various treatments applied to raw water to remedy undesirable characteristics, e.g., color, taste, odor, or turbidity, may affect the ultimate microbiological quality of the finished water. Microorganisms may be physically removed or the disinfectant demand of the water altered.

Presedimentation to remove suspended matter, coagulation with alum or other agents, and filtration reduce the organic material in the raw water and, thus, the disinfectant demand. Removal of ferrous iron similarly reduces the demand for oxidizing disinfectants as will aeration, which eliminates hydrogen sulfide. Prechlorination to a free chlorine residual is practiced early in the treatment sequence as one method to alter taste- and odor-producing compounds, to suppress growth of organisms in the treatment plant, to remove iron and manganese, and to reduce the interference of organic compounds in the coagulation process.

The necessity for these treatments or others is determined by the characteristics of the raw water. The selection of one of the various methods to achieve a particular result will be based upon cost-effectiveness in the particular situation. When chlorination is used, the application or point of application in the treatment sequence of some of the above-mentioned procedures can affect the undesirable THM content of the finished water.

Reduction of precursors in raw water by coagulation and settling prior to chlorination reduces final THM production (Hoehn et al., 1977; Stevens et al., 1975). The Louisville Water Company reduced THM concentrations leaving the plant by 40%–50% by shifting the point of chlorination from the presedimentation basin to the coagulation basin (Hubbs et al., 1977). The available information on these variations is limited, and a universally applicable procedure cannot be recommended in view of the diverse treatments required for different raw waters.

Particulates and Aggregates

To inactivate organisms in water, the active chemical species must be able to reach the reactive site within the organism or on its surface. Inactivation will not result if this cannot occur. Microorganisms may acquire physical protection in water as a result of their being adsorbed to the enormous surfaces provided by clays, silt, and organic matter or to the surfaces of solids created during water treatment, e.g., aluminum or ferric hydrated oxides, calcium carbonate, and magnesium hydroxide. Viruses, bacteria, and protozoan cysts may be adsorbed to these surfaces. Such particles, with the adsorbed microorganisms, may aggregate to form clumps, affording additional protection. Organisms themselves may also aggregate or clump together so that organisms that are on the interior of the clump are shielded from the disinfectant and are not inactivated. Organisms may also be physically embedded within particles of fecal material, within larger organisms such as nematodes, or, in the case of viruses, within human body cells that have been discharged in fecal material.

To disinfect water adequately, the water must have been pretreated, when necessary, to reduce the concentration of solid materials to an acceptably low level. The primary drinking water turbidity standard of 1 nephelometric turbidity unit (NTU) is an attempt to assure that the concentration of particulates is compatible with current disinfection techniques. Where it is possible to obtain lower turbidities, this is desirable.

Disinfection studies in which the complications of adsorbed organisms, aggregation, or embedment were thought to occur were excluded from this study. The conclusions in this report should not be extrapolated to such situations as the disinfection of turbid or colored waters.

The Importance of Residuals

Water supplies are disinfected through the addition or dosage of a chemical or physical agent. With a chemical agent, such as a halogen, a given dosage should theoretically impart a predetermined concentration (residual) of the active agent in the water. From a practical point of view, most natural waters exert a "demand" for the disinfectant, as discussed above, so that the residual in the water is less than the calculated amount based on the dosage. The decrease in residual, which is caused by the demand, is rapid in most cases, but it may be prolonged until the residual eventually disappears. In addition, the chemical agent may decompose spontaneously, thereby yielding substances having little or no disinfection ability and exerting no measurable residual. For example, ozone not only reacts with substances in water that exert a demand, but it also decomposes rapidly. To achieve microbial inactivation with a chemical agent, a residual must be present for a specific time. Thus, the nature and level of the residual, together with time of exposure, are important in achieving disinfection or microbial inactivation. Because the nature of the dosage–residual relationship for natural waters has not been and possibly cannot be reliably defined, the efficacy of disinfection with a chemical agent must be based on a residual concentration/time-of-exposure relationship.

Residual measurements are important and useful in controlling the disinfection process. By knowing the residual–time relationship that is required to inactivate pathogenic or infectious agents, one can adjust the dosage of the disinfecting agent to achieve the residual that is required for effective disinfection with a given contact time. Thus, the effectiveness of the disinfection process can be controlled and/or judged by monitoring or measuring the residual.

Following disinfection of a water supply at a treatment plant, the water is distributed to the consumers. A persistent residual is important for continued protection of the water supply against subsequent contamination in the distribution system. Accidental or mechanical failures in the distribution system may result in the introduction of infectious agents into the water supply. In the presence of a residual, disinfection will continue and, as a result, offer continued protection to the users. Physical agents such as radiation may provide effective disinfection during application, but they do not impart any persistent residual to the water.

The dosage of a chemical agent that is used to effect microbial inactivation should not be so great that it imparts a health hazard to the water consumer. From another point of view, the aesthetic quality of the finished water should not be impaired by the dosage of the chemical agent or the residual that is required for effective disinfection. These qualities might include discoloration of water from potassium permanganate ($KMnO_4$) or iodine or problems of taste and odor from excessive chlorine.

Application of the Disinfectant

Optimum inactivation occurs when the disinfectant is distributed uniformly throughout the water. To disperse the chemical disinfectant when it is added to the water, it must be mixed effectively to assure that all of the water, however small the volume, receives its proportionate share of the chemical. Additions of a disinfectant at points in a flowing water stream, e.g., from submerged pipes, is seldom adequate to assure uniform concentration. In such cases, mechanical mixing devices are needed to disperse the disinfectant throughout the water. Disinfection by radiation treatment also requires good mixing to bring all of the water within the effective radiation distance.

Microbiological Considerations[1]

Comparison of the biocidal efficacy of disinfectants is complicated by the need to control many variables, a need not realized in some early studies. Halogens in particular are significantly affected by the composition of the test menstruum and its pH, temperature, and halogen demand. For very low concentrations of halogen to be present over a testing period, halogen demand must be carefully eliminated. Different disinfectants may have different biocidal potential. In earlier work,

[1] Nomenclature in this report follows that recommended in the Eighth Edition of *Bergey's Manual of Determinative Bacteriology* (Buchanan and Gibbons, 1974). Thus, the name of an organism mentioned in the text may not be that used by the author of the work cited.

analytical difficulties may have precluded defining exactly the species present, but new techniques allow the species to be defined for most disinfectants. Information on the species of disinfectant actually in the test system should be included in future reports on disinfection studies.

Investigators studying efficacy have usually adopted one of two extremes. Some have conducted carefully designed laboratory experiments with controls for as many variables as possible. Certain of these investigators have reduced the temperature to slow the inactivation reactions. Although these experiments yield good basic information and can be used to determine which variables are important, they often have little quantitative relationship to field situations. The other extreme, a field study or reconstruction of field conditions, is difficult to control. Moreover, their results are often not repeatable.

In addition to the variables noted above, prereaction of chemicals in the test system, the culture history of the organism being used, and the "cleanup" procedures applied to it may also affect the observed results. Despite these problems, there have been some attempts to standardize efficacy testing.

MODEL SYSTEMS AND INDICATOR ORGANISMS

A major factor that influences the evaluation of the efficacy of a particular disinfectant is the test microorganism. There is a wide variation in susceptibility, not only among bacteria, viruses, and protozoa (cyst stage), but also among genera, species, and strains of the microorganism. It is impractical to obtain information on the inactivation by each disinfectant for each species and strain of pathogenic microorganism of importance in water. In addition, interpretation of the data would be confounded by the condition and source of the test microorganism (e.g., the degree of aggregation and whether the organisms were "naturally occurring" or laboratory preparations), the presence of solids and particulates, and the presence of materials that react with and consume the disinfectant.

The overwhelming majority of the literature on water disinfection concerns the inactivation of model microorganisms rather than the pathogens. These disinfectant model microorganisms have generally been nonpathogenic microorganisms that are as similar as possible to the pathogen and behave in a similar manner when exposed to the disinfectant. The disinfectant model systems are simpler, less fastidious, technically more workable systems that provide a way to obtain basic information concerning fundamental parameters and reactions. The information gained with the model systems can then be used to design key experiments in the more difficult systems. The disinfection model microorganism should be clearly distinguished from the indicator organism. The indicator microorganism, as defined in *Drinking Water and Health* (National Academy of Sciences, 1977), is a "microorganism whose presence is evidence that pollution (associated with fecal contamination from man or other warm-blooded animals) has occurred." Following are criteria for the indicator microorganism (Fair and Geyer, 1954):

1. The indicator should always be present when fecal material is present and absent in clean, uncontaminated water.
2. The indicator should die away in the natural aquatic environment and respond to treatment processes in a manner that is similar to that of the pathogens of interest.
3. The indicator should be more numerous than the pathogens.
4. The indicator should be easy to isolate, identify, and enumerate.

Only a restrictive application of the second criterion is necessary for a disinfection model. The response of the test microorganism to the disinfectant must be similar to that of the pathogen that it is intended to simulate. The disinfection model is not meant to function as an indicator microorganism.

During the latter part of the nineteenth century, investigators recognized the presence of a group of bacteria that occured in large numbers in feces and wastewater. The most significant member of this group (currently called the coliform group) is *Escherichia coli*. Since the late nineteenth century, this coliform group has served as an indicator of the degree of fecal contamination of water, and *E. coli* has been used routinely as a disinfection model for enteric pathogens. Butterfield and co-workers (Butterfield and Wattie, 1946; Butterfield *et al.*, 1943; Wattie and Butterfield, 1944) provided information on the inactivation of *E. coli* and other enteric bacterial pathogens with chlorine and chloramines. At pH values above 8.5, all strains of *E. coli* were more resistant to free chlorine than were *Salmonella typhi* strains. At pH values of 6.5 and 7.0, strains of *S. typhi* were more resistant. Only slight differences between the two genera were found when chloramines were used as the disinfectant. The bactericidal activity of chloramine was noticably less than that of free chlorine.

Bacteria of the coliform group, especially *E. coli*, have proved useful as an indicator and disinfection model for enteric bacterial pathogens but are poor indicators and disinfection models for nonbacterial pathogens. *E. coli* has been observed to be markedly more susceptible to chlorine than certain enteric viruses and cysts of pathogenic protozoa (Dahling *et al.*, 1972; Kruse, 1969).

The bacterial viruses of *E. coli* have received increased attention as possible disinfection models and indicators of enteric viruses in water and wastewater. At present, the data to justify the bacterial viruses as indicators for enteric viruses are limited and inconsistent. However, there is a growing body of knowledge on the utilization of bacterial viruses as disinfection models.

Hsu (1964) and Hsu *et al.* (1966) first reported the use of the f2 virus as a model for disinfection studies with iodine. They showed that inactivation of both the f2 virus and poliovirus 1 were inhibited by increasing concentrations of iodide ion and that both f2 RNA and poliovirus 1 RNA were resistant to iodination.

Dahling *et al.* (1972) compared the inactivation of two enteric viruses (poliovirus 1 and coxsackievirus A9), two DNA phages (T2 and T5), two RNA phages (f2 and MS2), and *E. coli* ATCC 11229 under demand-free conditions with free chlorine at pH 6.0. They found enteric viruses to be most resistant to free chlorine followed by RNA phages, *E. coli*, and the T phages.

Shah and McCamish (1972) compared the resistance of poliovirus 1 and the coliphages f2 and T2 to 4 mg/liter combined residual chlorine. The f2 virus was shown to be more resistant to this form of chlorine than poliovirus 1 and T2 coliphage.

Cramer *et al.* (1976) compared the inactivation of poliovirus 3 (Leon) and f2 with chlorine and iodine in buffered wastewater. Both viruses were treated together in the same reaction flask, thereby eliminating any inherent differences due to virus preparations and replicate systems. In wastewater effluent at pH 6.0 and 10.0 with a 30 mg/liter dosage of halogen under prereacted (halogen added to wastewater, allowed to react, viruses added at zero time) and dynamic (viruses added to wastewater, halogen added at zero time) conditions, f2 was, in each case, at least as or more resistant to chlorine and iodine than poliovirus 1. The f2 virus appears to be more sensitive to free chlorine but more resistant to combined chlorine than poliovirus 1 is.

Neefe *et al.* (1945) observed that the agent of infectious hepatitis was inactivated by breakpoint chlorination (free chlorine) but not completely inactivated by combined chlorine.

Engelbrecht *et al.* (1975) reported that the use of a yeast (*Candida parapsilosis*) and two acid-fast bacteria (*Mycobacterium fortuitum* and

Mycobacterium phlei) may provide suitable disinfection models. They observed that the yeast was more resistant to free chlorine than were poliovirus 1 and the enteric bacteria under all conditions tested. The acid-fast bacilli were most resistant.

There is no generally accepted disinfection model for protozoan cysts. In disinfection studies for protozoan diseases, investigators have used the pathogen or its cysts. Work with such systems is, however, generally difficult.

The use of disinfection models provides useful information that is helpful to the comparison of the relative efficiencies of various disinfectants in the laboratory and in controlled field investigations. Strains of *E. coli* have been used extensively as models for enteric pathogenic bacteria. While not as widely accepted, the bacterial viruses of *E. coli* are used as disinfection models for enteric viruses. The difficulty of available methods has limited the number of disinfection studies with protozoan cysts.

LABORATORY CULTURES VERSUS "NATURALLY OCCURRING" ORGANISMS

The resistance or sensitivity to disinfectants of some bacteria (e.g., *E. coli*) in the laboratory may bear very little resemblance to their responses in nature. This is true in spite of the fact that standardized procedures govern the conditions under which cells are grown, harvested, washed, etc., when they are used as inocula. Examples of such differences range from Gram-negative bacteria and their comparative resistance to disinfectants in general (Carson *et al.*, 1972; Favero *et al.*, 1971, 1975) to Gram-positive bacterial spores and heat resistance (Bond *et al.*, 1973) and to halogen resistance of *Entamoeba histolytica* cysts from simian hosts as opposed to those grown in *in-vitro* systems (Stringer *et al.*, 1975). Presumably, the mechanisms creating this phenomenon among these three groups vary widely.

The comparative resistance to disinfectants among Gram-negative bacteria varies greatly. A good example of this is the study of Favero and Drake (1966). They first applied the term "naturally occurring" to certain Gram-negative bacteria with the potential for rapid growth in water. They observed that *Pseudomonas alcaligenes,* a common bacterial contaminant in iodinated swimming pools, could grow well in swimming pool waters that had been sterilized by membrane filters and rendered free of iodine or chlorine. Starting with contaminated swimming pool water that contained a variety of bacteria, they isolated a pure culture of *P. alcaligenes* by an extinction–dilution technique in which filter-sterilized swimming pool water was used as the diluent and growth medium. Since these cells had been isolated in pure culture without exposure to conventional laboratory culture media, they were referred to as "naturally occurring" *P. alcaligenes*. Subsequent tests showed that these naturally occurring cells were significantly more resistant to free iodine than were cells of the same organism that had been subcultured one time on trypticase soy agar. In fact, standard disinfectant tests using the cells that had been subcultured on an enriched laboratory medium suggested that *P. alcaligenes* should never be found in pools that had been disinfected even minimally with iodine. This was obviously an erroneous assumption. The discovery that naturally occurring cells were extremely resistant to iodine explained the relatively high concentrations of *P. alcaligenes* that accumulated in pool water that had been iodinated for several weeks.

Subsequently, Favero *et al.* (1971, 1975) and Carson *et al.* (1972) published a series of papers showing that *Pseudomonas aeruginosa* could grow rapidly in distilled water, which they obtained from hospitals, and could reach high concentrations of cells that remained stable for a long time. Naturally occurring cells that were grown in distilled water reacted quite differently to chemical and physical stresses than did cells grown on standard laboratory culture media. For example, naturally occurring cells of *P. aeruginosa* were significantly more resistant to chlorine, quaternary ammonium compounds, and alkaline glutaraldehyde than were subcultured cells.

In halogen-disinfected waters, naturally occurring bacteria can be from one to two orders of magnitude more resistant to the disinfectant than cells of the same organism that had been subcultured on conventional laboratory culture media. Since standard disinfectant testing necessarily employs subcultured and washed bacterial cells, a false sense of confidence may be created if these data are used as an absolute criterion for the dilution of a disinfectant. These results could explain the frequent discrepancies between tests that are performed under laboratory conditions and those that are performed under field conditions.

If bacteria could be used in their naturally occurring state, one might explore the possibility of bridging the gaps between laboratory and field conditions by using this experimental system. The ability of some Gram-negative bacteria to grow in water makes it possible to produce and control large numbers of cells for such studies.

More difficult to answer is the more basic question of why naturally occurring cells of Gram-negative water bacteria become more sensitive to disinfectants when grown in a rich medium than the same strain when grown in water . One would expect the reverse to occur. Milbauer and Grossowicz (1959) showed that cells of *E. coli* were much more sensitive to chlorine when grown on a medium of glucose mineral salts than when grown on nutrient agar. Since Favero and Drake (1966) reported that filter-sterilized dehalogenated swimming pool water could be considered a minimal medium, one would expect that *P. alcaligenes* cells that were grown in this environment would be less resistant to iodine than those grown in trypticase soy broth. This phenomenon has not been explained. Evidently it is not primarily a genetic response since the extreme difference in iodine resistance occurs with one subpassage on trypticase soy agar.

Over the years various investigators have tried without success to "train" bacteria to become more resistant to chlorine and/or iodine (Favero, 1961; Favero *et al.*, 1964; Krusé, 1969). This failure is not surprising, because, if halogens are truly a general cytoplasmic poison that affects primarily the sulfhydryl groups of enzymes (see pp. 36–39), it would be very difficult for an organism to modify its physiology to the extent that it becomes resistant, very unlike the situation with antibiotics and bacteria. Consequently, the extreme resistance or differing resistances of naturally occurring bacteria can be attributed only to "environmental" factors and, perhaps, to the different compositions of cell walls and membranes. However, there have been no data to substantiate this hypothesis.

Despite the questions that have been raised by differences in the behavior of organisms under both laboratory and field conditions, valuable comparative information can be obtained from studies of disinfectants that are conducted in similar laboratory systems.

CHLORINE AND CHLORAMINES

Chlorine is a strong oxidizing disinfectant that has been used to treat drinking water supplies for more than 60 yr. The gas was named "chlorine" after the Greek word for green, "chloros," because of its characteristic color. About 1800, chlorine gas was used as a general disinfectant in both France and England. In the United States, electrolytically produced chlorine was first used directly for water disinfection for only a week or two in 1896 at the Louisville Experimental Station in Kentucky. The first continuous municipal application of chlorine (as sodium hypochlorite [NaOCl]) to water in the United States occurred in 1908 at Jersey City, New Jersey. This was followed in 1912 by the first full-scale use of liquid chlorine for water disinfection at Niagara Falls, New York, where solution-feed equipment was used. This use of chlorine successfully eliminated recurring outbreaks of typhoid fever. In 1913, improved solution-feed equipment was developed to measure chlorine gas, dissolve it in water, and apply the solution to the water supply. This equipment was first installed at Boonton, New Jersey, where it replaced the use of sodium hypochlorite. Other equally significant historical occurrences (Laubush, 1971; White, 1972) led to the eventual addition of chlorine to drinking water in most of the United States for disinfection to destroy or inactivate pathogenic microorganisms (see *Drinking Water and Health,* National Academy of Sciences, 1977).

Chemistry of Chlorine in Water

Chlorine has an atomic number of 17, a melting point of $-102°C$, a boiling point of $-35°C$, and an oxidation potential of -1.36 V at $25°C$ (i.e., $2 Cl^- \rightleftharpoons Cl_2 + 2 e^-$). It is a green–yellow gas at room temperature.

When chlorine is added to water, the following chemical reactions occur:

$$Cl_2 + H_2O \rightleftharpoons HOCl + H^+ + Cl^- \qquad (1)$$

$$HOCl \rightleftharpoons H^+ + OCl^- \qquad (2)$$

Extremely little molecular chlorine (Cl_2) is present at pH values greater than pH 3.0 and total chlorine concentrations of less than $\sim 1,000$ mg/liter (White, 1972). The hypochlorous acid (HOCl) that is produced further ionizes to form hypochlorite ion (OCl^-) and hydrogen ion (H^+) (Reaction 2). The dissociation of hypochlorous acid is dependent chiefly upon pH and, to a much lesser extent, temperature, with almost 100% hypochlorous acid present at pH 5 and almost 100% hypochlorite ion present at pH 10 (Figure II-1). Free available chlorine refers to the concentration of hypochlorous acid and hypochlorite ion, as well as any molecular chlorine existing in a chlorinated water.

CHLORAMINE FORMATION: INORGANIC CHLORAMINES

During chlorination of a water supply for disinfection, chlorine will react with any ammonia (NH_3) in the water to form inorganic chloramines.

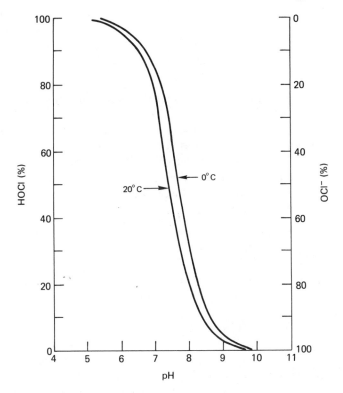

FIGURE II-1   Effect of pH on quantities of hypochlorous acid (HOCl) and hypochlorite ion (OCl⁻) that are present in water. Data from Fair *et al.*, 1948.

Furthermore, ammonia is sometimes deliberately added to chlorinated public water supplies to provide a combined available chlorine residual, i.e., inorganic chloramines. Chlorine will also react with organic amines. The organic chloramines that are produced (see below) are considered encompassed in the term "combined available chlorine."

Although inorganic chloramines are less effective oxidizing and disinfecting agents than hypochlorous acid and hypochlorite ion, they are more stable. Consequently, they will produce a residual in water that will persist for a longer time (Symons *et al.*, 1977).

Inorganic chloramines are formed when hypochlorous acid reacts with ammonia:

$$NH_3 + HOCl \rightleftharpoons NH_2Cl + H_2O \qquad (3)$$

$$NH_2Cl + HOCl \rightleftharpoons NHCl_2 + H_2O \qquad (4)$$

The chloramine that is formed in the reaction depends upon the ratio of ammonia to hypochlorous acid and the pH of the system. Dichloramine ($NHCl_2$) is the predominant form of chloramine at a 1:1 molar ratio of ammonia to chlorine at pH values of 5 and below, whereas at pH values of 9 and above, monochloramine (NH_2Cl) predominates. Figure II-2 shows the proportions of monochloramine and dichloramine formed for pH values of 4 to 9 and temperatures of 0°C, 10°C, and 25°C (Morris, 1978, personal communication).

ORGANIC CHLORAMINES

Chlorine is also known to combine slowly with organic or albumenoid nitrogen (amines) to form organic chloramines (Taras, 1953):

$$R{-}NH_2 + HOCl \rightleftharpoons R{-}NHCl + HOH \qquad (5)$$

Although the reaction between organic amines and chlorine is generally considered to be slow, organic chloramines may be formed, thereby producing a stable combined available chlorine residual after many hours of contact. It is generally accepted that most organic chloramines have little disinfecting capability, i.e., less than the inorganic chloramines (Feng, 1966; Nusbaum, 1952).

BREAKPOINT CHLORINATION

Hypochlorous acid and other chlorine compounds having disinfecting ability by virtue of their being oxidizing agents will oxidize sulfites (SO_3^{2-}), sulfides (S^-), and ferrous (Fe^{2+}) or manganous (Mn^{2+}) ions. The disinfecting species are reduced, and the products have no disinfecting activity. All of the interfering compounds that destroy the disinfecting ability of the added chlorine exert a "chlorine demand," which may be defined as the difference between the amount of chlorine applied and the quantity of free or combined available chlorine residual measured in the water at the end of a specified contact period. When chlorine is added to water with no chlorine demand, a linear relationship is established between the chlorine dosage and the free chlorine residual (Figure II-3).

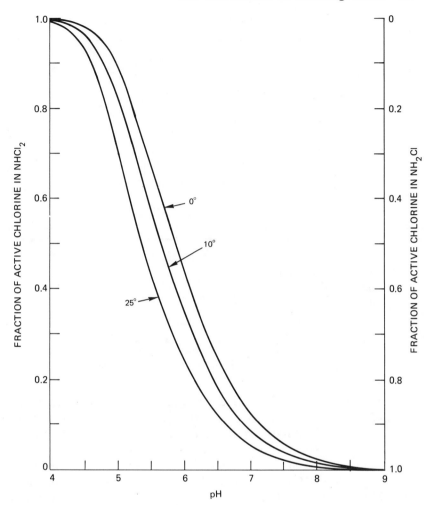

FIGURE II-2   Proportions of mono- and dichloramine (NH₂Cl and NHCl₂) in water chlorination with equimolar concentrations of chlorine and ammonia. Data from J.C. Morris, personal communication.

However, when increasing amounts of chlorine are added to water containing reducing agents and ammonia, the so-called breakpoint phenomenon occurs. The breakpoint is that dosage of chlorine that produces the first detectable amount of free available chlorine residual.

When chlorine is added to water, it reacts with any reducing agents and ammonia that are present. It is believed that chlorine reacts first with

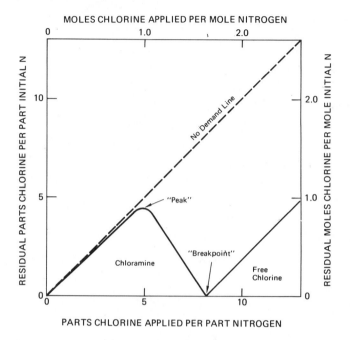

FIGURE II-3   Diagrammatic representation of completed breakpoint reaction. From Morris, 1978, personal communication.

the reducing agents. Since the chlorine is destroyed, no measurable
residual is produced. Following the oxidation of these reducing agents,
e.g., sulfides, sulfites, nitrites (NO_2^-), and ferrous ions, the chlorine will
react with ammonia to form inorganic chloramines. The quantity of
monochloramine and dichloroamine that is formed is determined
primarily by the pH of the water and the ratio of chlorine to ammonia.
When the ratio by weight is less than 5:1, or the molar ratio is less than
1:1, and the pH is in the range of 6.5 to 8.5, the combined available
chlorine residual is probably due primarily to monochloramine (Reaction 3). With additional chlorine, the ratio of chlorine to ammonia
changes with the result that the monochloramines are converted to
dichloramines (Reaction 4). When all of the ammonia has been reacted,
a free available chlorine residual begins to develop. As the concentration
increases, the previously formed chloramines are oxidized to nitrous
oxide (N_2O), nitrogen trichloride (NCl_3), and nitrogen (N_2). The
reactions leading to the formation of these oxidized forms of nitrogen
destroy the combined available chlorine residual so that the measurable
residual in the water actually decreases. Upon completion of the

oxidation of all the chloramines, the addition of more chlorine creates the breakpoint phenomenon. At the breakpoint dosage, some resistant chloramines may still be present, but at such small concentrations that they are unimportant.

As pointed out by Morris (1970), the occurrence of reactions giving rise to the "breakpoint" is most rapid in the pH range 7.0 to 7.5. At greater and lesser pH values, it becomes slower and less distinct, e.g., at pH's < 6 or > 9 the concept of "breakpoint" is not significant. In the pH range 7.0 to 7.5 the "breakpoint" is about half developed within 10 min at 15°C to 20°C and is then substantially completed within about 2 hr.

Analytical Methods and Their Evaluation

Standard Methods (1976) lists six acceptable methods for the determination of chlorine residuals in natural and treated waters: iodometric methods, amperometric titration, the stabilized neutral orthotolidine (SNORT) method, the ferrous diethyl-*p*-phenylenediamine (DPD) method, the DPD colorimetric method, and the leuco crystal violet (LCV) method.

The amperometric, LCV, DPD, and SNORT methods are unaffected by dichloramine concentrations in the range of 0 to 9 mg/liter (as Cl_2) in the determination of free chlorine. If nitrogen trichloride is present, it reacts partially as free available chlorine in the amperometric, DPD, and SNORT methods. Nitrogen trichloride does not interfere with the LCV procedure for free chlorine. The sample color and turbidity may interfere with all colorimetric procedures. Thus, a compensation must be made. Also, organic contaminants in the sample may produce a false-free chlorine reading in most colorimetric methods.

Standard Methods (1976) contains data on the precision and accuracy of the methods used in the measurement of chlorine. These data were obtained from participating laboratories by the Analytical Reference Service (1969, 1971), which then operated in an agency that preceded the Environmental Protection Agency. However, as noted in *Standard Methods* (1976), these results are valuable only for comparison of the methods tested, and many factors, such as analytical skill, recognition of known interferences, and inherent limitations, determine the reliability of any given method. Moreover, some oxidizing agents, including free halogens other than chlorine, will appear quantitatively as free chlorine. This is also true of chlorine dioxide. Also, some nitrogen trichloride may be measured as free chlorine. The actions of interfering substances should be familiar to the analyst because they affect a particular method.

Although orthotolidine (i.e., orthotolidine and orthotolidine arsenite) methods have been widely used in many disinfection studies, they are omitted from the 14th edition of *Standard Methods* (1976) primarily because of their inaccuracy and high overall (average) total error in comparison with other available methods.

Research studies on disinfection are restricted by the limitations that are inherent in the methods themselves or by poor selection of methods by the investigator. The chemical conditions of the test water have not always been well defined. The types of titratable chlorine, i.e., free (hypochlorous acid or hypochlorite ion) or combined (mono- or dichloramine) in the chlorinated water, have not always been differentiated, and the rates of microbial destruction or inactivation have not always been studied in experimental systems with little or no chlorine demand. In fact, reports prior to the 1940's have been especially difficult to interpret, because reliable test methods for distinguishing between free and combined chlorine, between hypochlorous acid and hypochlorite ion, and between mono- and dichloramine in solution were not developed until the 1950's. For example, many earlier researchers claimed to have tested mono- and dichloramine by controlling the pH and the ratio of chlorine to nitrogen. They used methods such as the orthotolidine or thiosulfate titrations to determine total chlorine residual. Much of this early work is now questionable, since it was not possible to detect free chlorine contamination in their chloramine solutions or the quantitative ratios between the mono- and dichloramine tested. In addition, these earlier studies had high chlorine demand in the test systems.

Some more contemporary studies have lacked quantitated information on chlorine residual and/or types of chlorine present in the test systems.

Biocidal Activity

In the absence of reducing agents, inorganic ammonia, and organic amines, the addition of chlorine to municipal water supplies will result in free available residual chlorine, represented by the hypochlorous acid or hypochlorite ion. The pH determines the relative amounts of each species. However, inorganic chloramines will be formed if the background level of ammonia in the water supply is significant or if ammonia is intentionally added during treatment. If such is the case, monochloramine would predominate due to the alkaline pH of most finished water (see Figure II-2).

In 1966, Feng proposed that the active forms of chlorine would exhibit disinfection properties in the following descending order:

$$Cl_2 > HOCl > OCl^- > NHCl_2 > NH_2Cl > R{-}NHCl$$

Butterfield *et al.* (1943) published the first treatise on the use of chlorine demand-free water for studies of water disinfection. They proposed that to study the disinfectant capacity of any chlorine species, the test medium must meet certain exacting criteria. It must be nontoxic to bacteria except for the variables under study such as chlorine and pH, well buffered at the desired pH, free of all ammonia and organic matter capable of forming chlorine-addition products, free of background chlorine, and of such a nature that calculated additions of chlorine are recoverable after 5 min without a loss in residual and that free chlorine must still be present several hours after contact.

Most studies of combined chlorine have dealt with poorly defined mixtures of mono- and dichloramine. Also, test conditions have often been inadequately defined, poorly controlled, or both.

EFFICACY AGAINST BACTERIA

Free Chlorine (HOCl and OCl⁻) Butterfield *et al.* (1943) studied percentages of inactivation as functions of time for *E. coli, Enterobacter aerogenes, Pseudomonas aeruginosa, Salmonella typhi,* and *Shigella dysenteriae.* They used different levels of free chlorine at pH values ranging from 7.0 to 10.7 and two temperature ranges—2°C to 5°C and 20°C to 25°C. Their work is of great importance, since very few other studies have been conducted that dealt with the action of disinfectants on pathogens. Generally, they found that the primary factors governing the bactericidal efficacy of free available chlorine and combined available chlorine were:

● the time of contact between the bacteria and the bactericidal agent, i.e., the longer the time, the more effective the chlorine disinfection process;
● the temperature of the water in which contact is made, i.e., the lower the temperature, the less effective the chlorine disinfecting activity; and
● the pH of the water in which contact is made, i.e., the higher the pH, the less effective chlorination.

Thus, the test bacteria will be killed more rapidly at lower pH values and at higher temperatures. Since hypochlorous acid would predominate at lower pH's (Figure II-1), the data of Butterfield *et al.* show that it is a better bactericide than the hypochlorite ion. For example, to produce a 100% inactivation of an initial inoculum of 8×10^5 *E. coli* in 400 ml of sterile chlorine demand-free water (2,000/ml) at 20°C–25°C with a chlorine level of 0.046 to 0.055 mg/liter, 1.0 min was required at pH 7.0, but at pH 8.5, 9.8, and 10.7, between 20 and 60 min of exposure were needed. At higher concentrations of chlorine, i.e., from 0.1 to 0.29 mg/liter, exposure of 1.0 min was required at pH 7.0, 10 min at pH 8.5, 20 min at 9.8, and 60 min at 10.7. A similar pH effect was noted for *S. typhi.*

Unfortunately, Butterfield *et al.* (1943) lifted their cells from agar slants but failed to wash them in demand-free water. The cells probably carried trace amounts of albumenoid nitrogen from the slants to the test flasks, thereby creating the small chlorine demand that the investigators had tried so carefully to avoid. The effect of such a trace amount of chlorine demand would be most apparent in test solutions with very low chlorine levels. In studies using approximately 0.1 mg/liter or less free chlorine at decreasing pH values, Butterfield *et al.* (1943) observed that the disinfection of the organisms required a very long time. This might indicate interference at the low levels due to the formation of combined chlorine.

Under very exact controlled test conditions of pH and temperature and using chlorine demand-free buffer systems, Scarpino *et al.* (1972) observed that at 5°C *E. coli* was 99% destroyed by 1.0 mg/liter hypochlorous acid at pH 6 in less than 10 s and at pH 10 by 1.0 mg/liter hypochlorite ion in about 50 s. Their studies, which totally eliminated any form of combined chlorine from the test solutions, indicated that hypochlorous acid was approximately 50 times more effective than the hypochlorite ion as a bactericide. Fair *et al.* (1948) and Berg (1966) analyzed the data of Butterfield *et al.* (1943) on the destruction of *E. coli.* They reported that hypochlorous acid was 70–80 times as bactericidal as hypochlorite ion.

Engelbrecht *et al.* (1975) investigated new microbial indicators of disinfection efficiency. In their chlorination studies, they noted the following decreasing order of resistance to free chlorine at pH values of 6, 7, and 10 and at 5°C and 20°C: acid-fast bacteria > yeasts > poliovirus > *Salmonella typhimurium* > *E. coli.*

Monochloramine (NH₂Cl) In 1948, Butterfield summarized previous results on the bactericidal properties of chloramines (and free chlorine) in water at pH values ranging from 6.5 to 10.7 and in two temperature ranges—2°C to 5°C and 20°C to 25°C. The test bacteria included strains of *Escherichia coli, Enterobacter aerogenes, Pseudomonas aeruginosa, Salmonella typhi,* and *Shigella dysenteriae.* Although he admitted that adequate tests for separate determination of free and combined chlorine forms were not used in these studies, the solutions were vigorously prepared to ensure the exclusions of free chlorine. Chloramines were determined using orthotolidine; readings made after 10 to 30 s at 20°C gave free chlorine levels, and those after standing for 10 min at 20°C were recorded as total residual chlorine. Since no free chlorine was reported (and should not have been found, according to the authors), the 10-min readings of total residual chlorine were also those of total chloramine levels. No distinction could be made between monochloramine and dichloramine. However, he estimated that at pH 6.5, 7.0, 7.8, 8.5, 9.5, and 10.5 the chloramines were present as monochloramine at 35%, 51%, 84%, 98%, 100%, and 100%, respectively. The balance was believed to be dichloramine.

Butterfield and his associates (Butterfield, 1948; Butterfield et al., 1946) found that chloramine disinfection was always slower than that for free chlorine. For example, in order to achieve a 100% inactivation of the initial number of bacteria tested after 60 min of contact time at 20°C, 0.6 mg/liter chloramine was required at pH 7.0 and 1.2 mg/liter at pH 8.5. At 4°C, a 100% inactivation required 1.5 mg/liter chloramine at pH 7.0 and 1.8 mg/liter at pH 8.5. However, only 0.03 to 0.06 mg/liter free chlorine was needed at pH ranges of 7.0 and 8.5 at either 4°C or 22°C to achieve 100% inactivation in 20 min.

The bactericidal effects of monochloramine alone were confirmed by Siders *et al.* in 1973. They found that at 15°C *E. coli* was 99% destroyed in approximately 20 min using 1.0 ppm monochloramine in pH 9 borate buffer. Since *E. coli* was less resistant to monochloramine than were the animal viruses tested, Siders *et al.* questioned the validity of using *E. coli* as an indicator organism for measuring the viral quality of a chlorinated water supply. Chang (1971) had previously calculated that 4 mg/liter monochloramine would be needed to give 99.999% reduction of *E. coli* bacterium in 10 min at 25°C.

Dichloramine ($NHCl_2$)   Chang (1971) calculated that 1.2 mg/liter dichloramine would be needed to give 99.999% reduction of enteric bacteria in 10 min at 25°C.

In carefully conceived studies, Esposito *et al.* (1974) examined the destruction rates of test organisms in contact with dichloramine in demand-free phthalate buffer at pH 4.5 and 15°C. Figure II-4 shows the comparisons that were made among enteroviruses (poliovirus 1 and

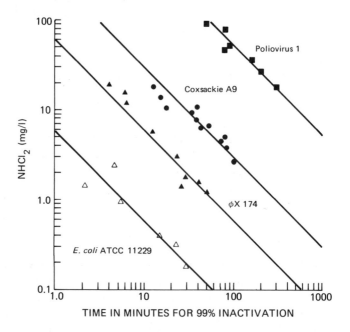

FIGURE II-4   Inactivation of various microorganisms with dichloramine ($NHCl_2$) at pH 4.5 and 15°C. From Esposito, 1974.

coxsackievirus A9), the bacteriophage ΦX-174, and *E. coli* (ATCC 11229).

From a review of the literature and an analysis of the data, Chang (1971) calculated that the relative bactericidal efficiency of dichloramine to monochloramine was 3.3:1. However, Esposito (1974) and Esposito *et al.* (1974) showed experimentally that Chang's estimate was conservative. They found that dichloramine was 35 times more bactericidal than was monochloramine, not 3.3. At 15°C, poliovirus 1 was 17 times more resistant than coxsackievirus A9, 83 times more resistant than ΦX-174, and 1,700 times more resistant than *E. coli* to dichloramine (Figure II-4). They observed that dichloramine was a better bactericide than monochloramine.

Organic Chloramines   These chlorine derivatives exhibit some bactericidal activity, but markedly less than either free chlorine or the inorganic chloramines (Feng, 1966; Nusbaum, 1952).

In summary, the bactericidal efficiency of hypochlorous acid, the hypochlorite ion, monochloramine, and dichloramine have been accurately defined in recent years by investigators using rigidly controlled test conditions. The order of disinfection efficiency presented by Feng (1966) has been confirmed. Comparative c · t values are shown in Table II-3 at the end of the section on chlorine.

EFFICACY AGAINST VIRUSES

In reviewing disinfection of enteroviruses in water, Clarke and Chang (1959) excluded all studies on the inactivation of viruses by chlorine that were conducted before 1946. Their justification for this exclusion was the failure of these studies to differentiate between free and combined chlorine. Furthermore, they attributed the irregular virucidal results of some studies to the use of animal inoculation methods for assaying virus concentrations. For these same reasons, those studies have been omitted in this report. The advent of viral propogation techniques using tissue cultures (Enders *et al.*, 1949) enabled research of a more exacting nature to be performed, resulting in more precise virus inactivation data.

Free Chlorine (HOCl and OCl⁻)   Generally, enteroviruses are more resistant to free chlorine than are the enteric bacteria (Chang, 1971; Clarke and Kabler, 1954; Scarpino *et al.*, 1972). For example, in what was probably the first well-defined study, Clarke and Kabler (1954) used purified coxsackievirus A2 to investigate viral inactivation in water by free chlorine. They carefully controlled their free chlorine residuals with a modified form of the orthotolidine test to determine total chlorine and an orthotolidine-arsenite method for free chlorine. (Combined chlorine was then calculated as the difference between "total" and "free" chlorine readings.) They measured virus recoveries by using suckling mice and the LD_{50} quantitation procedure. Their results indicated that inactivation times for the virus increased with increasing pH (6.9 to 9.0), decreasing temperatures (27°C–29°C to 3°C–6°C), and decreasing total chlorine concentration. They estimated that approximately 7 to 46 times as much free chlorine was required to obtain comparable inactivation of coxsackievirus A2 as was required for a suspension of *E. coli* cells (Butterfield *et al.*, 1943). For instance, Butterfield *et al.* (1943) found that at pH 7.0 and at 2°C to 5°C, 99.9% of *E. coli* cells were inactivated in 5 min with 0.03 mg/liter of free chlorine. At approximately the same pH and temperature ranges, Clarke and Kabler (1954) observed 99.6% inactivation of coxsackievirus A2 in 5 min with 1.4 mg/liter of free chlorine, i.e., 46 times as much free chlorine as that required to inactivate *E. coli* cells. At a pH of 8.5 at 25°C, 99.9% of *E. coli* cells were inactivated in 3 min with 0.14 mg/liter of free chlorine (Butterfield *et al.*,

1943), while at a pH of 9.0 at 27°C to 29°C, 99.6% of the virus was inactivated in 3 min by 1.0 mg/liter of free chlorine. Thus, Clarke and Kabler's work showed that 7 times as much free chlorine was required to inactivate the test coxsackievirus compared to the time necessary to kill the bacterium *E. coli*. In a subsequent study, Clarke *et al.* (1956) found that adenovirus type 3, *E. coli,* and *Salmonella typhi* were all inactivated or destroyed at approximately the same concentration of free chlorine.

In 1958, Weidenkopf reported his studies on the rate of inactivation of poliovirus 1 as a function of free available chlorine (HOCl and OCl⁻) and pH at 0°C. His results showed that 99% inactivation of poliovirus 1 was obtained with 0.10 mg/liter free chlorine in 10 min at pH 6.0 and of 0°C. At pH 6, most of the free chlorine should have been present as hypochlorous acid. Increasing the pH to 7.0 increased the time required for the same degree of inactivation by approximately 50%. At that pH, the free chlorine should have been a mixture containing predominantly hypochlorous acid and significant levels of hypochlorite ion. Both Weidenkopf (1958) and Clarke *et al.* (1956) indicated that an increase in pH (from 7.0 to 8.5, Weidenkopf; from 8.8 to 9.0, Clarke *et al.*) increased the inactivation time about sixfold. At these pH's, the free chlorine should have been present as mixtures of both hypochlorous acid and hypochlorite ion, but predominantly as the ion.

After comparing these studies, Clarke *et al.* (1964) concluded that at 0°C to 6°C poliovirus 1 and coxsackievirus A2 were considerably more resistant to hypochlorous acid than was *E. coli*, while adenovirus type 3 was more sensitive (Figure II-5). For 99% destruction of *E. coli*, a 99-s contact time was required when the system was dosed with 0.1 mg/liter free chlorine as hypochlorous acid. The same percentage of the adenovirus was inactivated in approximately one-third of that time by the same concentration of hypochlorous acid. Under the same conditions, 8.5 min was required to inactivate 99% of the poliovirus, i.e., approximately 5 times the contact time required for *E. coli*. Coxsackievirus required a contact time for 99% inactivation in excess of 40 min, more than 24 times that required for *E. coli*.

Clarke and Kabler (1954) and Clarke *et al.* (1956) reported that the time required for inactivation of coxsackievirus A2 and adenovirus increased with increasing pH, decreasing total chlorine concentrations, and decreasing temperatures. Clarke and Chang (1959) concluded from data in the literature that a 10°C increase in temperature increased the rate of virus inactivation by a factor of 2 to 3.

Kelly and Sanderson (1958) reported that each of six enteric viruses possessed a different sensitivity to chlorine. Their results suggested that the inactivation of enteric viruses in water at pH 7.0 and 25°C required a

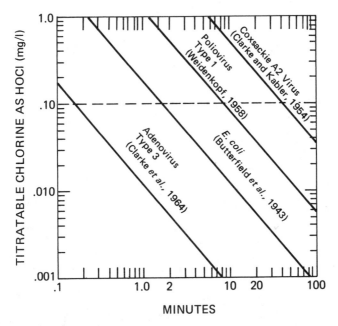

FIGURE II-5   Concentration-time relationship for 99% destruction of *E. coli* and several viruses by hypochlorous acid at 0°–6°C. From Clarke *et al.*, 1964.

minimum free residual chlorine concentration of 0.3 mg/liter with a contact time of at least 30 min. With combined chlorine in water, a concentration of at least 9.0 mg/liter was necessary for a 99.7% inactivation of poliovirus at 25°C and a pH of 7.0. Poliovirus 1 (strain MK 500) was the most resistant strain tested and coxsackievirus B5 the most sensitive. Poliovirus 1 (Mahoney strain), poliovirus 2, coxsackievirus B1, and poliovirus 3 were intermediate in resistance. The virucidal efficiency of hypochlorous acid was more than 50 times greater than that of the chloramines (Kelley and Sanderson, 1958, 1960).

Liu *et al.* (1971) studied the manner in which 20 strains of human enteric viruses responded to free chlorine. They used Potomac River water that had been partially treated by coagulation with alum and filtration through sand. Chlorine was added to the water at one dosage, 0.5 mg/liter. The final pH was 7.8. They stored the sample at 2°C. There was a wide range of resistance to chlorine by the viruses. The most sensitive virus was reovirus type 1, which required 2.7 min for inactivating 4 logs (99.99%) of the virus with 0.5 mg/liter of free chlorine. The most resistant, as judged by extrapolating the experimental data, was

TABLE II-1 Time Required for 99% Inactivation by Free Residual Chlorine at 5.0°C ± 0.2°C[a]

pH	Concentration of Free Chlorine, mg/liter[b]	Virus Strain	Minutes for 99% Inactivation	Rank Ordering
6.00	0.46-0.49	Coxsackie A9 (Griggs)	0.3	1
6.00	0.48-0.49	Echo 1 (Farouk)	0.5	2
6.00-6.02	0.48-0.51	Polio 2 (Lansing)	1.2	3
6.00-6.03	0.38-0.49	Echo 5 (Noyce)	1.3	4
6.00	0.47-0.49	Polio 1 (Mahoney)	2.1	5
6.00-6.06	0.51-0.52	Coxsackie B5 (Faulkner)	3.4	6
7.81-7.82	0.47-0.49	Coxsackie A9 (Griggs)	ND[c]	
		Echo 1 (Farouk)	1.2	1
		Polio 2 (Lansing)	ND[c]	
7.79-7.83	0.48-0.52	Echo 5 (Noyce)	1.8	3
7.80-7.84	0.46-0.51	Polio 1 (Mahoney)	1.3	2
7.81-7.82	0.48-0.50	Coxsackie B5 (Faulkner)	4.5	4
10.00-10.01	0.48-0.50	Coxsackie A9 (Griggs)	1.5	1
10.00-10.40	0.49-0.51	Echo 1 (Farouk)	96.0	6
9.89-10.03	0.48-0.50	Polio 2 (Lansing)	64.0	4
9.97-10.02	0.49-0.51	Echo 5 (Noyce)	27.0	3
9.99-10.40	0.50-0.52	Polio 1 (Mahoney)	21.0	2
9.93-10.05	0.50-0.51	Coxsackie B5 (Faulkner)	66.0	5

[a] Data from Engelbrecht et al., 1978.
[b] Range of measured free chlorine residual in the "test" reactor at the termination of each of three separate experiments.
[c] ND = not determined.

poliovirus 2, which required 40 min for the same degree of inactivation. Using actual experimental data, the most resistant virus was echovirus 12, which required a contact time of greater than 60 min for 99.99% inactivation. Liu *et al.* (1971) concluded from their extrapolated values that the reoviruses were the least resistant to chlorine treatment, that both adenoviruses and echoviruses were less resistant, and that the polioviruses and coxsackieviruses were the most resistant. However, assuming a 20-min contact time, most of the viruses tested at pH 7.8 and 2°C would have been 99.99% inactivated with a free chlorine residual of 0.5 mg/liter.

Using six of the same virus strains studied by Liu *et al.* (1971), Engelbrecht *et al.* (1978) investigated the effect of pH on the kinetics of chlorine inactivation at 5.0 ± 0.2°C. The suspending medium was buffered, chlorine demand–free, distilled–deionized water. Each virus stock was also prepared so as to be chlorine demand-free. Table II-1 summarizes the results, giving the chlorine levels used and the time required for two logs (99%) inactivation of the viruses at pH 6.0 and 7.8 in phosphate buffer and at pH 10.0 in borate buffer. Because of the use of two different buffer systems, i.e., at pH 6.0 and 10.0, virus inactivation was determined at pH 7.8 with each of the two buffer systems. The kinetics of inactivation of poliovirus 1 at pH 7.8, using both the phosphate and borate buffer, were the same. The results shown in Table II-1 indicate that there is a significant difference in the time required for two logs inactivation for the various viruses at pH 6.0 and 10.0. In every case, the rate of inactivation at pH 10.0 was significantly less than at pH 6.0. The rank ordering in Table II-1 shows that there is also a wide range of sensitivity of related viruses to chlorine disinfection. For example, at pH 10.0, coxsackie B5 was 40 times more resistant than coxsackie A9. There are several cases in which the relative sensitivity to chlorine was altered (rank ordering) between pH 6.0 and 10.0, suggesting important effects of pH on the virion as well as on the chlorine species, i.e., hypochlorous acid versus. hypochlorite ion. This observation can be seen more clearly in Table II-2 in which the time required for two logs of inactivation of the various viruses and the ratio of inactivation times at pH 6.0 and 10.0 are compared. Even at pH 7.8, differences in relative sensitivity appear when ranked and compared to results at pH 6.0 or 10.0 (Table II-1).

Combined Chlorine (NH$_2$Cl and NHCl$_2$)   Viral inactivation rates with chloramines have been found to be much slower than with free chlorine. For example, Kelly and Sanderson (1958) studied the effects of chlorine on several enteric viruses. They reported that at pH 7 at 25°C–28°C, 0.2–

TABLE II-2   Comparison of Virus Inactivation by Free
Residual Chlorine[a] at pH 6.0 and 10.0, at 5.0°C ± 0.2°C[b]

| Virus Strain | Minutes for 99% Inactivation | | |
	pH 6.0	pH 10.0	Ratio[c]
Coxsackie A9 (Griggs)	0.3	1.5	5
Echo 1 (Farouk)	0.5	96.0	192
Polio 2 (Lansing)	1.2	64.0	53
Echo 5 (Noyce)	1.3	27.0	21
Polio 1 (Mahoney)	2.1	21.0	10
Coxsackie B5 (Faulkner)	3.4	66.0	19

[a] Chlorine concentrations as noted in Table II-1 at pH 6.0 and 10.0.
[b] Data from Engelbrecht et al., 1978.
[c] $\dfrac{\text{Time required at pH 10.0}}{\text{Time required at pH 6.0}}$.

0.3 mg/liter free chlorine inactivated 99.9% of all test viruses in 8 min. At the same temperature and pH, combined chlorine at 0.7 mg/liter and at least 4 hr of contact time were needed to achieve 99.7% inactivation of the test viruses.

Although most viral inactivation studies with chloramines have not differentiated between mono- and dichloramine (Kelly and Sanderson, 1958; Lothrop and Sproul, 1969), Kelly and Sanderson (1958, 1960) noted that viral inactivation by chloramines proceeds more rapidly at pH 6–7 than at pH 8–10. This tendency indicates that dichloramine may be more virucidal than monochloramine since its proportion increases with increased hydrogen ion concentration.

In 1971, Chang proposed that 5.0 mg/liter dichloramine or 20 mg/liter monochloramine would be needed to inactivate enteroviruses by 99.99% in 10 min at 25°C. Subsequently, Siders et al. (1973) presented evidence of the first comparative studies on viral inactivation due solely to monochloramine. At pH 9 at 15°C, poliovirus 1 (Mahoney) was 10 times more resistant to monochloramine than was E. coli. Similarly, coxsackievirus A9 was approximately 4 times more resistant than E. coli. Siders' data can be compared to Chang's theory on the disinfectant capacity of monochloramine. Assume that poliovirus inactivation has a temperature coefficient for a 10°C rise (Q_{10}) of 3. Based on Chang's (1971) calculations that 20 mg/liter monochloramine at 25°C would be needed to achieve 99.999% reduction of enterovirus in 10 min, one would extrapolate that 3 × 20 or 60 mg/liter monochloramine would be needed at 15°C to achieve an equivalent reduction of poliovirus in 10 min. However, examination of the data of Siders et al. reveals that approximately 18 min were needed to achieve only 99% inactivation using 60 ppm monochloramine. Therefore, it appears that Chang slightly overestimated the virucidal capacity of monochloramine.

EFFICACY AGAINST PARASITES

Some studies, mostly in the field of wastewater treatment, have shown that ova and larvae of the helminth parasites that affect humans and that could occur in U.S. water supplies are resistant to current chlorination procedures. They can survive concentrations and exposure periods considerably in excess of those used in the treatment of municipal water supplies. In studies of various free-living nematodes, Chang et al. (1960) observed that 2.5 to 3.0 mg/liter of free chlorine for a 120-min contact period and 15 to 45 mg/liter of free chlorine for 1 min were not lethal. Free chlorine residuals as high as 95 to 100 mg/liter for 5 min killed only 40%–50% of the nematodes. Thus, it may be speculated that all the helminths, including their larvae, may approach the degree of resistance to chlorine that had been demonstrated by the free-living nematodes.

There have been a number of studies on the effectiveness of chlorine in destroying or inactivating cysts of the protozoan parasite, Entamoeba histolytica, in water, especially during the early 1940's (Brady et al., 1943; Chang, 1944b; Chang and Fair, 1941). Varied results reflect primarily the different experimental conditions and techniques that were used. The presence of organic matter, pH, and temperature, as well as the concentration and form of chlorine and exposure period, have been shown to exert an influence on disinfection. However, the consensus is that, compared with bacteria, these cysts are rather resistant to current chlorination procedures, but are much less resistant than helminths.

Brady et al. (1943) conducted field-simulated studies with cysts in raw water that had been treated with calcium hypochlorite (CaOCl), resulting in pH levels ranging from approximately 7.5 to 8.0. They found that at temperatures of 23°C–26°C, exposures of 20 min and longer to residuals of 3 to 4 mg/liter were required to produce an estimated 99% cyst destruction as judged via a culture technique. Chang (1944b), also using a culture technique, studied the cysticidal effectiveness of calcium hypochlorite solution, chloramines, and gaseous chlorine in tap water as well as the effects of pH and organic matter on the biocidal activity. At contact periods of up to 30 min, gaseous chlorine was the most powerful, hypochlorite solution slightly less so, and chloramines the least. Increase in pH and organic matter reduced cysticidal efficacy. For comparison with Brady et al. (1943), the "lethal" residual concentration in tap water at 18°C and pH 6.8–7.2 ranged from 2.8 to 3.2 mg/liter at 15 min, and from 1.8 to 2.2 mg/liter at 30 min (as estimated from a graph in Chang, 1944b).

Recently, Stringer et al. (1975) reported on comparative studies of the cysticidal efficacy of chlorine, bromine, and iodine as disinfectants. Using chlorine gas bubbled into buffered distilled water as stock, they obtained 99.9% cyst inactivation (as measured by excystment capability) after 15 min exposure to 2 mg/liter free chlorine in "clean water" at pH 6. However at pH 8 a contact time exceeding 60 min was required to achieve 99% mortality. In "secondary treated sewage effluent," Stringer et al. considered 13.7 mg/liter chlorine at pH 8 to be ineffectual as a cysticide.

In keeping with these findings, it is unlikely that the chlorine residuals generally maintained in distribution systems provide much protection against E. histolytica cysts in the event of contamination because of cross-connections, seepage, etc.

During the past 10 yr, a number of outbreaks of waterborne infections from Giardia lamblia (another intestinal protozoan) have been reported (National Academy of Sciences, 1977). Most incidents in the United States that were traced to municipal water supplies involved surface water sources where disinfection appeared to be the only treatment. The cysts of this parasite are thought to be as resistant to chlorine as those of E. hystolytica. However, there seem to be no studies of the resistance of this parasite to chlorine or other disinfectants.

Mechanism of Action

One of the earliest references to the mechanism of inactivation of microorganisms by chlorine resulted from the work of Chang (1944a,b). While studying the inactivation of E. histolytica cysts by chlorine, he observed greater uptake of chlorine and less survival at low pH than at high pH. This observation was associated with the increased inactivation efficiency of the undissociated hypochlorous acid. Supportive evidence for the hypothesis that permeability of the uncharged chlorine species is important in determining sensitivity to chlorine has been provided by Skvortsova and Lebedeva (1973), Kaminski et al. (1976), and Dennis (1977). Chang (1944a) also noted that the inactivation of amoebic cysts was accompanied by microscopic damage to the cell nucleus, which was dependent on chlorine penetration.

The importance of penetration and/or damage to the permeability barrier of the cell membrane as a result of exposure to chlorine has been observed by several investigators. In 1945, Rahn suggested that the inactivation of bacteria by chlorine was due to multiple injuries to the cell surface. From their work with bacterial spores, Kulikovsky et al. (1975) implicated permeability damage as a mechanism of chlorine inactivation. Studies with Escherichia coli have shown that chlorine causes leakage of cytoplasmic material, first protein, then RNA and DNA, into the suspending menstruum. It also inhibits the biochemical activities that are associated with the bacterial cell membrane (Venkobachar, 1975; Venkobachar et al., 1977). Friberg (1957) observed that E. coli also loses nondialyzable phosphorus following exposure to chlorine. In a recent study, Haas (1978) demonstrated that chlorine caused certain bacteria and yeast to release organic matter or UV-absorbing material, presumably protein or nucleic acid or their precursors. This investigator also noted that chlorine affected the uptake and retention of potassium by these same microorganisms.

Green and Stumpf (1946) and Knox et al. (1948) indicated that destruction of bacteria by chlorine was caused by an inhibition of the mechanism of glucose oxidation. Specifically, they suggested that chlorine affected the aldolase enzyme of E. coli by oxidizing the sulfhydryl group that is associated with the enzyme. Venkobachar et al. (1977) recently reported that chlorine significantly inhibits both oxygen uptake and oxidative phosphorylation. The latter effect was attributed to inhibition of the respiratory enzyme rather than to a deficiency in phosphate uptake. However, it is unclear whether free or combined chlorine was used in these studies. Haas (1978) also observed chlorine to affect the respiration of bacteria as well as the rate of synthesis of protein and DNA. Others have also noted that chlorine affects the nucleic acids or physically damages DNA (Bocharov, 1970; Bocharov and Kulikovskii, 1971; Fetner, 1962; Rosenkranz, 1973; Shih and Lederberg, 1976a,b).

It appears that chlorine, having penetrated the cell wall, encounters the cell membrane and alters its permeability. Simultaneously or subsequently, the chlorine molecules may enter the cytoplasm and interfere with various enzymatic reactions. It should be noted that permeases and respiratory enzymes are associated with the cytoplasmic membrane of bacteria.

Chang (1971) supported the hypothesis that the rapid destruction of vegetative bacteria by chlorine was due to the extensive destruction of metabolic enzyme systems. He also addressed the subject of virus inactivation, commenting that viruses are generally more resistant to chlorine than bacteria. He associated this observation with the fact that viruses completely lack a metabolic enzyme system. He speculated that inactivation of viruses by chlorine probably result from the denaturation of the capsid protein. Furthermore, since protein denaturation is more difficult to achieve than destruction of enzymatic R—S—H bonds by oxidizing agents, it is understandable why greater levels of chlorine are required to inactivate viruses than bacteria. However, from their experimental work with the bacterial virus f2, Olivieri et al. (1975) concluded that chlorine caused initial lethal damage to the viral genome and that the capsid protein was affected after the virus was inactivated. Dennis (1977) reported that the incorporation of chlorine into the f2 bacterial virus is dependent on pH and that the higher rates of incorporation occur at lower pH values.

There is limited information in the literature on the mechanism of inactivation of microorganisms by chloramines. Nusbaum (1952) proposed that since low levels of inorganic chloramines were effective in inactivating bacteria, the mechanism of action must be essentially the same as that of hypochlorous acid on enzymes. Ingols et al. (1953) showed that monochloramine was not able to immediately and irreversibly oxidize sulfhydryl groups. Such oxidation would have resulted in the rapid inactivation of the bacteria. They hypothesized that since monochloramine required higher concentrations and longer contact times to destroy bacteria completely and could not readily and irreversibly oxidize the sulfhydryl groups of the glucose oxidation enzymes, its ability to inactivate microorganisms should be attributed to changes in enzymes that may not be involved in the inactivation of the organism by hypochlorous acid. Thus, while the sulfhydryl group may be the most vulnerable to a strong oxidant like hypochlorous acid, changes in other groups produced by the weaker oxidant, monochloramine, may lead also to microbial inactivation. More recent information indicates that the destructive effects of chloramine might be associated with the effects of chloramine on nucleic acids or DNA of cells (Fetner, 1962; Shih and Lederberg, 1976a,b).

Nusbaum (1952) suggested that the disinfective activity of dichloramine occurs by a mechanism similar to monochloramine, but there do not appear to be any data to support this contention.

Considering the mechanism of destruction or inactivation of microorganisms by chlorine and associated compounds, it is interesting to note that Fair et al. (1948) speculated that there might be three or four "targets" or points of attack and that perhaps all must be affected before there is death. This "multiple hit" concept supported the observation that monochloramine must alter groups other than the sulfhydryl group to be effective in the destruction of microorganisms.

Thus, the action of chlorine on microbes such as bacteria and amebic cysts may involve some or all of the steps in the following sequence: penetration of the disinfectant through the cell wall followed by attack on the cell membrane (the site of cellular respiration in bacteria) and disruption of permeability of the cell membrane, which leads to a loss of cell constituents, thereby disrupting metabolic functions within the cell including those involving nucleic acids. Changes in viability may result from this process. Experimental studies on virus (Olivieri et al., 1975) demonstrated that chlorine caused initial damage on the viral nucleic acid while leaving the capsid protein unaffected until after the virus was inactivated.

Summary

Chlorine is the most widely used water supply disinfectant in the United States. Depending upon the predominant species of chlorine, hypochlorous acid, and/or hypochlorite ion, disinfection with chlorine can achieve greater than 99.9% destruction of bacteria. For example, a chlorine residual of 0.2 to 1.0 mg/liter and a contact time of 15 to 30 min will inactivate 99.9% of E. coli (Walton, 1969). According to Walton, a properly designed, constructed, and operated water treatment plant, consisting of chemical coagulation, sedimentation, filtration, and disinfection, can remove or destroy more than 99.999% of the coliform bacteria that are present. Although most investigations on the removal or destruction of bacteria have used E. coli, there is evidence that the bacterial pathogens, e.g., Salmonella typhi, respond somewhat similarly to E. coli.

Laboratory studies have demonstrated that that there is limited virus inactivation after the added chlorine has reacted with any ammonia that is in the water. Most inactivation probably occurs in the first few seconds before the chlorine has completed its reaction with ammonia (Olivieri et al., 1971).

Table II-3 displays c · t values for E. coli and poliovirus inactivation for the various species of free and combined chlorine.

Research Recommendations

Recent reports of enhanced chlorine resistance of certain viral and bacterial strains should be investigated and the mechanism of increased resistance elucidated, if the reports are corroborated.

TABLE II-3 Dosages of Various Chlorine Species Required for 99% Inactivation of *Escherichia Coli* and Poliovirus 1

Test Microorganism	Disinfecting Agent	Concentration, mg/liter	Contact Time, min	c•t[a]	pH	Temperature, °C	References
E. coli	Hypochlorous acid (HOC1)	0.1	0.4	0.04	6.0	5	Scarpino et al., 1974
	Hypochlorite ion (OCl⁻)	1.0	0.92	0.92	10.0	5	Scarpino et al., 1974
	Monochloramine (NH₂Cl)	1.0	175.0	175.0	9.0	5	Siders et al., 1973 Dorn, 1974
		1.0	64	64.0	9.0	15	Siders et al., 1973 Dorn, 1974
		1.2	33.5	40.2	9.0	25	Siders et al., 1973 Dorn, 1974
	Dichloramine (NHCl₂)	1.0	5.5	5.5	4.5	15	Esposito, 1974 Esposito et al., 1974

Poliovirus 1						
Hypochlorous acid (HOC1)	1.0	1.0	1.0	6.0	0	Weidenkopf, 1958
	0.5	2.1	1.05	6.0	5	Engelbrecht et al., 1978
	1.0	2.1	2.1	6.0	5	Scarpino et al., 1974
	1.0	1.0	1.0	6.0	15	Brigano et al., 1978
Hypochlorite ion (OCl$^-$)	0.5	21	10.5	10.0	5	Engelbrecht et al., 1978
	1.0	3.5	3.5	10.0	15	Brigano et al., 1978
Monochloramine (NH$_2$Cl)	10	90	900	9.0	15	Siders et al., 1973; Dorn, 1974
	10	32	320	9.0	25	Siders et al., 1974; Dorn, 1974
Dichloramine (NHCl$_2$)	100	140	14,000	4.5	5	Esposito, 1974; Esposito et al., 1974
	100	50	5,000	4.5	15	Esposito, 1974; Esposito et al., 1974

[a] Concentration of compound times contact time.

Other recommendations, applicable to other agents as well as to chlorine, are included after the evaluations of the other methods of disinfection.

OZONE

Chemistry of Ozone in Water

Ozone has the molecular formula O_3, a molecular weight of 48 g/mol, and a density, as a gas, of 2.154 g/liter at 0°C and 1 atm. It is approximately 13 times more soluble in water than is oxygen. At saturation in water at 20°C, a 2% weight mixture of ozone and oxygen contains about 11 mg of ozone and 40 mg of oxygen per liter.

Ozone has a half-life in pure distilled water of approximately 40 min at pH 7.6, but this decreases to 10 min at pH 8.5 (Stumm, 1958) at 14.6°C. Rising temperatures increase the rate of decomposition. Because its half-life is so short, ozone must be generated on the site where it is to be used.

Ozone is a powerful oxidant that reacts rapidly with most organic and many inorganic compounds. It does not convert chloride to chlorine under test conditions (U.S. Environmental Protection Agency, 1976), nor does it react extensively with ammonia (NH_3) (Singer and Zilli, 1975). However, bromide and iodide are oxidized to bromine and iodine. Singer and Zilli (1975) reported that oxidation of ammonia was pH-dependent. At pH 7.0, 9% of a 29 mg/liter ammonia nitrogen (NH_3-N) solution was oxidized in 30 min, but at pH 9.0 70% of a 24.4 mg/liter solution was oxidized in the same time. During disinfection, only minor amounts of ammonia are oxidized when ozone is used. Ozone's limited reaction with ammonia is desirable, but its fast reaction rate with most organic and many inorganic compounds further shortens its persistence in water.

Production and Application of Ozone

Ozone is produced on site from a stream of clean dry air or oxygen by passing an electrical discharge between electrodes that are separated by a dielectric. Approximately twice the percent of ozone by weight is obtained if oxygen, rather than air, is used as the feed stream. Power requirements are about 13 to 22 kWh/kg of ozone that is generated from air and approximately half that when oxygen is used (Rosen, 1972). Compressors and dryers may increase these requirements by 20% to 50%. Other factors affecting efficiency are the rate of gas flow, applied voltage, and the temperature of the gas. The heat that is produced during the process must be removed by cooling with either air or water.

The ozone gas stream must be fed into the water to effect the transfer of ozone. The usual methods are to inject the ozone gas stream through an orifice at the bottom of a co- or countercurrent contact chamber or to aspirate the gas into a contact chamber where it is mixed with the water mechanically. Successful design and operation of the contactor system is necessary to minimize costs of the operation.

Commercial equipment is available in a wide range of capacities— from a few grams of ozone per day to more than 40 kg/day. Larger capacities are obtained by adding additional units. Successful delivery of ozone to the water to be treated requires a dependable power supply and reasonably maintenance-free ozonization equipment.

Ozone has been used in a great number of water treatment plants throughout the world. However, in small institutions and private residences, its use appears limited, because it requires dependable power supplies and, usually, a second disinfectant to furnish a disinfecting residual in the system. The maintenance and repairs that are required for the specialized ozone generation equipment provide further barriers against the use of ozone by small institutions.

Analytical Methods

The disinfection process is usually controlled in one of two ways: by the dosage of a specified amount of ozone or by the maintenance of a specified minimum residual for a given time. Residual measurements in both the gas stream and water are sometimes required. *Standard Methods* (1976) contains descriptions of the measurement of ozone in water by the iodometric, orthotolidine–manganese sulfate, and orthotolidine–arsenite methods. Of these methods the iodometric method, which is subject to the fewest interferences, is the method of choice. Determinations must be made immediately since ozone decomposes rapidly.

In all three methods, the oxidant compounds that result from the reaction of ozone with contaminants in water may react with the test reagents, thereby indicating a higher concentration of ozone than is actually present. This is particularly true in the presence of organic matter, which results in the formation of organic peroxides. In the iodometric method this interference and others are minimized by stripping the ozone from the sample with nitrogen or air and absorbing it from this gas stream in an iodide solution. These and other methods are described in *Standard Methods*.

Schecter (1973) developed a UV spectrophotometric method to

measure the triiodide that is formed by the oxidation of iodide by ozone. She reported a better sensitivity at low ozone concentrations (0.01 to 0.3 mg/liter) than achieved with the normal titration method. The effects of interferences on the direct measurement of ozone without sparging the ozone to a separate iodide solution were not indicated. These effects are noted in *Standard Methods*.

Analytical determination of ozone in water in the presence of other oxidants is poor. Considerable work in this area is needed.

Residual

As discussed above, ozone is unstable in water with a half-life of approximately 40 min at pH 7.6 and 14.6°C. Many regard the half-life in water supplies at higher ambient temperatures to be 10 to 20 min.

In a recent review of the literature, Peleg (1976) concluded that the possible species to be found in an ozone solution were ozone, hydroxyl radicals ($\cdot OH$), hydroperoxyl radicals ($HO_2 \cdot$), oxide radicals ($O \cdot$), ozonide radicals ($O_3 \cdot$), and, possibly, free oxygen atoms ($\cdot O \cdot$). Hydrogen peroxide (H_2O_2) may also be present by dimerization of the hydroxyl radicals. There have been no studies on the disinfecting activities of these individual species except for those on hydrogen peroxide, which is a poor biocide (when compared to chlorine). Peleg concluded that evidence indicates that the dissociation species are better disinfectants than ozone.

Biocidal Activity

EFFICACY AGAINST BACTERIA

Wuhrmann and Meyrath (1955) found that 99% of *Escherchia coli* were inactivated in 21 s with 0.0125 mg/liter residual ozone, in 62 s with 0.0023 mg/liter residual ozone, and in 100 s with 0.0006 mg/liter residual ozone at pH 7.0 and 12°C. Spores of a *Bacillus* species were much more resistant, requiring 2 min with 0.191 mg/liter residual ozone and 5 min with 0.049 mg/liter residual ozone for 99% inactivation. These data were obtained at pH 7.2 and 22°C. The observed ozone residuals were reported as being constant throughout the test periods.

Katzenelson *et al.* (1974) found that an initial residual ozone concentration of 0.04 mg/liter in demand-free water inactivated approximately 3 logs of *E. coli* in 50 s, while a concentration of 1.3 mg/liter achieved the same degree of inactivation in 5 s. They obtained their inactivation data from experiments in which the loss of initial ozone residuals did not exceed 20%. Their work was conducted at 1°C and pH 7.2. The ozone was determined by the method of Schecter (1973).

Using washed cells of *E. coli, Bacillus megaterium,* and *Bacillus cereus,* which were suspended in deionized water with 10^6 cells/ml, and different concentrations of ozone up to 0.71 mg/liter, Broadwater *et al.* (1973) demonstrated that the inactivation of all three test organisms gave an "all-or-none" response. They measured the ozone by stripping it into iodide at the end of the contact period. Consequently, any demand should have used up whatever ozone was needed. They did measure what they presumed to be ozone and not some breakdown product. Thus, they appear to have eliminated the ozone demand problem as much as is possible with present techniques. However, it is possible that their results reflect some effect or artifact not yet understood. With the constant contact time of 5 min, no inactivation of vegetative cells of *E. coli* or *B. megaterium* occurred until the initial residual concentration of ozone was 0.19 mg/liter, when the density of viable cells of both species decreased to "near zero." With the vegetative cells of *B. cereus,* an initial ozone residual of 0.12 mg/liter was required before any inactivation occurred, and then it was nearly complete. Spores of *B. megaterium* and *B. cereus* were not inactivated until the ozone residual reached approximately 2.29 mg/liter, when the spores of both organisms showed an "all-or-none" response. All of the inactivation experiments were performed at 28°C, but the pH was not reported.

Burleson *et al.* (1975) determined that *E. coli, Staphylococcus aureus, Salmonella typhimurium, Shigella flexneri, Psuedomonas fluorescens,* and *Vibrio cholerae* were all reduced by 7.5 logs in 15 s after exposure to approximately 0.5 mg/liter of ozone at 25°C in phosphate-buffered saline. The pH was not reported. In this study, the bacteria were placed in unozonized water (no initial residual), and the ozone was then sparged into the water. After 15 s the ozone concentration in solution reached approximately 0.5 mg/liter. This technique does not render quantitative data. Ozone was determined by spectrophotometric measurement of iodine that was released from iodide without stripping of the ozone.

The inactivation of *E. coli* with initial counts of about 5×10^5/ml in buffered demand-free water at 11°C was measured by Ross *et al.* (1976). For 99% inactivation with 0.1 mg/liter of initial ozone residuals, contact times of 16.5 and 21 s were required at pH 6 and 10, respectively. Ozone was measured by the diethyl-*p*-phenylenediamine (DPD) method.

Farooq (1976) and Farooq *et al.* (1977a,b,c) studied the effects of pH and temperature in ozone inactivation studies with *Mycobacterium fortuitum* and *Candida parapsilosis* (a yeast). They concluded that if the ozone residual remains constant, the disinfection capability will not be affected by a change in pH. They also demonstrated that for a given dosage a rise in temperature increases the rate of inactivation, even though the ozone residual was decreased. (Ozone was less soluble at higher temperature). Vorchinskii (1963) concluded that whereas the bactericidal dose of ozone at 4°C to 6°C was unity, the corresponding dose at 18°C to 21°C was 1.6 and at 36°C to 38°C was 3.6.

The work of Farooq and his colleagues is in agreement with that of Morris (1976), who observed that the disinfection capability of ozone does not change significantly with pH, at least over the normal pH range (6 to 8.5) of water supplies.

EFFICACY AGAINST VIRUSES

Katzenelson et al. (1974) investigated the inactivation of poliovirus 1 at 5°C and pH 7.2. A 99% inactivation of the virus occurred in less than 8 s with 0.3 mg/liter of initial residual ozone. Their experimental methods were the same as those described above for bacteria. They also observed that inactivation resulted from two distinct stages (rates) of action. The first stage of inactivation, less than 8 s long, produced a virus inactivation of from 99% to 99.5%, depending upon the ozone residual. The second stage, which lasted from 1 to 5 min, still left some viruses infective. Additional work showed that the slower second-stage inactivation apparently involved the inactivation of viruses that were clumped together. The single virus particles were inactivated during the first stage. After ultrasonic treatment, 99.5% of the virus was inactivated within 8 s and more than 99.99% within 3 min at an initial ozone residual of 0.1 mg/liter.

Coin et al. (1964) investigated the inactivation of poliovirus 1 (Mahoney) in a batch system in which a measured amount of ozone was introduced into a virus suspension in distilled and filtered river water. In distilled water, nearly 1 log of the virus was inactivated in 4 min at a 4-min ozone residual of approximately 0.23 mg/liter. In river water, the inactivation was in excess of 99.99% in 4 min when the ozone concentration, also measured at 4 min, exceeded 0.3 mg/liter. The ozone was measured by the iodide titration without stripping of the ozone. Rather large ozone demands existed in this system. An initial 5 mg/liter residual ozone concentration in the distilled water decreased to about 0.6 to 0.8 mg/liter in 4 min. The same initial residual in river water decreased to between 0.2 to 0.6 mg/liter. Temperature and pH were not reported.

Keller et al. (1974) studied ozone inactivation of viruses in a water supply by using both batch tests and a pilot plant with a 38 liter/min (10

TABLE II-4   Ozone Required for Inactivation of Viruses in 10 Minutes at pH 7.0 and 25°C[a]

| | Ozone Required, mg/liter | |
Virus	99.9% Inactivation	99% Inactivation
Coxsackie B3	0.6	0.095
Polio 3	0.22	0.082
Polio 1	0.095	0.042
Echo 1	0.086	0.044
Coxsackie B5	0.076	0.053
Polio 2	0.052	0.039

[a] Data from Evison, 1977.

gal/min) flow rate. Inactivation of poliovirus 2 and coxsackievirus B3 in 5 min was greater than 99.9% in the batch tests when the ozone residual was between 0.8 and 1.7 mg/liter at the end of the 5-min contact period. Initial ozone residuals varied from 1.6 to 2.8 mg/liter. At the pilot plant, greater than 99.999% inactivation of coxsackievirus B3 could be achieved with an ozone dosage of 1.45 mg/liter, which provided an ozone residual of 0.28 mg/liter after 1 min in lake water. Temperature and pH conditions were not reported. Ozone was measured by the iodide method without prior stripping of the ozone.

Burleson et al. (1975) obtained inactivations of >99.9% for vesicular stomatitis virus, >99.99% for encephalomyocarditis virus, and 99.99% for GD VII virus in 15 s with an ozone residual of approximately 0.5 mg/liter of ozone. The experiment was conducted in the same manner as that described above for their studies with bacteria. Evison (1977) reported data for the inactivation of a number of viruses in buffered water at pH 7.0 and 25°C (Table II-4).

The reported ozone concentrations were evidently those measured initially and maintained by the addition of ozone during the experiment. Ozone was measured by a colorimetric version of Palin's DPD technique. The Evison data show that more ozone or a longer time are required for inactivation than do the data of other workers. This may have resulted from the virus purification used. Her viruses were purified by low-speed centrifugation and filtration through an 0.2-μm membrane filter. These cleanup procedures are neither as complete nor as thorough as those used by other investigators. The unremoved cell debris and organic matter offer protection to the virus. Either higher ozone residuals or longer contact times would be required to inactivate such preparations to the same extent as clean virus. Other data showed that the inactivation of coliphage 185 was relatively unaffected by pH's ranging from 6.0 to 8.0 at ozone concentrations exceeding 0.05 to 0.10 mg/liter. Evison (1977) also concluded that the rate of inactivation of the coliphage 185 by ozone was much less affected by temperature than was the inactivation by chlorine.

Farooq (1976) observed a 99% inactivation of 10^5/ml poliovirus 1 in 30 s in distilled water at an initial ozone residual concentration between 0.23 and 0.26 mg/liter at 24°C and pH 7.0. In this study, ozone was measured by the Schecter (1973) method.

Sproul et al. (1978) reported total inactivation in 10 s of poliovirus 1 (Sabin), which had initial concentrations of 1.3×10^2 to 2.4×10^3 plaque-forming units (PFU)/ml. The initial ozone residual of 0.012 to 0.085 mg/liter decreased by approximately one-third in 40 s. The experiments were conducted with the Sharpe dynamic reactor. Ozone was measured by the Schecter (1973) method.

EFFICACY AGAINST PARASITES

No studies on the efficacy of ozone as an antihelmintic agent appear to have been reported.

Ozone may have application as an antiparasitic agent in the treatment of water supplies but only limited information is available. Newton and Jones (1949) reported that ozone, with 5-min residuals as low as 0.3 mg/liter, inactivated from 98% to >99% of *Entamoeba histolytica* cysts that were suspended in water. Initial ozone residuals that were required to obtain 5-min residuals of 0.3 mg/liter varied from 0.7 mg/liter to 0.9 mg/liter. With the ozone concentrations used, the cysticidal action was not affected by temperatures from 10°C to 27°C nor by pH's between 6.5 to 8.0. Ozone was measured by titration of iodine, which was released from iodide directly in the reactors without removal of ozone by sparging.

Mechanism of Action

Investigations of the inactivation of bacteria by ozone have centered on the action of ozone on the cell membrane. Scott and Lesher (1963) concluded from their work with *E. coli* that the primary attack of ozone occurred on the double bonds of the fatty acids in the cell wall and membrane and that there was a consequent change in the cell permeability. Cell contents then leaked into the water. This was confirmed by Smith (1967). Prat *et al.* (1968), examining extracts from ozonized *E. coli*, reported that thymine was more sensitive to ozone attack than were cytosine and uracil.

Riesser *et al.* (1977) showed that ozone attacked the protein capsid of poliovirus 2 in such a manner that the virus was not taken up into susceptible cells. An electrophoretic study showed complete loss of viral proteins in a poliovirus 2 sample that had showed an inactivation of 7 logs in 20 min.

Summary and Conclusions

Inactivation with ozone at specified ozone residuals is relatively insensitive to pH's between 6.0 and 8.5. Moreover, ozone does not react with ammonia over this same range when short detention times are used. The data on temperature are not sufficiently firm to permit conclusions concerning its effect on disinfection. Ozone must be generated on site, and the process is relatively energy intensive. To make economic comparisons of ozone with other disinfectants, the cost of local power must be ascertained.

Available kinetic data on ozone inactivation are presented in Table II-5. The c · t product for 99% inactivation of *E. coli* appears to be approximately 0.006 at near-neutral pH values and at temperatures of ≤ 10°C. There was less consistency for the c · t products of poliovirus 1. These values varied from <0.005 to 0.42 at pH 7 and at temperatures from 5°C to 25°C.

The c · t products vary over a broad range. These variations illustrate the difficulty of doing quantitative experimentation with ozone and microorganisms in water. Among other reasons, these difficulties are caused by undetected ozone demand in the water, poor analytical techniques for residual ozone, and nonuniformity of microorganisms from one laboratory to another. As an example of the latter, different strains of poliovirus with different inactivation rates are used, but the inactivation data are frequently not reported as strain-specific. Furthermore, viruses frequently exist in an undetected clumped state rather than in the presumed single discrete particle state. Higher c · t products are required for the clumped viruses than for the unclumped ones.

Because of ozone's relatively short half-life in water, another disinfectant must be added to maintain a disinfection capability in the

TABLE II-5 Concentration of Ozone and Contact Time Necessary for 99% Inactivation of *Escherichia coli* and Polio 1 Virus

Test Microorganism	Ozone, mg/liter	Contact Time, min	c·t[a]	pH	Temperature, °C	References
E. coli	0.07	0.083	0.006	7.2	1	Katzenelson et al., 1974
	0.065	0.33	0.022	7.2	1	Katzenelson et al., 1974
	0.04	0.50	0.02	7.2	1	Katzenelson et al., 1974
	0.01	0.275	0.027	6.0	11	Ross et al., 1976
	0.01	0.35	0.035	6.0	11	Ross et al., 1976
	0.0006	1.7	0.001	7.0	12	Wuhrmann and Meyrath, 1955
	0.0023	1.03	0.002	7.0	12	Wuhrmann and Meyrath, 1955
	0.0125	0.33	0.004	7.0	12	Wuhrmann and Meyrath, 1955
Polio 1	<0.3	0.13	<0.04	7.2	5	Katzenelson et al., 1974
	0.245	0.50	0.12	7.0	24	Farooq, 1976
	0.042	10	0.42	7.0	25	Evison, 1977
	<0.03	0.16	<0.005	7.0	20	Sproul et al., 1978

[a] Concentration of ozone times contact time.

distribution system. The most effective disinfectant, its optimum concentration, and method of addition must be determined. The disinfection process with ozone will probably be controlled by specifying the ozone residual at the beginning and end of a given contact time.

Research Recommendations

Future research studies with ozone should be conducted to:

- provide data on the inactivation of enteric pathogens;
- provide more data on the inactivation of protozoan cysts, especially those of *Giardia lamblia*;
- provide analytical methods that are specific for ozone;
- provide additional definitive data on bacteria and viruses, and eliminate discrepancies; and
- provide operating data from full-scale drinking water plants to demonstrate reliability of operation, operating costs, ozone dosages, residuals, contact times, and disinfection results.

CHLORINE DIOXIDE

Chlorine dioxide (ClO_2) was first prepared in the early nineteenth century by Sir Humphrey Davey (1811). By combining potassium chlorate ($KClO_3$) and hydrochloric acid (HCl), he produced a greenish-yellow gas, which he named "euchlorine." Later, this gas was found to be a mixture of chlorine dioxide and chlorine. The bleaching action of chlorine dioxide on wood pulp was recognized by Watt and Burgess (1854).

Large quantities of chlorine dioxide are produced each day in the United States. Although its primary application has been the bleaching of wood pulp, it is also used extensively for bleaching and dye stripping in the textile industry and for bleaching flour, fats, oils, and waxes (Gall, 1978).

In the United States, chlorine dioxide was first used in 1944 at the water treatment plant in Niagara Falls, New York, to control phenolic tastes and odors arising from the presence of industrial wastes, algae, and decaying vegetation (Synan *et al.*, 1945). Granstrom and Lee (1958) surveyed water treatment plants believed to be using chlorine dioxide.

The majority of respondents (956 plants) were using it for taste and odor control. Other uses reported were algal control (7 plants), iron and manganese removal (3 plants), and disinfection (15 plants).

Sussman (1978) compiled a partial listing of plants using chlorine dioxide. He reported that the compound is used primarily to control taste and odor in the United States. In England, Italy, and Switzerland, it is used for disinfection of water supplies.

The Chemistry of Chlorine Dioxide in Water

Chlorine dioxide reacts with a wide variety of organic and inorganic chemicals under conditions that are usually found in water treatment systems (Stevens *et al.*, 1978). However, two important reactions do not occur. Chlorine dioxide per se does not react to cause the formation of trihalomethanes (THM's) (Miltner, 1976). However, THM's will be formed if the chlorine dioxide is contaminated with chlorine. Such a situation may occur when chlorine is used in the preparation of chlorine dioxide.

Chlorine dioxide does not react with ammonia, but will react with other amines (Rosenblatt, 1978). The amine structure determines reactivity. Tertiary amines are more reactive with chlorine dioxide than secondary amines, which, in turn, are more reactive than primary amines.

Production and Application

Chlorine dioxide condenses to form an unstable liquid. Both the gas and liquid are sensitive to temperature, pressure, and light. At concentrations above 10% in air, chlorine dioxide may be explosive, and at 4% in air, it can be detonated by sparks (Gall, 1978; Sussman, 1978). As a result, the preparation and distribution of chlorine dioxide in bulk have not been deemed practical. It has been generated and used on site.

Sodium chlorate ($NaClO_3$) or sodium chlorite ($NaClO_2$) may be used to generate chlorine dioxide. The method of production will depend upon the amount of chorine dioxide that is required. The reduction of sodium chlorate is the more efficient process and is generally used when large volumes and high concentrations of chlorine dioxide are needed. Commercial processes that are used in North America for large-scale production of chlorine dioxide are based on the three reactions listed below. To reduce the sodium chlorate, each process uses a different agent: sulfur dioxide (SO_2), methanol (CH_3OH), and the chloride ion (Cl^-).

$$2NaClO_3 + H_2SO_4 + SO_2 \rightarrow 2ClO_2 + 2NaHSO_4 \tag{6}$$

$$2NaClO_3 + CH_3OH + H_2SO_4 \rightarrow$$
$$2ClO_2 + HCHO + Na_2SO_4 + 2H_2O \tag{7}$$

$$NaClO_3 + NaCl + H_2SO_4 \rightarrow ClO_2 + \frac{1}{2}Cl_2 + Na_2SO_4 + H_2O \tag{8}$$

All of these processes are used in the pulp and paper industry. They can also be used to prepare chlorine dioxide for the large waterworks that might require several metric tons per day. Small quantities of chlorine are formed during the side reactions and intermediate reactions in these processes. A more detailed review of the chemistry that is involved in the production of chlorine dioxide from chlorate is given by Gall (1978) and Gordon et al. (1972).

Chlorine dioxide can be prepared from chlorine and sodium chlorite through the following reactions:

$$Cl_2 + H_2O \rightarrow HOCl + HCl \tag{9}$$

$$HOCl + HCl + 2NaClO_2 \rightarrow 2ClO_2 + 2NaCl + H_2O \tag{10}$$

The theoretical weight ratio of sodium chlorite to chlorine is 1.00:0.39 (Dowling, 1974). With available sodium chlorite (80%), the weight ratio is 1:0.30. In practice, Gall (1978) recommended a chlorite to chlorine ratio of 1:1. The excess chlorine lowers the pH, thereby increasing the reaction rate and optimizing the yield of chlorine dioxide. Dowling (1974) reported that the maximum theoretical yield of chlorine dioxide was produced when the ratio was normally maintained at a minimum of 1.0:0.5.

Alternatively, chlorine dioxide may be prepared from sodium hypochlorite (NaOCl) and sodium chlorite. The sodium hypochlorite is acidified to yield hypochlorous acid (HOCl), and the chlorine dioxide is generated according to Reaction 10. Each of the methods produces a solution containing both chlorine and chlorine dioxide.

Chlorine dioxide may also be prepared by the addition of a strong acid, such as sulfuric acid (H_2SO_4) or hydrochloric acid, to sodium chlorite as shown in the following reactions:

$$10NaClO_2 + 5H_2SO_4 \rightarrow 8ClO_2 + 5Na_2SO_4 + 2HCl + 4H_2O \qquad (11)$$

$$5NaClO_2 + 4HCl \rightarrow 4ClO_2 + 5NaCl + 2H_2O \qquad (12)$$

Although some investigators have claimed that this method produces chlorine-free chlorine dioxide, Feuss (1964) and Schilling (1956) reported that chlorine is also formed. Dowling (1974) indicated that chlorine was formed even when sulfuric acid was used.

Analytical Methods

Chlorine dioxide is one of the few stable nonmetallic inorganic free radicals (Rosenblatt, 1978). It does not contain available chlorine in the form of hypochlorous acid or hypochlorite ion (OCl^-). However, concentrations of chlorine dioxide are often reported in terms of available chlorine. The chlorine atom in chlorine dioxide has a valance of $+4$. A reduction to chloride results in a gain of five electrons. In terms of available chlorine, chlorine dioxide has 263% or more than 2.5 times the oxidizing capacity of chlorine.

$$\frac{5e^- \times 35.45}{67.45} \times 100 = 263\% \qquad (13)$$

The weight ratio of chlorine dioxide to available chlorine is 67.45 to 35.45 or 1.9. However, in water treatment practices this increased oxidizing capacity is rarely realized. The reduction of chlorine dioxide depends heavily on pH and the nature of the reducing agent. At neutral or alkaline pH, chlorine dioxide is reduced to chlorite, a net gain of one electron. Thus, only one-fifth or 20% of its oxidizing capacity is utilized. At low pH, the chlorite (ClO_2^-) is reduced to chloride (Cl^-) releasing the remaining four available electrons.

Chlorine dioxide may be determined iodometrically (*Standard Methods*, 1976), amperometrically (Haller and Listek, 1948; *Standard Methods*, 1976), spectrophotometrically (Gordon et al., 1972), and colorimetrically (Aston, 1950; Hodgen and Ingols, 1954; Masschelein, 1966; Palin, 1957, 1960, 1967, 1970, 1974, 1975; Post and Moore, 1959; *Standard Methods*, 1976).

Several studies contain comparisons of various analytical methods and procedures for the measurement of chlorine dioxide. Adams *et al.* (1966) compared the H-acid, tyrosine, amperometric, and diethyl-*p*-phenylene-diamine (DPD) procedures for free chlorine, chlorine dioxide, and chlorite. They reported DPD to be the most reliable, as did Dowling (1974), Miltner (1976), and the U.S. Public Health Service (Miltner, 1976). Myhrstad and Samdal (1969) noted that the DPD method (Palin, 1957, 1960) yielded consistently higher residual measurements for chlorine dioxide than those that are produced with other analytical methods. After analysis with acid chrome violet K (Masschelein, 1966), chlorine dioxide was not observed in the water of the distribution system; however, chlorite was found. The residuals that were previously interpreted as chlorine dioxide were apparently due to chlorite.

Recently, more sophisticated procedures were suggested for the determination of chlorine dioxide. Moffa *et al.* (1975) reported the use of electron spin resonance, and Issacsson and Wettermark (1976) described a chemiluminescent method for active chlorine compounds. Stevenson *et al.* (1978) reviewed electrochemical methods and presented preliminary results for a membrane amperometric probe. Under development is a sensor that shows a linear response region from about 0.5 to 10 mg/liter. The response to hypochlorous acid and chloramines was low, and the sensor does not measure chlorite or other ionized species.

No one procedure appears to possess the necessary sensitivity, selectivity, and simplicity to permit reliable determinations in the treatment of water. Each of the titration methods are prone to error because of volatilization. They are time-consuming and particularly complex when differentiation of chlorine and oxychloro species are necessary. The colorimetric procedures require strict control of pH, temperature, and reaction times and will be affected by turbidity. In addition, the selectivity of the indicators for chlorine dioxide is questionable. The direct spectrophotometric determination of chlorine dioxide at 360 nm is selective and rapid but is not sufficiently sensitive for use in water. Limited experience with the more recent procedures (chemiluminescence and membrane amperometric probe) does not permit an evaluation.

In practice, the principal distinction that must be made is that between the active biocidal species (hypochlorous acid, the hypochloride ion, and chlorine dioxide), the moderately biocidal species (monochloramine [NH_2Cl], dichloramine [$NHCl_2$], and nitrogen trichloride [NCl_3]), and the relatively nonbiocidal species (chlorite and chlorate [ClO_3^-] ions). This is imperative when the primary purpose for the addition of chlorine dioxide is the inactivation of microorganisms. Furthermore, when the formation of THM's is to be considered, the distinction between free chlorine and chlorine dioxide becomes important.

Biocidal Activity

EFFICACY AGAINST BACTERIA

Experimental data on the efficacy of chlorine dioxide as a disinfectant became available in the early 1940's. McCarthy (1944, 1945) reported that chlorine dioxide was an effective bactericide in water with a low organic content. When the levels of organic material in the water were high, chlorine dioxide was less effective.

Ridenour and Ingols (1947) reported that chlorine dioxide was at least as effective as chlorine against *Escherichia coli* after 30 min at similar residual concentrations. Both chlorine and chlorine dioxide residues were determined by the orthotolidine–arsenite (OTA) method. The bactericidal activity of chlorine dioxide was not affected by pH values from 6.0 to 10.0. Ridenour and Armbruster (1949) extended their observation to other enteric bacteria. The common waterborne pathogens were similarly inactivated with chlorine dioxide. They also reported that the efficiency of chlorine dioxide decreased as the temperature decreased from 20°C to 5°C.

Ridenour *et al.* (1949) found chlorine dioxide to be more effective than chlorine (based on OTA residuals) against bacterial endospores. They indicated that less weight of chlorine dioxide than chlorine is required to inactivate the spores of *Bacillus mesentericus* in either demand-free water or in waters containing ammonia. In the waters containing ammonia, chlorine had to be applied beyond breakpoint before efficient sporicidal activity was observed.

The work of Ridenour and colleagues is not discussed in depth because the small amounts of free chlorine that are produced during the generation of chlorine dioxide are not distinguished from the chlorine dioxide by the OTA method that they used for both stock solutions and residual determination. In their 1947 paper (Ridenour and Ingols, 1947), the survival measurements were ± and not quantitative. In their 1949 paper (Ridenour and Armbruster, 1949), the survival measurement was quantitative, but only one contact time was used, 5.0 min. Since chlorine dioxide is a rapidly acting disinfectant, c · t products may be misleading using this contact time.

Russian investigators (Bedulevich *et al.*, 1953; Trakhtman, 1946) found chlorine dioxide to be a more effective or at least as effective a bactericide as chlorine. Additional data were reported for *Bacillus anthracis.* They observed that the efficiency of chlorine dioxide decreased as the pH of the system containing the *B. anthracis* increased.

Early studies on disinfectant activity are difficult to interpret because the methods of preparing chlorine dioxide invariably included the addition or production of chlorine. Analytical procedures were not sufficiently advanced to differentiate between chlorine dioxide and other oxychloro species. Thus, the quantitative analyses of stock solutions and reports of dose and residual chlorine dioxide may be in error. This suggests that the initial and residual concentrations of chlorine dioxide were probably lower than reported values and that the comparative bactericidal efficiency would suffer accordingly. In addition, the older investigations did not take into account the volatility of chlorine dioxide. Depending upon concentration and length of exposure, losses of 7% to 30% can occur within an hour.

Many of the difficulties that were encountered during the early studies were overcome in a series of studies reported by Benarde and co-workers during the mid-1960's. Their work on disinfection was based heavily on the improved methods of preparing and analyzing chlorine dioxide, which were reported by Granstrom and Lee (1958). They prepared chlorine dioxide by oxidizing sodium chlorite with persulfate ($S_2O_8^{2-}$) under acid conditions. The resulting chlorine dioxide was swept to a collection vessel by high purity nitrogen gas. Chlorine dioxide was measured spectrophotometrically at 357 nm.

Bernarde *et al.* (1965) compared the bactericidal effectiveness of chlorine with that of chlorine dioxide at pH 6.5 and 8.5 in a demand-free buffered system. At pH 6.5, both chlorine and chlorine dioxide inactivated a freshly isolated strain of *E. coli* in less than 60 s. Chlorine was slightly more effective at the lower dosages at the lower pH. At pH 8.5, chlorine dioxide was dramatically more effective than chlorine. Greater than 99% inactivation of *E. coli* was observed in 15 s with 0.25 mg/liter chlorine dioxide, while, under the same conditions, chlorine required almost 5 min for similar inactivation. Chlorine dioxide was significantly more efficient than chlorine in the presence of high levels of organic and nitrogenous material. Bernarde *et al.* (1967a) also reported that temperature affects the rate of inactivation of bacteria with chlorine dioxide. A decrease in disinfectant activity was observed as temperature decreased from 30°C to 5°C. For 99% inactivation of *E. coli* with 0.25 mg/liter of chlorine dioxide, 190, 74, 41, and 16 s were required at 5°C, 10°C, 20°C, 30°C, respectively. More recent work by Cronier (1977) in a clean system also demonstrated the excellent bactericidal activity of chlorine dioxide. Results of both studies are shown in Table II-6.

TABLE II-6   Concentrations of Chlorine Dioxide and Contact Times
Necessary for 99% Inactivation of *Escherichia coli*

Test Microorganism	Chlorine Dioxide, mg/liter	Contact Time, min	c·t[a]	pH	Temperature, °C
E. coli	0.25	1.8	0.45	6.5	5
(freshly	0.50	0.83	0.41	6.5	5
isolated	0.75	0.50	0.38	6.5	5
from feces)[b]	0.25	1.2	0.30	6.5	10
	0.50	0.47	0.24	6.5	10
	0.75	0.3	0.23	6.5	10
	0.25	0.68	0.17	6.5	20
	0.50	0.35	0.18	6.5	20
	0.75	0.25	0.19	6.5	20
	0.25	0.27	0.07	6.5	32
	0.50	0.22	0.11	6.5	32
	0.75	0.15	0.11	6.5	32
E. coli	0.30	1.8	0.54	7.0	5
(ATCC 11229)[c]	0.50	0.98	0.49	7.0	5
	0.80	0.58	0.41	7.0	5
	0.30	1.3	0.39	7.0	15
	0.50	0.75	0.38	7.0	15
	0.80	0.47	0.38	7.0	15
	0.30	0.98	0.29	7.0	25
	0.50	0.55	0.28	7.0	25
	0.80	0.35	0.28	7.0	25

[a] Concentration of chlorine dioxide times contact time.
[b] Data from Bernarde *et al.*, 1967a.
[c] Data from Cronier, 1977.

EFFICACY AGAINST VIRUSES

In the mid-1940's, there were also investigations on the virucidal activity of chlorine dioxide. Ridenour and Ingols (1946) reported that chlorine dioxide was as effective as chlorine against a mouse-adapted strain of poliovirus (Lansing). Again, their comparison was based upon OTA-determined residual levels of each disinfectant. Hettche and Ehlbeck (1953) found chlorine dioxide to be more effective against poliovirus than either chlorine or ozone. In addition to the difficulties that are associated with the preparation and measurement of chlorine dioxide and chlorine, the early virus studies were also saddled with difficult and time-consuming virus test systems.

The first definitive work on the virucidal activity of chlorine dioxide was done in Göteborg, Sweden. Warriner (1967) showed that the rate of inactivation of poliovirus 3 increased with increasing pH at pH values of 5.6 to 8.5 (see Table II-7). Similar to the action on bacteria, the viral inactivation occurred rapidly. When chlorine and chlorine dioxide were combined, the inactivation was synergistic. The inactivation with the two chlorine species together was more efficient at lower pH, but the presence of chlorine dioxide enhanced inactivation by chlorine at the higher pH.

Cronier (1977) compared the inactivation of $E.$ $coli$ (ATCC 11229), poliovirus 1, and coxsackievirus A9. All of the microorganisms that were tested were sensitive to low concentrations ($<$1 mg/liter) of chlorine dioxide. Poliovirus 1 and coxsackievirus A9 were more resistant than $E.$ $coli.$ Similar to its bactericidal activity, chlorine dioxide was more effective as a virucide at higher pH. Cronier also reported that on a weight basis, it was similar to hypochlorous acid and better than hypochlorite ion, monochloramine, and dichloramine.

The effect of bentonite ($AlO_3 \cdot 4SiO_2 \cdot H_2O$) (added to the test as a model for turbidity) on disinfection with chlorine dioxide was studied by Scarpino et $al.$ (1977). At turbidity levels below 2.29 nephelometric turbidity units (NTU) at 25°C, no protection was afforded to poliovirus 1 by the bentonite. However, at 3.22 and 14.1 NTU's, poliovirus inactivation was noticeably decreased. The bentonite at these levels appeared to offer protection to the virus.

EFFICACY AGAINST PARASITES

The data that are available on the efficacy of chlorine dioxide on helminths or protozoan cysts do not appear to be suitable for comparison with the action of other disinfectants.

COMPARATIVE BIOCIDAL ACTIVITY

The data presented in Tables II-6 and II-7 were collected for demand-free systems within the last 15 yr, when relatively reliable chemical methods and/or quantitative biocidal assay procedures were used. Table II-6 shows the concentration of chlorine dioxide necessary for 99% inactivation of $E.$ $coli$ strains. Even at 5°C and chlorine dioxide concentrations of 0.25 to 0.30 mg/liter, less than 2 min was required for 99% inactivation. Increases in chlorine dioxide concentration and/or

TABLE II-7   Concentrations of Chlorine Dioxide and Contact Times Necessary for 99% Inactivation of Viruses

Test Microorganism	Chlorine Dioxide, mg/liter	Contact Time, min	c·t[a]	pH	Temperature, °C
Poliovirus 3[b]	0.5	5.0	2.5	5.6	20
	0.5	5.0	2.5	7.2	20
	0.5	0.25	0.125	8.5	20
	1.6	5.0	8.00	5.6	20
	1.6	1.0	1.60	7.1	20
	1.6	0.25	0.40	8.0	20
Poliovirus 1[c]	0.3	16.6	5.0	7.0	5
	0.5	12.0	6.0	7.0	5
	0.8	6.8	5.4	7.0	5
	0.3	4.2	1.3	7.0	15
	0.5	2.5	1.25	7.0	15
	0.8	1.7	1.4	7.0	15
	0.3	3.6	1.08	7.0	25
	0.5	2.0	1.0	7.0	25
	0.8	1.5	1.2	7.0	25
Coxsackievirus A9	0.3	1.2	0.4	7.0	15
	0.5	0.05	0.34	7.0	15
	0.8	0.25	0.20	7.0	15

[a] Concentration of chlorine dioxide times contact time.
[b] Data from Warriner, 1967a.
[c] Data from Cronier, 1977.

temperature markedly reduced the contact time that was necessary. Table II-7 presents similar data for viruses. Increased chlorine dioxide concentration, temperature, and pH decreased the contact time that was required to produce 99% inactivation of the viruses. The amount of inactivation depended on the virus that was tested.

Mechanism of Action

There is little information concerning the mode of action by which chlorine dioxide inactivates bacteria and viruses. Ingols and Ridenour (1948) suggested that the bactericidal effectiveness of chlorine dioxide is due to its adsorption on the cell wall with subsequent penetration into the cell where it reacts with enzymes containing sulfhydryl groups.

Benarde *et al.* (1967b) demonstrated that chlorine dioxide abruptly inhibited protein synthesis. The incorporation of ^{14}C-labeled amino acids into protein by whole cells stopped within a few seconds after the addition of chlorine dioxide. Subsequently, Olivieri (1968) reported a dose–response in the inhibition of protein synthesis in bacteria that had been treated with chlorine dioxide. The site of action was localized in the soluble portion (enzymes) of the cell extracts of treated cells without affecting the integrity of the ribosomes' function in protein synthesis.

Conclusion

Chlorine dioxide is an effective bactericide and virucide under the pH, temperature, and turbidity that are expected in the treatment of potable water. It should be noted that the U.S. Environmental Protection Agency (1978) has set an interim Maximum Contaminant Level of 1 mg/liter on chlorine dioxide (U.S. Environmental Protection Agency, 1978) because of the unresolved questions on its health effects (Symons *et al.*, 1977).

Research Recommendations

A simple, selective, and sensitive test for chlorine dioxide should be developed to monitor residual concentration.

Chlorine dioxide is currently used at several plants. A review of plant records and field studies on the stability and effectiveness of chlorine dioxide in the distribution system should be undertaken.

Studies should be directed toward evaluating the inactivation of protozoan cysts.

More information should be obtained on the mode of action by which chlorine dioxide inactivates bacteria, viruses, and cysts.

IODINE

The use of iodine as a biocide has had a long history, primarily as an antiseptic for skin wounds and mucous surfaces of the body and, to a lesser degree, as a powerful sanitizing agent in hospitals and laboratories (Gershenfeld, 1977). The use of iodine as a disinfectant of drinking and swimming pool water has not been extensive, mainly because of the costs and problems that are involved in applying the dosage.

Aside from the emergency iodination of small volumes for field and emergency drinking water and limited experience with swimming pool

TABLE II-8   Hydrolysis of Iodine at 25°C Showing the Percentage of
Iodine Species at Different pH's[a]

pH	Percentage of Iodine Species by Concentration of Iodine								
	0.5 mg/liter			5.0 mg/liter			50.0 mg/liter		
	I_2	HOI	OI^-	I_2	HOI	OI^-	I_2	HOI	OI^-
5	99	1	0	100	0	0	100	0	0
6	90	10	0	99	1	0	100	0	0
7	52	48	0	88	12	0	97	3	0
8	12	88	0.005	52	48	0	86	14	0

[a] Data from Chang, 1958.

disinfection (Black *et al.*, 1959), the only substantial experience with
iodine disinfection of piped water system is that of Black *et al.* (1965,
1968). Two water systems serving three prisons in the state of Florida
were disinfected satisfactorily with 1 mg/liter of iodine. A persistent
residual was maintained throughout the distribution system despite a
finished water pH of 8.0 to 9.5. No adverse effects on health were
observed among those consuming the water.

Chemistry of Iodine in Water

Iodine is the only common halogen that is a solid at room temperature,
and it possesses the highest atomic weight (126.91). Of the four common
halogens, it is the least soluble in water, has the lowest standard
oxidation potential for reduction to halide, and reacts least readily with
organic compounds.

$$I_2 + H_2O \rightleftharpoons HOI + H^+ + I^- \qquad (14)$$

Diatomic iodine (I_2) reacts with water to form hypoiodous acid (HOI)
and iodide ion (I^-). The effect of pH on this reaction is shown in Table
II-8.

The distribution of chemical species of iodine given in Table II-8 was
taken from the calculations that were made by Chang (1958) from the
equilibrium expression:

$$\frac{[HOI][H]^+[I]^-}{[I_2]} = K_h \qquad (15)$$

The value of K_h, the hydrolysis constant, is given by Wyss and Strandskov (1945) as 3×10^{-12} at 25°C. With iodine residuals at 0.5 mg/liter, which are expected in water systems, and a pH of 5, approximately 99% of the total iodine residual is present as iodine and only 1% as hypoiodous acid. At pH 7, the two forms are present in almost equal concentrations. At pH 8, only 12% is present as elemental iodine and 88% as hypoiodous acid, which can be converted to hypoiodite ion (OI⁻).

$$HOI \rightleftharpoons H^+ + OI^- \qquad (16)$$

$$\frac{[H^+][OI^-]}{[HOI]} = K_a = 4.5 \times 10^{-13} \qquad (17)$$

$$[H^+] = K_a \frac{[HOI]}{[OI^-]} \qquad (18)$$

$$\frac{[HOI^-]}{[OI^-]} = \frac{H^+}{K_a} \qquad (19)$$

The dissociation constant, K_a, of hypoiodous acid (at 20°C) is 4.5×10^{-13}. Consequently, the dissociation of hypoiodous acid, which occurs at high pH's, is not important for practical purposes. However, as confirmed by the field studies in Florida, hypoiodous acid can form iodate ion by autooxidation at pH values above 9.

$$3HOI + 2OH^- \rightleftharpoons HOI_3 + 2H_2O + 2I^- \qquad (20)$$

The iodate ion possesses no disinfecting ability (Marks and Strandskov, 1950).

Production and Application

Iodine may be added to a municipal water supply by several procedures. One method is to employ nonhazardous solvents and solubilizing agents such as ethyl alcohol (C_2H_5OH) and potassium iodide (KI) to overcome the low concentration of aqueous iodine stock for solution feeders. Another method produces the required concentration of iodine by passing water through a bed of crystalline iodine (saturator). This has been used in many small, semipublic and private home water systems. Since the maximum concentration is limited by solubility to 200–300 mg/liter at the ambient temperatures that are expected for drinking water, some physical complications would accompany the introduction of this method into the large waterworks system in view of the large saturation beds required. The iodinated anion exchange resin bed and the vaporization technique are not sufficently developed to be considered for use in public water supplies.

In certain circumstances, potassium iodide might be combined with an oxidation reaction to release iodine. The chemistry is simple, and the persistence of the iodine that is generated may be much better than chlorine. This method has been used in swimming pools and for dechlorination purposes where a chlorine residual may be exchanged for an iodine residual, or an iodine residual may be provided where ozone is the primary disinfectant.

Analytical Methods

Both amperometric titration and leuco crystal violet (LCV) colorimetric methods give acceptable results when used to measure free iodine in drinking water. Waters containing oxidized forms of manganese interfere with the LCV method. Also, when iodide ion exceeds 50 mg/liter and chloride ion exceeds 200 mg/liter, the amperometric method is preferred. Under unusual situations, where mixtures of chlorine, bromine, and ozone occur along with iodine, the problem of separation is difficult (*Standard Methods*, 1976).

Biocidal Activity

Table II-9 shows the relative resistance of bacteria, viruses, and cysts to inactivation by iodine.

EFFICACY AGAINST BACTERIA

Chang and Morris (1953), summarizing the development of a universal water disinfectant tablet for the military, concluded that iodine concentrations of 5 to 10 mg/liter were effective against bacterial pathogens. Iodine was less dependent than chlorine upon the pH, temperature, contact time, and secondary reactions with nitrogenous impurities in the water. As a cysticide, iodine was poor in water with a high pH. Consequently, the tablet that was formulated contained an acid buffer to lower the pH of the water. The tablet, called "Globaline," released 8

TABLE II-9   Comparative Values from Confirmed Experiments on Disinfecting Water with Iodine at 23°C to 30°C, at pH 7.0[a]

Organism	Iodine mg/liter	Minutes for 99% Inactivation	c·t[b]
Coliform bacteria	0.4	1	0.4
Poliovirus 1	20	1.5	30.0
f_2 Virus	10	3.0	30.0
Simian cysts	15	10.0	150.0

[a] References to these values appear in the text.
[b] Concentration of iodine times contact time.

mg/liter of iodine, which is extremely high compared to the amount that is possibly needed for public water supplies. The tablet is not widely accepted, since color, taste, and odor problems are fairly common (O'Connor and Kapoor, 1970).

Chambers et al. (1952) investigated the effect of iodine concentration, pH, exposure time, and temperature on 13 enteric bacteria in a clean system. Their results are not completely quantitative in that the reported iodine concentration is that required to inactivate all test organisims plated out after 1, 2, and 5 min of contact. This was equivalent to approximately 99.9% activation with the procedure that they followed. There was definitely an observed pH effect. At 2°C to 5°C, some bacterial species required 3 to 4 times as much iodine for similar inactivation at pH 9.0 as was required at pH 7.5. For 5 min of exposure, the required dosage for ≥99.9% bacterial inactivation in high pH water at 20°C–26°C was always less than 1 mg/liter. A summary of their work with E. coli is given in Table II-10. This is the best available information on iodine as a bactericide.

EFFICACY AGAINST VIRUSES

Studies on the efficacy of iodine on viruses have shown that viruses are more resistant to disinfection than are vegetative cells of bacteria. Krusé (1969) compared virus and bacterial inactivation. At an iodine dose of 10 mg/liter in 0.048 mM potassium iodide at room temperature and pH 7.0,

TABLE II-10   Concentrations of Iodine and Contact
Times Necessary for 99% Inactivation of *Escherichia coli*[a]

Iodine, mg/liter	Contact Time, min	c·t[b]	pH	Temperature °C
1.3	1	1.3	6.5	2-5
0.9	2	1.8	6.5	
1.3	1	1.3	7.5	
0.7	2	1.4	7.5	
0.8	1	0.8	7.5	
0.6	2	1.2	7.5	
0.8	1	0.8	8.5	
0.9	2	1.8	8.5	
1.8	1	1.8	9.1	
1.2	2	2.4	9.1	
0.35	1	0.35	6.5	20-25
0.20	2	0.40	6.5	
0.45	1	0.20	7.5	
0.30	2	0.60	7.5	
0.45	1	0.45	8.5	
0.40	2	0.80	8.5	
0.45	1	0.20	9.1	
0.30	2	0.60	9.1	

[a] Data from Chambers *et al.*, 1952.
[b] Concentration of iodine times contact time.

E. coli was inactivated more rapidly than f2 virus but both were reduced by 4 logs in less than 1 min. However, when the potassium iodide concentration was raised to 0.5 *M*, bacterial inactivation was 4 logs in 1 min while virus inactivation was only 0.5 log in 1 hr (Figure II-6).

Berg *et al.* (1964) measured the dynamics of survival for poliovirus, coxsackievirus, and echovirus that were iodinated at pH 6.0 and at temperatures of 5°C, 15°C, and 25°C. The work of the Johns Hopkins group from 1962 to 1969 (Krusé, 1969) was primarily with the virus model f2, although some comparative poliovirus 1 work was done. Cramer *et al.* (1976) have shown that the mode of inactivation of these two viruses by iodine is similar. Data on the inactivation of virus by iodine are summarized in Table II-11 for both polio and f2. The results of inactivation studies by the various groups compare very favorably. At pH 6.0, iodine approaches the order of magnitude of virucidal activity of

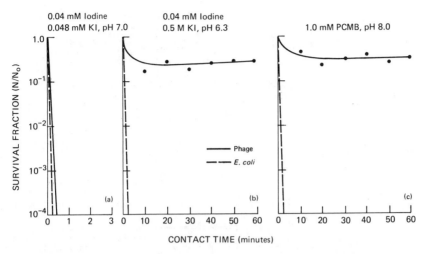

Figure II-6   Survival of *E. coli* and f_2 bacteriophage reacted with 0.04 m*M* iodine containing (a) 0.048 m*M* potassium iodide (KI) at 37°C and (b) 0.5 m*M* potassium iodide at 0°C, and survival obtained with (c) 1 m*M* of a sulfhydryl reacting agent, *p*-chloromercuribenzoic acid (ClHgC$_6$H$_4$COOH). From Krusé, 1969, with permission.

hypochlorous acid (HOCl). At the pH's likely to be maintained in the distribution system (pH 8.0), iodine is a vastly more effective virucide than combined chlorine and is not far removed from the activity range of free chlorine.

EFFICACY AGAINST PARASITES

Many studies on cyst inactivation have been reported, but there are discrepancies in their results due mainly to differences in the test systems that were used. The dose, pH, and temperature that were used in many of the studies are in doubt as are the different sources, cleaning methods for cysts, number of cysts used per test, and determination of viability. Stringer (1970) compared the resistance to iodine disinfection of *Entamoeba histolytica* cysts obtained from *in-vitro* culturing with those harvested from a human carrier and mixed amoebic cysts from monkeys. In water at room temperature at pH 6.5, 3 times the iodine dose was required in 10 min of exposure for 99% inactivation with wild (naturally formed) cysts compared to the cultured cysts. Large numbers of amoebic cysts from simian hosts were more readily available than cysts from

68

TABLE II-11 Concentrations of Iodine and Contact Times Necessary for 99% Inactivation of Polio and f_2 Viruses with Flash Mixing

Test Microorganism	Iodine, mg/liter	Contact Time, min	c·t[a]	pH	Temperature,°C	References
f_2 Virus	13	10	130	4.0	5	Kruse, 1969
f_2 Virus	12	10	120	5.0		Kruse, 1969
f_2 Virus	7.5	10	75	6.0		Kruse, 1969
f_2 Virus	5	10	50	7.0		Kruse, 1969
f_2 Virus	3.3	10	33	8.0		Kruse, 1969
f_2 Virus	2.7	10	27	9.0		Kruse, 1969
f_2 Virus	2.5	10	25	10.0		Kruse, 1969
f_2 Virus	7.6	10	76	4.0	25-27	Kruse, 1969
Poliovirus 1	30	3	90	4.0		Kruse, 1969
f_2 Virus	64	10	64	5.0		Kruse, 1969
f_2 Virus	4.0	10	40	6.0		Kruse, 1969
Poliovirus 1	1.25	39	49	6.0		Berg et al., 1964
Poliovirus 1	6.35	9	57	6.0		Berg et al., 1964
Poliovirus 1	12.7	5	63	6.0		Berg et al., 1964
Poliovirus 1	38	1.6	60	6.0		Berg et al., 1964
Poliovirus 1	30	2.0	60	6.0		Cramer et al., 1976
f_2 Virus	3.0	10	30	7.0		Kruse, 1969
Poliovirus 1	20	1.5	30	7.0		Kruse, 1969
f_2 Virus	2.5	10	25	8.0		Kruse, 1969
f_2 Virus	2.0	10	20	9.0		Kruse, 1969
f_2 Virus	1.5	10	15	10.0		Kruse, 1969
Poliovirus 1	30	0.5	15	10.0		Cramer et al., 1976

[a] Concentration of iodine times contact time.

human stools. They served as a reliable model for human *E. histolytica*.

The most extensive and reliable data on the cysticidal properties of iodine are found in the work of Chang and Stringer and their co-workers (Change and Baxter, 1955; Chang *et al.*, 1955; Stringer, 1970; Stringer and Krusé, 1971; Stringer *et al.*, 1975). The only quantitative comparative study of the cysticidal properties of chlorine, bromine, and iodine believed to be published is that of Stringer, who reported a 99.9% inactivation. The earlier studies of others involved "total kills" and are quite dependent on the cyst density that was used.

All investigators more or less agree that iodine is an excellent cysticide in low pH waters ($<$pH 4.0), suggesting that molecular iodine (I_2), rather than hypoiodous acid, is the active agent. Chang (1958) observed that when the titratable iodine dosages exceed 20 mg/liter in the presence of iodide ion, the triiodide ion (I_3^-) has a cysticidal efficiency that is equal to 1/11, 1/8, and 1/7 that of I_2 at 6°C, 25°C, and 35°C. He further calculated relative cysticidal efficiency of hypoiodous acid to be one-third that of I_2 at 6°C and one-half that of I_2 at 20°C.

There may be the problem of ineffective iodine residual in the distribution system where cross-connection introduction of cyst contamination is a possibility. This is due to the practice (for corrosion control) of maintaining water in the distribution system at approximately pH 8.0. At the low halogen residual levels that are usually maintained, the most cysticidal form, I_2, would be less prevalent than hypoiodous acid. Water at 25°C and pH 8.0 with a total iodine residual of 0.5, 1.0, and 2.0 mg/liter would contain only 0.06, 0.2, and 0.62 mg/liter of molecular iodine. Table II-12 shows the time in minutes required for 90% inactivation of simian cysts with residuals of bromine, chlorine, and iodine in water at pH 6.0, 7.0, and 8.0 and a temperature of 30°C. At pH 8.0, iodine is inferior to free bromine and chlorine. However, in the presence of excess ammonia, with which the halogens could react, bromine appears to be more effective at pH 8.0 than do similar dosages of iodine or chlorine. Residual iodine in water at pH 8.0 has the ability to persist.

The kinetics of iodine as a cysticide in water at 20°C to 30°C have been assembled and compared. The cultured *E. histolytica* cyst data of Chang and co-workers (Chang and Baxter, 1955; Chang and Morris, 1953; Chang *et al.*, 1955) and the results of Stringer *et al.* (1975) present a consistent picture. For cultured cysts in water at pH 5 the c · t values for 99% inactivation calculated by Chang were 200 at 3°C, 130 at 10°C, and 65 at 23°C (Chang and Morris, 1953). Stringer *et al.* (1975) extended the cultured cyst data at 30°C for a range of pH given below:

TABLE II-12 Contact Times Necessary for Low Residual Bromine, Chlorine, and Iodine in Water at 30°C to Effect 99% Inactivation of Cysts from Simian Stools[a]

| | Contact Time Required, min, by 10-min Halogen Residual Concentration, mg/liter | | | | | | | | |
| | 0.5 mg/liter | | | 1.0 mg/liter | | | 2.0 mg/liter | | |
pH	Br_2	Cl_2	I_2	Br_2	Cl_2	I_2	Br_2	Cl_2	I_2
Buffered water									
6.0	10	10	20	4	4	10	3	3	5
7.0	12	14	40	8	12	20	4	5	7
8.0	15	20	ND[b]	10	15	80	5	10	20
Buffered water in presence of excess ammonia									
6.0	10	65	20	8	35	10	4	22	5
7.0	30	120	40	10	55	20	7	35	7
8.0	35	ND[b]	ND[b]	13	80	80	9	50	20

[a] Data from Stringer et al., 1975. The proportions of the molecular species present in the test system depend upon the halogen, the pH, and the presence or absence of ammonia.
[b] ND = not determined.

pH	c · t for 99% inactivation
6.0	40
7.0	50
8.0	100
8.5	200

These c · t values from Stringer *et al.* (1975) were approximately one-half the values they obtained with *E. histolytica* cysts from human stools and for mixed cysts from simian stools.

Mechanism of Action

The failure of a strong commercial iodine disinfectant to inactivate poliovirus (Wallis *et al.*, 1963) led to interest in the responsible mechanism, especially the role of pH and iodide ion. Berg *et al.* (1964) claimed that iodine inactivation of coxsackievirus resulted from biomolecular reaction with a single iodine molecule and that clumping of virions played a role in resistance to disinfection. Fraenkel-Conrat (1955) pointed out inconsistencies in the literature regarding the virucidal properties of iodine. Hsu (1964) and Hsu *et al.* (1965) clarified the mechanism of iodine on cells and virus. Hsu extracted fully active transforming DNA from iodine-inactivated *Haemophilus parainfluenzae* cells and just as much infectious RNA from f2 bacterial virus that had been inactivated (5 logs) by iodine as from noniodinated controls. Iodine inactivation, unlike the action of chlorine, appears to be attributable to a reaction with vital amino acids in proteins. Further experiments were conducted to determine whether sulfhydryl, tryptophanyl, histidyl, or tyrosyl groups were involved. With bacterial cells, there was a striking similarity between the kinetics of inactivation with iodine and the application of *p*-chloromercuribenzoic acid, a sulfhydryl reacting agent. While the active chemical species of iodine is not known, Hughes (1957), Allen and Keefer (1955), Bell and Gelles (1951), and Hsu (1964) hypothesized that the hydrated cationic iodine species (H_2OI^+) attacks the base, first against the sulfhydroxyl groups, and is not materially affected by the presence of iodide ion as was tyrosine. When sulfhydroxyl groups are the site of inactivation, a low pH should favor the reaction. With the viruses, the sulfhydroxyl group is not involved. Evidence of tyrosine's involvement came from parallel experiments showing similar patterns of inactivation curves between iodination of f2 virus and L-tyrosine. Li (1942, 1944) had shown that the presence of iodide ion and low pH iodine (I_2) inhibited the iodination of tyrosine. Both poliovirus and f2 virus inactivation with iodine was inhibited by the iodide ion

(Cramer *et al.*, 1976). At pH 4.0, both polio and f2 viruses survived iodination whereas at pH 10 inactivation was complete. Although iodine decomposes rapidly to iodate (IO_3^-) and iodide at pH 10, flash mixing of iodine (yielding hypoiodous acid) overcomes this difficulty effectively, and the virus inactivation is complete in less than 1 min (Longley, 1964). Therefore, there is evidence that iodine action, with little or no iodide present, is effected by the modification of protein without destroying DNA or RNA (Brammer, 1963; Hsu, 1964). The mode of action of iodine in cyst penetration and inactivation has not been studied.

Conclusions

Iodine has many features that are comparable to free chlorine and bromine as a water disinfectant, but iodamines are not formed. Free iodine is an effective bactericide over a relatively wide range of pH. Field studies on small public water systems have shown that low levels of 0.5 to 1 mg/liter of free iodine can be maintained in distribution systems and that the magnitude of residual is sufficient to produce safe drinking water with no adverse effects on human health. Like other halogens, the effectiveness of iodine against bacteria and cysts is significantly reduced by high pH, but unlike bromine and chlorine it is much more effective against viruses because of the enhanced iodination of tyrosine. Currently, its use is restricted primarily to emergency disinfection of field water supplies because of its high cost and because it is difficult to apply to large systems. The possible adverse health effects of increased iodide intake for susceptible individuals in the population must also be considered.

Research Recommendations

Studies should be conducted to determine the consequences for human health of the long-term consumption of iodine in drinking water with special regard for more susceptible subgroups of the population.

BROMINE

Chemistry of Bromine in Water

Bromine was first applied to water as a disinfectant in the form of liquid bromine (Br_2) (Henderson, 1935), but it can also be added as bromine chloride gas (BrCl) (Mills, 1975) or from a solid brominated ion exchange resin (Mills, 1969). Oxidation of bromide (Br^-) to bromine can also be accomplished either chemically or electrochemically. Oxidation with aqueous chlorine gives either bromine or hypobromous acid (HOBr), depending on the ratio of chlorine to bromide. Both bromine (Liebhafsky, 1934) and bromine chloride (Kanyaev and Shilov, 1940) hydrolyze to hypobromous acid:

$$Br_2 + H_2O \rightarrow HOBr + H^+ + Br^- \qquad (21)$$

$$BrCl + H_2O \rightarrow HOBr + H^+ + Cl^- \qquad (22)$$

Molecular bromine exists in water at moderately acid pH and high bromide concentrations since the equilibrium constant of Reaction 21 is 5.8×10^{-9} at 25°C. Like chlorine, bromine chloride has a much higher hydrolysis constant than this, so it does not exist as the molecular form in appreciable concentrations under conditions of water treatment. The ratio of molecular bromine to hypobromous acid depends on both pH and bromide concentration. From the equilibrium expression for Reaction 21:

$$\log \frac{(Br_2)}{(HOBr)} = \log(Br^-) - pH + 8.24 \qquad (23)$$

Thus, for a solution containing 10 mg/liter bromide and a pH of 6.3, 1% of the bromine is Br_2, while at lower bromide concentrations or higher pH aqueous bromine occurs almost entirely as hypobromous acid, which is a very weak acid with a dissociation constant (for Reaction 24) of 2×10^{-9} at 25°C (Farkas and Lewin, 1950).

$$HOBr \rightleftharpoons H^+ + OBr^- \qquad (24)$$

The hypobromite ion (OBr^-) becomes the major form of bromine above pH 8.7 at 25°C. Lower temperature decreases both of the above equilibrium values, thereby increasing the pH range where hypobromous acid is the major chemical form of bromine in water.

Bromine and bromine chloride also react with basic nitrogen compounds to form combined bromine or bromamines (Galal-Gorchev and Morris, 1965; Johannesson, 1958; Johnson and Overby, 1971):

$$HOBr + NH_3 \rightarrow NH_2Br + H_2O \tag{25}$$

$$NH_2Br + HOBr \rightarrow NHBr_2 + H_2O \tag{26}$$

$$NHBr_2 + HOBr \rightarrow NBr_3 + H_2O \tag{27}$$

The observed breakpoint for ammonia (NH_3) solutions that have been treated with bromine is similar to that seen with chlorine. For bromine, this point corresponds to 17 mg/liter bromine for 1 mg/liter of ammonia nitrogen (NH_3-N). At this point, a minimum of bromamine stability occurs (Inman et al., 1976) as ammonia nitrogen is oxidized to nitrogen gas:

$$3HOBr + 2NH_3 \rightarrow N_2 + 3HBr + 3H_2O \tag{28}$$

At bromine-to-ammonia ratios higher than this and in the acid pH range, nitrogen tribromide (NBr_3) is stable. It is the most abundant bromamine in such aqueous solutions. At lower bromine concentrations, dibromamine ($NHBr_2$) can be present, but it is quite unstable. Only at alkaline pH values and very high ammonia concentrations such as those found in wastewater are significant quantities of monobromamine (NH_2Br) formed. Organic bromamines are also formed, but there is little information on their forms or stability.

Production and Application

Bromine is produced by oxidation of bromide-rich brines (that contain between 0.05% and 0.6% bromide) with chlorine. Bromine is then stripped with steam or air and is collected as liquid Br_2.

Bromine chloride is produced by mixing equal molar quantities of pure bromine and chlorine (Mills, 1975). It condenses to liquid bromine chloride below 5°C at 1 atm pressure or above 30 psig at 25°C. In the liquid phase, more than 80% of the liquid is bromine chloride, and the remainder is Br_2 and Cl_2. In the gas phase, 40% of the bromine chloride dissociates to Br_2 and Cl_2 at 25°C.

Bromine has been applied to water as liquid Br_2. The difficulties that are encountered when handling the liquid and its corrosive nature, especially when wet, have encouraged the use of bromine chloride. Liquid bromine chloride is removed from cylinders under moderate pressure. It is then vaporized, and the gas is metered in equipment that is similar to that used for chlorine. Like chlorine, bromine chloride is shipped as the dry liquid in steel containers. Gas feeders must be made of Teflon, Kynar, or Viton plastics because bromine chloride is more reactive than chlorine with polyvinylchloride plastics.

Analytical Methods

Bromine concentrations can be measured iodometrically by procedures that are identical to those used to measure total chlorine residuals (*Standard Methods*, 1976). None of these procedures is capable of distinguishing free bromine (Br_2, HOBr, OBr^-) from combined bromine (bromamines) or other oxidants that are capable of reacting with iodide under the slightly acid conditions used in these procedures. However, bromate does not interfere except at low pH (Kolthoff and Belcher, 1957). UV spectroscopy can be used to measure the bromamines selectively in the presence of one another and without interference from free bromine because none of the free bromine forms except Br_3^- has strong UV absorptivities (Johnson and Overby, 1971).

Biocidal Activity

Since residual bromine was rarely measured in the studies cited here, c • t (concentration, mg/liter, times contact time, min) products have generally been calculated using the dosage of bromine added to the system.

EFFICACY AGAINST BACTERIA

The efficacy of bromine inactivation of bacteria has been summarized by Farkas-Hinsley (1966). Vegetative cells are readily inactivated by bromine, but reports often leave the type of bromine compound and its residual concentration as uncertain. Consequently, it is difficult to make quantitative comparisons with other disinfectants. Tanner and Pitner (1939) reported that the concentrations of hypobromous acid that are required to give "complete kill" in 30 min are 0.15 mg/liter for *Escherichia coli* and 0.6 mg/liter for *Salmonella typhi*. Spores of *Bacillus subtilis* required more than 150 mg/liter of bromine. Krusé *et al.* (1970) found that 4 mg of bromine per liter as hypobromous acid gave 5 logs of disinfection of *E. coli* in 10 min at 0°C. At pH 4.5, where significant Br_2 was present, 2 mg/liter bromine at 0°C gave 4 logs of *E. coli* disinfection in 3 min. However, Krusé also reported that 0.1 *M* bromide decreased *E. coli* disinfection to 2 logs of inactivation from 4.5 logs at 0.001 *M* bromide, using 4 mg/liter bromine at pH 7.5 and 0°C in each case. This is in conflict with observations made at low pH, since high bromide should also produce bromine. The data at pH 4.5 showed 4 logs inactivation with a c · t of 6 compared to 5 logs inactivation from a c · t of 40 for hypobromous acid. Even these data, the best available, are based on the concentrations of bromine added to the solution. It is difficult to compare the various studies on disinfection by bromine, since the chemical species of bromine present in most instances have not been measured or reported.

The effect of the formation and decomposition of the bromamines on the efficacy of bacterial disinfection was first discussed by Johannesson (1958). He reported that 0.28 mg/liter of monobromamine expressed as bromine resulted in 99% inactivation in less than 1 min, while the same concentration of N-bromodimethylamine $[N(CH_3)_2Br]$ required 12 min for 99% inactivation of *E. coli*. The measurements of the halogen remaining after the experiments showed very little loss.

The efficacy of bromine inactivation of spores of *Bacillus metiens* and *B. subtilis* has been studied by Marks and Strandskov (1950) and Wyss and Stockton (1947). Both pairs of investigators found that the activity was markedly pH-dependent at low pH values where molecular bromine predominates. The activity increased rapidly from pH 4 to pH 3, the lowest that was tested. The c · t required for 99% inactivation was 20–25 at 25°C and pH 3.0. At pH 6 to 8, the c · t was 225 to 375 (Wyss and Stockton, 1947). At pH 9, where the hypobromite ion starts to predominate, the c · t increased to more than 500.

Marks and Strandskov (1950) also determined that at pH 7 and 25°C monobromamine was one-half as effective as hypobromous acid against *B. metiens* spores. *N*-bromosuccinimide was 1/17, and *N*-bromopiperidine was 1/800 as effective. Wyss and Stockton (1947) showed the effect of changing chemical form and concentration by increasing the concentration of ammonia that was added to a 20 mg/liter bromine solution at pH 7 containing *B. subtilis* spores. Table II-13 shows the measured residual and the time required for 99% inactivation. Before the ammonia is added to the solution, hypobromous acid is the major chemical form. When the ammonia nitrogen reaches 1 mg/liter, nitrogen tribromide predominates. At 2 mg/liter ammonia nitrogen, the break-point occurs with rapid loss of combined bromine residual. At 10 and 30 mg/liter ammonia nitrogen, dibromamine is present and is less stable and effective than hypobromous acid. At 1,000 mg/liter ammonia nitrogen, monobromamine has a c · t value for 99% inactivation that is as effective as nitrogen tribromide and hypobromous acid.

The effect of temperature on the efficacy of hypobromous acid

TABLE II-13   The Effect of Ammonia on Bromine
Concentrations Required for 99% Inactivation of *Bacillus
subtilis* Spores at 20 mg/liter, pH 7, 25°C[a]

Ammonia, mg NH$_3$-N/liter	10-min Residual, mg/liter[b]	Contact Time, min	c·t[c]
0	20	14	280
1	16	19	304
2	2	> 100	> 200
10	8	85	680
30	9	70	630
100	14	18	252
1,000	19	14	266

[a] Data from Wyss and Stockton, 1947.
[b] Initial bromine concentration 20 mg/liter.
[c] Concentration of bromine times contact time.

inactivation of *B. subtilis* spores is shown in Table II-14 (Wyss and Stockton, 1947). The activity increases approximately 2.3 times for each 10°C rise in temperature. After measuring washed vegetative cells of *B. subtilis*, Wyss and Stockton also found them to be 500 times less resistant. They reported no temperature data for their vegetative cell studies.

EFFICACY AGAINST VIRUS

Krusé *et al.* (1970) reported that 4 mg/liter of bromine as hypobromous acid at pH 7 and 0°C gave 3.7 logs of inactivation of f2 *E. coli* phage virus in 10 min. At higher bromide concentrations and lower pH, where Br$_2$ becomes the principal form of bromine, the rates of inactivation increased. A c · t of 40 was required for 3.7 logs inactivation at pH 7.0 and 0°C compared to a c · t of 1 for 4.5 logs inactivation at 0°C and pH 4.8. At pH 7.5 and with a concentration of 0.1 *M* bromide at 0°C, a c · t of 12 yielded 5.5 logs inactivation. In these studies the residual concentrations of bromine were probably not significantly different from those in solutions that did not contain added salts. In the presence of added bromide, amines were difficult to quantify. After 2 hr, Krusé and his colleagues found no viable virus in a solution of 4 mg/liter bromine, starting from an initial titer of 1.7×10^9 plaque-forming units (PFU)/ml at 0°C and pH 7.5, when excess ammonia was present. However, the

TABLE II-14   The Effect of Temperature on Bromine
Concentrations Required for 99% Inactivation of *Bacillus
subtilis* Spores with 25 mg/liter Bromine at pH 7.0[a]

Temperature, °C	Contact Time, min	$c \cdot t$[b]
35	4	100
25	10	250
20	16	400
15	21	525
10	37	925
5	54	1,350

[a] Data from Wyss and Stockton, 1947.
[b] Concentration of bromine times contact time.

addition of bromine to phage solutions that contained excess methyl-
amine (CH_3NH_2) and glycine (H_2NCH_2COOH) essentially stopped
disinfection under these conditions. This may be due either to the
formation of the *N*-bromo compounds or to the reduction of bromine.

Taylor and Johnson (1974) used $\Phi x174$ *E. coli* phage and measured
concentrations of the disinfecting species in constant residual solutions.
They reported that 0.32 mg/liter hypobromous acid required only 1.1
min or a c · t of 0.35 to inactivate 99% of this phage at 0°C. Compared
to hypobromous acid, molecular bromine was approximately 3 times as
fast, requiring Br_2 at c · t of 0.1. Nitrogen tribromide was less potent,
requiring a c · t of 1.0 for 99% inactivation of this phage at 0°C.

The effect of temperature on $\Phi x174$ inactivation was measured for 0.16
mg/liter of hypobromous acid expressed as bromine at pH 7. The
Arrhenius plot of ln k against $1/T$ (where T is temperature) from 273°K
to 303°K gave a slope equivalent to 37 kcal/mol or an increase in rate of
inactivation of 1.9 times for a rise in temperature from 15°C to 25°C.

Sharp's group (Floyd *et al.*, 1976, 1978; Sharp *et al.*, 1975, 1976) has
made careful studies with measured, controlled residual concentrations.
They demonstrated that even under these controlled chemical conditions
the degree of aggregation or clumping had a marked effect on the
apparent, observed inactivation rates with reovirus and type 1 poliovirus
(Sharp *et al.*, 1975). Reoviruses, as single particles, required only 1 s for 3
logs of inactivation at pH 7 and 2°C with hypobromous acid at 0.46
mg/liter bromine. Aggregated samples gave much slower rates, especially at high levels of inactivation. At 3 logs of inactivation, the time

required doubled for the same concentration conditions (Sharp *et al.*, 1976). Poliovirus 1 was also rapidly inactivated by hypobromous acid when single virus particles were studied (Floyd *et al.*, 1976). At 2°C and pH 7, only 3.5 mg/liter bromine or a c · t of 0.2 was required for 2 logs of inactivation. However, the rate of inactivation did not increase linearly with concentration at this temperature. Higher concentrations were much less efficient than longer exposures. At 1 mg/liter hypobromous acid, 7 s were required for 1 log of inactivation or a c · t of 0.23 for 2 logs of inactivation at 2°C and pH 7 with hypobromous acid. The inactivation rate increased only slightly with temperature at this concentration. At 10°C a c · t of 0.21 for 2 logs of inactivation and at 20°C a c · t of 0.06 was required for 99% inactivation with hypobromous acid.

The inactivation of single poliovirus particles in buffered, distilled water and constant residual concentrations for the other major bromine chemical forms have also been studied by Floyd *et al.* (1978). Table II-15 gives the calculated c · t required to yield 99% inactivation for these different forms near 1 mg/liter expressed as bromine. The values in Table II-15 depend on concentration except for Br_2, for which time and concentration were inversely related as normally assumed from the Watson–Chick relationship (Morris, 1975). Floyd *et al.* (1978) also demonstrated that dibromamine, nitrogen tribromide, and hypobromous acid were less efficient at higher concentrations while the hypobromite ion became more effective as the concentration increased. The rate for the hypobromite ion is rapid compared to the other bromine compounds. This is interesting in light of the fact the hypochlorite ion (OCl^-) is generally considered to be a much poorer disinfectant than hypochlorous acid (HOCl).

EFFICACY AGAINST PARASITES

There appears to be no information regarding the effectiveness of bromine as a disinfectant against eggs or larvae of helminth parasites in water.

With protozoa that are important to public health, attention appears to have been devoted primarily to the efficacy of bromine in destroying cysts of *Entamoeba histolytica*. Most relevant information has been provided by Stringer *et al.* (1975) as a result of their studies on the comparative cysticidal efficacies of various halogens (shown in Table II-12 in the section on iodine). They used bromine stock solutions that were prepared by bubbling nitrogen through bottles of elemental bromine. Concentrations were determined by a colorimetric bromocresol purple

TABLE II-15 Exposure $(c \cdot t)^{a}$ to Various Bromine Compounds Required for 99% Inactivation of Poliovirus 1, Mahoney[b]

Chemical Form	$c \cdot t$	Temperature, °C	pH
Dibromamine (NHBr$_2$)	1.2	4	7.0
Nitrogen tribromide (NBr$_3$)	0.19	5	7.0
Bromine (Br$_2$)	0.03	4	5.0
Hypobromite ion (OBr$^-$)	0.01	2	10.0
Hypobromous acid (HOBr)	0.24	2	7.0
Hypobromous acid	0.21	10	7.0
Hypobromous acid	0.06	20	7.0

[a] Concentration of compound times contact time.
[b] Data from Floyd et al., 1978.

test. Cyst survival was evaluated by the excystation method that these investigators had developed.

In dose–response experiments in distilled water for exposures of 10 min and at pH levels from pH 4 to pH 10, bromine was found by Stringer et al. (1975) to be the most effective and fastest acting of the halogens tested over the widest pH range. At pH 4, 99.9% cyst mortality was obtained with 1.5 mg/liter of free bromine residual; whereas 2 mg/liter of chlorine and 5 mg/liter of iodine were required to attain the same mortality. Furthermore, increases in pH seemed to have less effect on the cysticidal efficacy of bromine as compared with the other halogens. At pH 10, 99.9% mortality was obtained with residuals of 4 mg/liter of bromine, 12 mg/liter of chlorine, and 20 mg/liter of iodine.

In studies more nearly simulating usual water treatment procedures, "flash mixing" of halogens at a dosage of 2 mg/liter with the cyst suspensions was used. In buffered distilled water, bromine again proved to be the most effective: 99.9% inactivation was obtained at pH 6 and pH 8 after 15 min of contact. Longer exposures at the lower pH were required for the other halogens in order to provide even less inactivation than this.

An interesting aspect of the study of Stringer et al. (1975) was that ammonia bromamines were nearly as cysticidal as free bromine except in waters of high pH (Table II-12).

Thus, under conditions likely to be found during the treatment of natural water supplies, free and combined bromine appear to be a practical, effective cystide, at least as far as cysts of *E. histolytica* are concerned.

Mechanisms of Action

The pattern of bromine disinfection appears to be similar to that of chlorine. After comparing the activity of chlorine, bromine, and iodine against spores, Marks and Strandskov (1950) noted that Br_2 was 9 times more effective than hypobromous acid and that the hypobromite ion and tribromide ion (Br_3^-) had very low activity. They noted that a high degree of polarity contributed to the inactivity of the ionic forms and the reduced activity of the hypohalous acid compared to the free molecular halogen. They also found that "the killing rates of bacterial spores for the hypohalous acids and probably for the molecular halogens decrease in the [following] order: chlorine, bromine, iodine."

Many workers attribute this decrease to the greater oxidation potential of the halogens with lower molecular weight. However, the polarity and perhaps the sizes of the halogens may be important in getting the disinfectants to the vital site.

Olivieri *et al.* (1975) demonstrated that bromine was effective in inactivating both naked viral RNA and intact virus. The primary site of inactivation of f2 phage more likely involves the reaction of bromine with the protein coat of the virus, because inactivation of RNA that was prepared from bromine-treated virus lagged significantly behind the inactivation of intact virus. The mechanism of inactivation with bromine, as with the other halogens, involves moving the disinfectant to the vital site, mass transport, and the reactivity of the bromine with that site, oxidation. The effectiveness of bromamines as disinfectants may be explained by their relatively low polarity and high reactivity. The effectiveness of the hypobromite ion as a virucide may be due to the fact the high pH's of the solutions make the virus more sensitive to the ion. Or, it could be attributed to Olivieri's observation that bromine acts primarily on the protein coat of viruses.

Summary and Conclusions

Laboratory tests show that bromine is an effective bactericide and virucide. It is more effective than chlorine in the presence of ammonia.

As a cysticide, it is highly active. Bromine is active over a relatively wide range of pH, and it retains some of its effectiveness as hypobromous acid to above pH 9.

The major disadvantage of bromine as a disinfectant is its reactivity with ammonia or other amines that may seriously limit its effectiveness under conditions that are encountered in the treatment of drinking water. Data on the effectiveness of bromine against bacteria are complicated by this reactivity and the lack of characterization of the residual species in disinfection studies.

Research Recommendations

Further research is required to quantitate the effectiveness of the various species of bromine and the bromamines, both organic and inorganic, against bacteria, viruses, and cysts, particularly with bacteria.

The reactivity of bromine and the dosages that are required to maintain effective residual in natural water systems should be investigated.

The effectiveness of various technologies for application of bromine or bromine chloride to intended drinking water should be evaluated.

FERRATE

Ferrates are salts of ferric acid (H_2FeO_4) in which iron is hexavalent. Fremy (1841) first synthesized potassium ferrate (K_2FeO_4) in the mid-nineteenth century. Since then, a wide variety of metallic salts have been prepared. However, only a few of the preparations yield ferrates of sufficient purity and stability for use in the treatment of water. Ferrates are strong oxidizing agents that have a redox potential of -2.2 V or 0.7 V in acid and base, respectively (Wood, 1958).

The Chemistry of Ferrate in Water

Aqueous solutions of potassium ferrate are unstable and decompose to yield oxygen (O_2), hydroxide (OH^-), and insoluble hydrous iron oxide [FeO(OH)]:

$$2FeO_4{}^{2-} + 3H_2O \rightarrow 2FeO(OH) + 1\tfrac{1}{2} O_2 + 4OH^- \qquad (29)$$

The hydrous iron oxide is a coagulant that is commonly used in water treatment. Initial ferrate concentration, pH, temperature, and the surface character of the resulting hydrous iron oxide affect the rate of decomposition (Schreyer and Ockerman, 1951; Wagner et al., 1952; Wood, 1958). Ferrate solutions are most stable in strong base (>3 M or at pH 10 to 11). Schreyer and Ockerman (1951) reported that dilute aqueous solutions of ferrate are more stable than concentrated solutions. The presence of other inorganic ions also affects ferrate stability in aqueous solutions.

Ferrate reacts rapidly with reducing agents in solutions (Murmann, 1974). It will also oxidize ammonia (NH_3). The rates for this reaction increase with pH (optimum pH range 9.5–11.2), molar ratio of ferrate to ammonia, and temperature (Strong, 1973). The oxidation of ammonia by ferrate below pH 9 is markedly slower than that observed for chlorine. Some information is available on the reaction of ferrates with various organic compounds (Audette et al., 1971; Becarud, 1966; Zhdanov and Pustovarova, 1967).

Preparation

Concentrated solutions of sodium ferrate (Na_2FeO_4) may be prepared electrochemically from the more common iron forms. Scrap iron can be converted to ferrate iron with a 40% efficiency (Murmann, 1974). Potassium ferrate may be prepared by wet oxidation of Fe(III) with potassium permanganate ($KMnO_4$). Subsequent recrystallization yields a crystalline solid with greater than 90% purity (Schreyer et al., 1950). Ferrate salts are not commercially available. Consequently, sufficient quantities for pilot or full-scale testing would have to be especially prepared.

Analytical Methods and Residuals

Aqueous ferrate solutions have a characteristic violet color that is similar to permanganate and a wavelength maximum at 505 nm in the visible portion of the electromagnetic spectrum. The molar extinction coefficient at 505 nm in 10^{-4} M sodium hydroxide (NaOH) was $1,070 \pm 30$ 1 M^{-1} cm^{-1} (Wood, 1958). Since ferrates are unstable, residual cannot be maintained.

Biocidal Activity

EFFICACY AGAINST BACTERIA

Gilbert *et al.* (1976) reported the inactivation of a pure culture of *Escherichia coli* at pH 8.0. Increased ferrate concentrations from 1.2 to 6.0 mg/liter yielded increased rates of inactivation of *E. coli.* They observed 99% inactivation at 6.0 mg/liter, pH 8.0, and 27°C in approximately 8.5 min. The rates of inactivation of *E. coli* with ferrate appear to be of the same order of magnitude as monochloramine (NH_2Cl). Waite (1978a,b) extended Gilbert's disinfection studies to include enteric pathogens and Gram-positive bacteria and evaluated the effects of pH and temperature. The rate of *E. coli* inactivation by ferrate increases as pH decreases from pH 8.0 to pH 6.0. At the lower pH value, the rate of ferrate decomposition is increased, and little inactivation was observed after 5 min. Several inconsistencies at low ferrate concentrations (0.12 mg/liter) were observed, but low-level inactivations (<50% inactivation) are difficult to interpret. At lower temperatures, the biocidal activities of ferrate appear to increase as temperature increases. At higher temperatures, the ferrate decomposition becomes an important factor. *Salmonella typhimurium* and *Shigella flexneri* were inactivated in a manner similar to that of *E. coli.* However, considerably higher dosages of ferrate (>12 mg/liter) were necessary for inactivation of *Streptococcus faecalis.* Ferrate concentrations of 12 mg/liter and 60 mg/liter required 5 min and 15 min, respectively, for 99% inactivation at pH 8.0. Other Gram-positive bacteria tested (*Bacillus cereus, Streptococcus bovis*, and *Staphylococcus aureus*) were noticeably more resistant to ferrates than were the enteric bacteria. Higher doses of ferrate (15–20 mg/liter) were also necessary to inactivate 99% to 99.9% of the bacteria in the presence of organic material in wastewater.

EFFICACY AGAINST VIRUSES

Waite (1978a,b) reported that the inactivation of the RNA bacterial f2 virus with ferrate appeared to be more dependent on pH than was bacterial inactivation. Considerably more viral inactivation was observed at pH 6.0 than at pH 8.0. At 1.2 mg/liter ferrate, just under 4 min were required for 99% inactivation, while for similar conditions 13 min were necessary at pH 8.0.

The disinfection efficacy of ferrate is summarized in Table II-16. The ferrate dose is given in the table, since ferrate residuals were not reported. Ferrate decomposes rapidly in aqueous solution, and the dose

TABLE II-16   Concentrations of Ferrate (FeO_4^{2-}) and Contact Times Necessary for 99% Inactivation of *Escherichia coli, Streptococcus faecalis,* and f_2 Virus[a]

Test Microorganism	Ferrate Dosage, mg/liter	Contact Time, min	$c \cdot t$[b]	pH	Temperature, °C
Escherichia	1.2	4.6	5.52	7.0	20
coli	6.0	2.5	15.0		
Streptococcus	1.2	365	438	7.0	20
faecalis	6.0	4.0	24		
f_2 Virus	1.2	3.7	4.4	6.0	20
	6.0	1.5	9		

[a] Data from Waite, 1978b.
[b] Concentration of ferrate times contact time.

represents an overestimate of ferrate concentration. Nevertheless, the c · t products (concentration, mg/liter, times contact time, min) indicate the difference in efficacy relative to the test microorganism and provide a crude idea of the c · t product for ferrate.

Mechanism of Action

No studies have elucidated the mechanism of inactivation caused by ferrate.

Conclusions

While not as biocidal as the free halogens, chlorine dioxide, or ozone, ferrate appears to be similar to or slightly better than the chloramines as a bactericide and more active as a virucide than the chloramines. The combined application of ferrate as a disinfectant and a coagulant makes it an attractive alternate biocide. Far more information on the feasibility of large-scale preparation of ferrate and its biocidal activity (particularly under water treatment conditions) are necessary before ferrate can be given consideration as a water disinfectant for public systems.

HIGH pH CONDITIONS

High pH values are obtained when drinking water is softened by the commonly used precipitation method, which removes calcium (Ca^{2+}) and magnesium (Mg^{2+}) ions that cause water hardness. In such cases, calcium hydroxide [$Ca(OH)_2$] is the usual source of hydroxide that is used to raise the pH. In this process, pH values as high as 10.5 are reached and maintained up to 6 hr. Low pH conditions are not used in water treatment processes. Therefore, while low pH's are lethal to most microorganisms, they are of less interest in this report than high pH conditions, which might have potential for disinfection through modification of current practices.

Attainment of Elevated pH

High pH values in water are obtained by using either calcium hydroxide or sodium hydroxide (NaOH). Sodium hydroxide is a by-product of the production of chlorine by the electrolysis method. Calcium hydroxide is prepared by reacting calcium oxide (CaO) with water. The calcium oxide is produced by heating calcium carbonate ($CaCO_3$) to drive off the carbon dioxide (CO_2). The calcium oxide is normally prepared off the site of the water treatment plant. However, it is often slaked on site at all but the smallest plants, which purchase calcium hydroxide and use it directly. A few, very large water treatment plants produce their own calcium hydroxide by calcining their water-softening sludge.

Hydroxide (OH^-) is added to water as a water slurry containing calcium hydroxide or as a water solution of sodium hydroxide. In the usual water-softening technique, the water is flocculated for 10–30 min to promote the precipitation reactions. The precipitates are then removed by sedimentation with retention times from 1 to 6 hr.

Disinfection with high pH is readily accomplished, but the required pH values are so high that the pH must be reduced before the water is consumed. In a full-scale water treatment plant, this is accomplished in the recarbonation stage, which is a normal component of the water-softening process. However, for small institutions or private residences the pH reduction requirement would mitigate against the use of this disinfection technique.

Analytical Methods and Process Control

The pH can be reliably measured with the glass electrode at pH values of approximately 7 and at room temperatures. Special care must be taken to obtain accurate values at other temperatures and at the elevated pH values that are necessary for disinfection with this process.

Residual

The hydroxide that is used to obtain the necessary pH values enters into few side reactions in natural water after the initial formation of metallic hydroxides and the reactions with carbon dioxide. The amounts of hydroxide for these reactions can be readily computed after the water has been chemically analyzed. There is a slow additional loss of hydroxide from the water by reaction with carbon dioxide entering from the atmosphere. However, this is not a serious problem.

Biocidal Activity

The microbial inactivation under consideration in this chapter is that caused solely by high pH. When the pH of water is raised, the opportunity exists for precipitation of many compunds associated with carbonates, oxides, and hydroxides, among many others. Even in distilled water, calcium carbonate may precipitate if calcium hydroxide is used to raise the pH and if sufficient carbon dioxide enters the water during the experiment. These precipitates provide opportunities for adsorption and coagulation of microorganisms and will cause an increased removal over that obtained from the pH effect alone without the precipitate. The research cited below, unless otherwise noted, was conducted with procedures that obviated this problem or that made its effect insignificant.

EFFICACY AGAINST BACTERIA

Wattie and Chambers (1943) determined the times required to obtain 100% inactivation of several bacterial species at initial concentrations of approximately 1,500 organisms/ml in 20°C to 25°C dechlorinated tapwater, using calcium hydroxide for pH adjustment (see Table II-17). The inactivation was significantly less at each pH for each organism between 0°C to 1°C. At a pH of 11.5, the time for 100% inactivation of *Escherichia coli* was increased from 210 min between 20°C to 25°C to 355 min between 0°C to 1°C. The time for 100% inactivation of

TABLE II-17 Contact Times Necessary for High pH Conditions to Effect 100% Inactivation of Initial Concentrations of 1,500 Organisms/ml[a]

| pH | Contact Time Required for 100% Inactivation by High pH Conditions, min | | | | |
	Escherichia coli	Enterobacter aerogenes	Pseudomonas aeruginosa	Salmonella typhi	Shigella dysenteriae
9.01-9.5	> 540	—	—	> 540	—
9.51-10.0	> 600	> 600	420	> 540	> 300
10.01-10.5	> 600	> 600	300	> 540	> 300
10.51-11.0	600	> 540	240	240	180
11.01-11.5	300	> 600	120	120	75

[a] Data from Wattie and Chambers, 1943. Experiments were conducted at 20°-25°C.

TABLE II-18   Inactivation of *Escherichia coli* by High pH Conditions at 25°C in a Dilution Medium[a]

pH	Contact time, min	Inactivation, %
11.55	50	~10
11.70	50	~90
11.81	35	96
12.01	10	99.8
12.04	6	97

[a] Data from Berg and Berman, 1967.

Salmonella typhi was increased from 75 min to 270 min for the same temperature change. No mention was made of difficulties from the formation of precipitates.

Riehl *et al.* (1952) reported *E. coli* inactivations of 95% in 8 hr at pH 10.5 and 5°C, 100% in 2 hr at pH 10.5 and 15°C, and 100% in approximately 30 min at pH 10.5 and 25°C in distilled water. Calcium hydroxide was used for pH adjustment. Inactivations of 50% and 55% in 10 hr were noted for *Salmonella montevideo* and *S. typhi*, respectively, at 2°C and pH 10.6 in distilled water. Initial concentrations of organisms were approximately 1,000/ml. They also observed that higher temperatures gave more inactivation at the same pH and contact time and that the composition of the water did not markedly influence the bacterial survival.

Berg and Berman (1967) determined the inactivation of *E. coli* at 25°C in the dilution water medium that is described in the 11th edition of *Standard Methods* (1960) (see Table II-18). Sodium hydroxide was used to adjust the pH.

EFFICACY AGAINST VIRUSES

Wentworth *et al.* (1968) reported that little or no poliovius 1 was inactivated in distilled water at pH 11.2 at room temperature in 90 min when calcium hydroxide or sodium hydroxide was used to increase the pH. For poliovirus 1 in distilled water without added salts, Sproul *et al.* (1970) showed that no inactivation occurred in 90 min at pH values of 10.5 or less when calcium hydroxide and sodium hydroxide furnished the hydroxide. Their work was done at 21°C to 22°C. Sproul (1975) obtained

TABLE II-19 Inactivation of Echovirus 7 by High pH
Conditions at 25°C in a Dilution Medium[a]

pH	Contact time, min	Inactivation, %
11.23	7	99.98
11.49	4	99.99
11.79	4	99.5
11.92	1.5	99.9

[a] Data from Berg and Berman, 1967.

poliovirus 1 inactivations in 30 min of 7% at pH 11.5, 59% at pH 11.9 in 30 min, 94% at pH 12.1 in 20 min, and 99.83% at pH 12.5 in 5 min. He used distilled water with 100 mg/liter of sodium chloride (NaCl) at 22°C to 23°C.

Berg and Berman (1967) showed the inactivation of echovirus 7 AGKP8A1 at 25°C in a dilution water medium (*Standard Methods*, 1960). They used sodium hydroxide to adjust pH (see Table II-19). From his work with the f2 bacteriophage, Donovan (1972) suggested that a calcium–virus complex was formed and that a large part of the observed decrease in titer at pH 11.5 was caused by an aggregation of the virus. Electron micrographs and chemical evidence supported the observation.

EFFICACY AGAINST PARASITES

The susceptibility of protozoa or helminths to inactivation by high pH conditions does not appear to have been studied.

Mechanisms of Action

The inactivation mechanism of high pH on bacteria has not been examined. There is ample evidence to show that the poliovirus is inactivated by the disruption of the capsid and a loss of the RNA to the water (Boeye and Van Elsen, 1967; Maizel *et al.*, 1967; Van Elsen and Boeye, 1966). Boeye and Van Elsen (1967) suggested that, at pH 10 and at elevated temperatures ($\geq 30°C$), the RNA was released from the capsid in a degraded form or that it was quickly and extensively broken down after release. The applicability of this mechanism to enteroviruses other than poliovirus is unknown.

Conclusions

The utilization of high pH conditions for disinfection of water is feasible, but higher pH values than are normally used in water treatment and long contact times are required. At pH values of approximately 10.5, bacteria are inactivated in up to 600 min, but viruses are probably unaffected. A pH value of 12.0 to 12.5 and a contact time of approximately 30 min can probably yield 99.0% to 99.9% inactivation of most bacteria and of certain viruses. This process has a drawback: the pH that is necessary for effective disinfection must be reduced before the water can be consumed. Use of the high pH as the sole means of disinfection is not recommended. In many situations where water is softened by the precipitation process and where the water is of poor biological quality, the disinfection potential of this process could be used by increasing the pH above its present values.

Research Recommendations

Although this method has not been used deliberately for disinfection in the past, additional work on this method may be warranted since high pH conditions are attained in many treatment plants. Studies are needed to determine the pH values required for inactivation of protozoans, a broader and more representative group of viruses, and a larger group of enteric bacteria.

HYDROGEN PEROXIDE

Hydrogen peroxide (H_2O_2) is a strong oxidizing agent that has been used for disinfection for more than a century. Its instability and the difficulty of preparing concentrated solutions have tended to limit its use. However, by 1950 electrochemical and other processes were developed to produce pure hydrogen peroxide in high concentration, which is known as stabilized hydrogen peroxide (Schumb et al., 1955). This product has been subjected to increased study and application. Most recently it has been used to disinfect spacecraft (Wardle and Renninger, 1975), foods (Toledo, 1975), and contact lenses (Gasset et al., 1975; Spaulding et al., 1977). Although there has been some interest in using hydrogen peroxide as a disinfectant for wastewater (Taki and Hashimoto, 1977), it has been used more for control of bulking in the activated sludge waste treatment process (Sezgin et al., 1978). Its use in drinking water disinfection appears minimal.

Analytical Methods

Analytical methods for hydrogen peroxide are based on oxidation or reduction with potassium permanganate ($KMnO_4$), potassium iodide (KI), or ceric sulfate [$Ce(SO_4)_2$] (Chadwick and Hoh, 1966). A colorimetric procedure based on the oxidation of titanium sulfate ($TiOSO_4$) (Snell and Snell, 1949) is sensitive to about 1 mg/liter in the absence of other oxidizing agents.

Production and Application

Commercially produced hydrogen peroxide is available in aqueous solution, usually ranging from 30% to 90%. It is stabilized during manufacture by addition of such compounds as sodium pyrophosphate ($Na_4P_2O_7$), acetophenetidin ($CH_3CONHC_6H_4OC_2H_5$), or acetanilide ($CH_3CONHC_6H_5$). As the concentration of hydrogen peroxide is decreased, the concentration of stabilizers is typically increased. Experience in the waterworks industry using hydrogen peroxide is nonexistent. However, hydrogen peroxide is widely used as a bleaching agent in making cotton textiles or in wood pulping (Chadwick and Hoh, 1966). Presumably, a concentrated solution would be diluted and applied with a chemical metering pump. Careful attention to safety in handling would be required because of the possibility of fire or explosion.

Biocidal Activity

The few pre-1965 references on disinfection by hydrogen peroxide have been summarized by Yoshpe-Purer and Eylan (1968). Although its bactericidal activity was indicated, a need for catalytic Fe^{2+} or Cu^{2+} was reported. Yoshpe-Purer and Eylan (1968) worked with *Escherichia coli*, *Salmonella typhi*, and *Staphylococcus aureus* in pure culture and as a mixture of bacteria. They also studied the effect of hydrogen peroxide concentrations (from 30 to 60 mg/liter), contact time (10 to 420 min), and initial concentration of organisms. Without ever measuring residuals, they concluded that bacterial inactivations were relatively slow, that *E. coli* was more resistant to hydrogen peroxide than *S. typhi* or *S. aureus*, and that the required inactivation time was increased as the initial concentration of organisms was increased. Regardless of the hydrogen peroxide concentration or the type of organism used , all tests were claimed to be "sterile" in 24 hr. Table II-20 summarizes some of these data.

Toledo *et al.* (1973) studied inactivation of *S. aureus* and spores of

TABLE II-20   Contact Times Necessary for Hydrogen Peroxide (H_2O_2) to Effect 99% Inactivation of Various Concentrations of *Escherichia coli, Salmonella typhi,* and *Staphylococcus aureus*[a]

Test Microorganism	Initial Concentration, bacteria/ml	Contact Time Required for 99% Inactivation by Hydrogen Peroxide, min		
		30 mg/liter	60 mg/liter	90 mg/liter
Escherichia	10^2	b	b	~360
coli	10^4	b	b	b
	10^6	b	b	~360
Salmonella	10^2	~60	>30 <45	<10
typhi	10^4	>300	>45 <60	30
	10^6	>300	>60	>45 <60
Staphylococcus	10^2	c	b	>15 <30
aureus	10^4	c	b	~60
	10^6	c	b	~180

[a] Data from Yoshpe-Purer and Eylan, 1968. Organism grown on nutrient agar (24-hr culture), suspended in saline, and exposed to varying concentrations of hydrogen peroxide in 1 liter of tap water, pH $\approx$ 6.5, at room temperature (not specified).
[b] Inactivation in 300 min was less than 90%.
[c] No data reported.

several species of *Bacillus* and *Clostridium* with 25.8% (258,000 mg/liter) hydrogen peroxide. The time to reduce *S. aureus* by 6 logs was 1 min, whereas reduction of spores by 99% required from less than 1 min to approximately 17 min, depending on the species. Increasing the hydrogen peroxide concentration up to 41% (or 410,000 mg/liter) or increasing temperature from 24°C to 76°C significantly reduced the required inactivation time.

Several studies on virus inactivation by hydrogen peroxide have been reported. Lund (1963) obtained a 99% inactivation of poliovirus (Saukett strain) in about 6 hr with 0.3% (3,000 mg/liter) hydrogen peroxide. Mentel and Schmidt (1973) worked with rhinovirus (types 1A, 1B, and 7). They found that while a 1.5% (15,000 mg/liter) concentration required approximately 24 min for 99% inactivation, equivalent inactivation occurred in 4 min with a concentration of 3% (30,000 mg/liter).

Information is lacking on the effect of hydrogen peroxide on protozoa and helminths in water.

In none of the studies cited above is there any indication that the dosage of hydrogen peroxide was measured other than by the volumetric addition of hydrogen peroxide. No measurements of residual were reported, although Yoshpe-Purer and Eylan (1968) claimed that a residual was present for up to 13 days as indicated by inactivation of added doses of bacteria.

Mechanism of Action

No studies have specifically identified the mechanism of action of hydrogen peroxide. Spaulding *et al.* (1977) believed that the hydrogen peroxide molecule itself was not responsible for the action but, rather, that the free hydroxyl radical (HO·) that it produced was the specific inactivating agent. They claimed that the catalytic effect of iron or copper ions supported this theory. Yoshpe-Purer and Eylan (1968) also reported that free radicals were important but that sufficient catalyzing metal ions were available either from the tap water that they used or from the bacterial cells themselves.

Conclusions

Because of its relatively high cost and the high concentrations that are required to achieve disinfection in reasonable time, hydrogen peroxide is not a generally satisfactory disinfectant for drinking water.

Research Recommendations

If further research is to be conducted, the stability of hydrogen peroxide and its residual effect in the presence of organic material and other substances in water or distribution systems should be investigated. Parallel studies using chlorine and hydrogen peroxide, separately and in conjunction, should be conducted.

IONIZING RADIATION

Ionizing radiation may be electromagnetic or particulate. As used for disinfection or sterilization, electromagnetic radiation may be UV, gamma, or X rays, and the particles may be alpha or beta or neutrons, mesons, positrons, or neutrinos. This discussion is limited to gamma rays and beta particles (or electrons).

Although there is extensive literature on the use of ionizing radiation in the preservation of food and other materials (Silverman and Sinskey, 1977), little information is available on water treatment.

Application

Laboratory studies of destruction of microorganisms are generally conducted by exposing small containers holding the test suspensions to the shielded source of ionizing radiation. However, in a practical application, the shielded source must be designed to permit relatively thin sheets of flowing liquid to be exposed. This is particularly important for high-energy electrons that have a less penetrating power than gamma rays. The MIT study (Massachusetts Institute of Technology, 1977) included a field demonstration in which a plant treating approximately 380,000 liters/day (minimum dosage of 400,000 rads) was designed and operated. The energy source was a 50-kW electron accelerator operated at 850,000 V. Sludge was pumped under the electron beam through a drum system that produced a layer that was 1.2-m wide and 2-mm thick. The entire operation was conducted in a concrete vault to shield the operators against X rays, which are produced incidentally. Shielding of workers is a major requirement both for gamma ray and high-energy electron sources.

Analytical Methods and Residual

No residual is produced by ionizing radiation. Consequently, dosage has been measured exclusively. The MIT (1977) report and Silverman and Sinksey (1977) summarized analytical methods including calorimetry, photoluminescent dosimetry, colorimetry, and the use of ionization chamber instruments.

Biocidal Activity

EFFICACY AGAINST BACTERIA

The first study of ionizing radiation in the treatment of water was reported by Dunn (1953). In addition to reviewing the literature and providing some discussion on ionizing radiation, he studied the use of a 1,000-Ci source of cobalt-60 (providing gamma rays) and a Van de Graaff generator (providing high-energy electrons). Working with natural waters and wastewaters that were not chemically or bacteriologically characterized or controlled, he exposed samples to a constant radiation flux (2,000 R/min from the cobalt-60 or electrons from 3-MV

TABLE II-21   Dosages of Cobalt-60 Irradiation
Necessary for 99% Inactivation of Microorganisms in
Distilled Water[a]

Test Microorganism	Dosage Required, rad
Bacillus subtilis var *niger*	3.5×10^5
Mycobacterium smegmatis	1.4×10^5
Escherichia coli	6.5×10^4
Micrococcus pyogenes var *aureus*	5.8×10^4
E. coli phage T3	3.2×10^4

[a] Data from Lowe *et al.*, 1956.

operation of the Van de Graaff generator). Varying only the time of exposure, Dunn found that it took 0.125 min (dosage 250,000 R) with the cobalt-60 source to reach 95.4% to 99.999% inactivation of total initial numbers of bacteria (as measured by a plate count at 37°C).

Ridenour and Armbruster (1956) studied the effect of a 10-kCi source of cobalt-60 (3,000 R/min) on a variety of natural waters, wastewaters, and pure cultures (approximately 2×10^7 organisms per milliliter) of 10 different organisms. They found that a dosage of 100,000 roentgen equivalent physical (rep) reduced the count of all species tested by $\geq 99\%$. (In order of increasing resistance, the species were: *Enterobacter aerogenes, Escherichia coli, Shigella flexneri, Salmonella typhi, S. sonnei, Salmonella* sp., *Staphylococcus aureus, S. paratyphi* B, *Streptococcus faecalis*, and *Bacillus subtilis*.) With river water, a dosage of from 50,000 to 100,000 rep reduced the total bacterial count and the coliform index by at least 99%, but 150,000 rep were required to reduce the streptococcus index by 99%. Varying the pH (5.0, 7.0, and 8.5) had no effect on the rate of inactivation.

Also using cobalt-60 (1,100 Ci), Lowe *et al.* (1956) exposed pure cultures of bacteria that were suspended in double distilled water and sterile settled sewage. The concentration of microorganisms was approximately 1×10^6/ml. Although they did not report exposure time, they summarized their exposure data in rads (radiation absorbed dose). (See Table II-21).

There have been more studies on the disinfection of wastewater than on disinfection of drinking water. Ballantine *et al.* (1969) and Compton *et al.* (1970) considered ionizing radiation not as good as other available methods but, with increased emphasis on water reclamation (Eliassen and Trump, 1973) and the use of high-energy electrons (Massachusetts Institute of Technology, 1977; Wright and Trump, 1956), the prospects for practical application seem improved. In the MIT (1977) study, which is the most systematic one conducted to date, washed cells or spores were suspended in 0.067-M phosphate buffer (1 × 10⁸ cells/ml) and exposed to high-energy electrons from a Van de Graaff generator. The approximate dosages, in rads, required for a 99% inactivation of the organisms tested were: *Escherichia coli* (K12), 38,000; *Salmonella typhimurium* (LT2), 24,000; *Micrococcus* sp., 35,000; *Aspergillus niger* (spores), 78,000; *S. typhimurium* (24), 100,000; *Streptococcus fecalis*, 300,000; and *Clostridium perfringens* (spores), 400,000. The investigators found that the solids in the wastewater had no effect on disinfection.

Of the factors affecting disinfection, oxygen was most important. For example, for *E. coli* K12, the dosage required for 99% inactivation was more than doubled when an atmosphere of air was replaced by one of nitrogen, and almost halved when the air was replaced by an oxygen-rich atmosphere.

EFFICACY AGAINST VIRUSES

The inactivation of viruses does not appear to be influenced by the source of the ionizing radiation (Lea, 1955). It is affected by factors that are similar to those described above for bacterial inactivation (Ballentine et al., 1969). Lowe et al. (1956) found that 32,000 rads were required for 99% inactivation of *E. coli* phage T3 (see Table II-21). In the MIT study (1977), from 300,000 to 420,000 rads were required for 99% inactivation of coxsackievirus B3, poliovirus 2, echovirus 7, reovirus 1, and adenovirus 5 (in order of increasing sensitivity), each suspended in 0.05 M glycine at pH 7.0.

EFFICACY AGAINST PARASITES

The MIT study (1977) appears to be the only one in which the effect of ionizing radiation on both protozoa and helminths was investigated; however, no quantitative data were reported. Brannan et al. (1975) found that to attain a 90% reduction of embryonation of *Ascaris lumbricoides* eggs, a dosage of approximately 30,000 rads was required.

Mechanism of Action

In a review of the literature, Silverman and Sinskey (1977) summarized the mode of action of disinfection by ionizing radiation. Two effects are recognized: the direct effect, in which the primary cellular target is DNA that is damaged by the energy released from the ionizing radiation, and the indirect effect, which is associated with the production of such substances in the cell menstruum as hydrogen peroxide (H_2O_2), organic peroxides, and free radicals. Oxygen is important because it reacts with electrons and radicals, which in turn react to form hydrogen peroxide or ozone (O_3).

Conclusions

Ionizing radiation can disinfect water effectively; however, the large source, shielding, and relatively thin exposure layers that are required create difficult engineering and safety problems. The complex technology may limit application to large facilities that can provide for adequate safeguards. The absence of residual disinfection is also restrictive.

Research Recommendations

Any further research should address practical methods of delivering the ionizing radiation to the water mass. Basic engineering design, construction, and operation data should be developed.

POTASSIUM PERMANGANATE

Potassium permanganate ($KMnO_4$) is a strong oxidizing agent, which was first used as a municipal water treatment chemical by Sir Alexander Houston of the London Metropolitan Water Board in 1913. In the United States, it was used in Rochester, New York, in 1927 and in Buffalo, New York, in 1928. Since 1948, it has been used more widely in waterworks as an algicide (Fitzgerald, 1964; Kemp et al., 1966), as an oxidant to control tastes and odors (Spicher and Skrinde, 1963; Welch, 1963), to remove iron and manganese from solution (American Water Works Association, 1971; Shull, 1962), and, to a limited extent, as a disinfectant (Cleasby et al., 1964).

The relatively limited information concerning disinfection with potassium permanganate is subject to criticism, because there have been no studies of the effects of organic constituents of the medium (test system) or destruction of a variety of organisms, especially pathogens.

Analytical Methods and Residual

Concentrations of potassium permanganate can be determined readily by iodometric titration using sodium thiosulfate ($Na_2S_2O_3$) as a titrant or by direct titration with ferrous sulfate. Manganese can be determined by atomic absorption spectrophotometry, or the permanganate ion (MnO_4^-) can be measured colorimetrically (*Standard Methods*, 1976). The minimum detectable concentration of manganese by the colorimetric procedures, using a 100-ml sample, is 50 μg/liter. A concentration of 0.05 mg/liter or greater can be detected visually by the pink color that is imparted to the water (Welch, 1963).

Production and Application

Crystalline potassium permanganate is highly soluble in water (2.83 g/100 g at 0°C). In waterworks, it is prepared usually as a dilute solution (1% to 4%) and applied with a chemical metering pump (American Water Works Association, 1971). It also may be added as a solid using conventional dry-feed equipment.

Reduction of the permanganate ion produces insoluble manganese oxide (Mn_3O_4) hydrates. To prevent distribution of turbid water or of water that will cause unsightly staining of plumbing fixtures, potassium permanganate most often is applied as a pretreatment that is followed by filtration. For example, addition of potassium permanganate to a finished water to maintain a residual in a distribution system is unacceptable because of the pink color of the compound itself or the brown color of the oxides.

Biocidal Activity

Cleasby *et al.* (1964) and Kemp *et al.* (1966) summarized the few scientific references to disinfection by potassium permanganate that were published earlier than 1960. Although some bactericidal activity was indicated, no quantitative data were presented, and the early reports disagreed as to its value.

The most systematic study of disinfection by potassium permanganate has been made by Cleasby *et al.* (1964). They worked exclusively with *Escherichia coli* (prepared as a lactose broth culture) and studied the effect of potassium permanganate at doses of 1 to 16 mg/liter at pH values of 5.9, 7.4, and 9.2, temperatures of 0°C and 20°C, and contact times of 4 to 120 min. They concluded that bacterial inactivation was relatively ineffective, but slightly better at the higher temperature, and

TABLE II-22 Concentrations and Contact Times Necessary for Potassium Permanganate to Effect 99% Inactivation of a 48-Hr *Escherichia coli* Lactose Broth Culture[a]

Contact Time Required for 99% Inactivation by Potassium Permanganate, min							
1 mg/liter	2 mg/liter	4 mg/liter	8 mg/liter	12 mg/liter	16 mg/liter	pH	Temperature, °C
45	45	c	c	10	5	5.9	0
b	c	c	c	b	115	7.4	
c	c	c	c	c	c	9.2	
95	45	15	15	10	5	5.9	20
b	c	b	80	80	25	7.4	
c	c	c	c	c	b	9.2	

[a] Data from Cleasby et al., 1964.
[b] Inactivation in 120 min was less than 90%.
[c] No data reported.

that increasing pH decreased disinfection rates. Table II-22 summarizes in tabular form their data, which were presented originally in graphic fashion.

At least two patent applications involve the use of potassium permanganate as a disinfectant for water in swimming pools (Heuston, 1972; Seidel, 1973). Seidel's patent covered use of a concentration of 0.1 to 0.2 mg/liter in a recirculating system including filtration through quartz gravel. She claimed removal of bacteria and algae, but the specific merit of potassium permanganate in her system cannot be determined from the patent application. Heuston (1972) proposed a tablet containing 0.001 g of potassium permanganate per 0.2 g tablet to give a dose of 1 mg/liter. Because the tablet includes potassium iodide (KI) and other oxidizing agents, it is impossible to assess the specific killing action of potassium permanganate.

A number of studies on inactivation by potassium permanganate have been reported. However, these dealt largely with the mode of action of potassium permanganate in viral inactivation (Lund, 1963, 1966) or at efforts to control human diseases (Peretts et al., 1960; Schultz and Robinson, 1942; Wagner, 1951), animal diseases (Derbyshire and Arkell, 1971), or plant diseases (Eskarous and Habib, 1972; Hughes and Steindl, 1955). They provide few clear-cut quantitative data on biocidal activity of the compound.

Information is lacking on the effect of potassium permanganate on protozoans and helminths in water.

Mechanism of Action

The mechanism of action of potassium permanganate has not been definitively identified. From the studies that have been conducted (Lund, 1963, 1966) it may be presumed that it exerts its disinfection activities by oxidizing compounds that are involved in essential cellular functions. However, Lund (1963) questioned the suggestion that the oxidative process was the mechanism for poliovirus inactivation, but was unable to exclude it as a possibility.

Conclusions

The relatively high cost, ineffective bactericidal action, and aesthetic unsuitability of maintaining a residual in the distribution system make potassium permanganate a generally unsatisfactory disinfectant for drinking water.

Research Recommendations

Additional studies on potassium permanganate are hardly warranted, but in the unlikely event that further research on its biocidal activities is conducted, it would be desirable to study the effect of organic material on its disinfection and the effect of the compound on organisms other than *E. coli*. To relate disinfection efficiency to more conventional practices, parallel studies using chlorine should be conducted.

SILVER

Silver as a metal has been known for millennia, and its use as a water disinfectant dates back to the Persian king Cyrus. The term oligodynamic, which describes the killing effect of small concentrations, was coined by von Naegeli in 1893, but it is unscientific and its use should be rejected. The antibacterial action of silver and silver nitrate ($AgNO_3$) was noted first by Raulin in 1869. Since the late nineteenth century, but especially since World War II, there have been considerable efforts to exploit the use of silver as a disinfectant, particularly for individual (home) water systems and swimming pools. Silver has been used both as a salt, most commonly silver nitrate, or as metallic silver, either bound in filter beds, generated by electrolytic devices, or applied as a colloidal suspension.

The relatively limited information concerning disinfection with silver has been seriously criticized because accurate measurement of low concentrations, i.e., <200 µg/liter, has been difficult; a suitable neutralizing agent has not always been incorporated in test protocols; and adsorption of silver on surfaces of test vessels has confounded some studies. Despite these limitations, silver has been used in parts of Europe and Japan as a water disinfectant.

Production and Application

In water treatment, silver has been applied principally by dissolving the metal or by incorporating a silver compound in a filter medium, often an activated carbon filter. Romans (1954) has described older processes and patents. Davies (1976) reviewed processes for treating swimming pool water in which silver was added as a soluble salt and the silver ions were kept oxidized by the addition of persulfate; metallic silver was deposited on an activated carbon filter; silver was released from solid silver electrodes, which were alternately made anodic and cathodic; silver was released from an activated carbon filter containing silver and supplemented by passing the water through anodic silver screens; and silver was released from a pair of silver–copper alloy electrodes by applying a low reversing voltage.

During the past 6 yr, dozens of patents have been issued in Germany, Spain, South Africa, India, and the United States for devices or systems for adding silver to home drinking water systems or swimming pools. The home systems are most frequently combinations of activated carbon to remove tastes and odors and silver to prevent bacterial growth on the filter.

Because of the low solubility of silver, the dose is usually less than 50 μg/liter. Presumably this is reduced rapidly because of the adsorption of silver to surfaces, but there is no information on the silver residual in treated water. However, the maximum contaminant level (MCL) is 0.05 mg/liter (U.S. Environmental Protection Agency, 1975).

Analytical Methods

Until recently there have been no satisfactory techniques for measuring silver at the μg/liter level. Using a dithizone colorimetric method, the minimum detectable quantity of silver is 200 μg/liter (*Standard Methods*, 1976). Using an atomic absorption spectrophotometric method, the detection limit is 10 μg/liter (U.S. Environmental Protection Agency, 1974), and, if a heated graphite furnace is used, the detection limit is reduced to 0.005 μg/liter (Rattonetti, 1974).

Biocidal Activity

One of the earliest studies was conducted by Just and Szniolis (1936), who found that 100 μg of silver per liter disinfected water within 3 to 4 hr, that silver nitrate and metallic silver were equally effective, and that histopathological changes occurred in rats that were given water containing 400–1,000 μg silver/liter for 100 days. Other systematic studies of silver disinfection have been conducted by Renn and Chesney (1953–1956), Wuhrmann and Zobrist (1958), and Chambers and Proctor (1960). These studies have been summarized by Woodward (1963). Table II-23, adapted from Wuhrmann and Zobrist (1958), shows that in the concentrations used, silver acted slowly, but that there were increases in the rate of bacterial inactivation with increasing temperature and pH. Chambers and Proctor (1960) obtained similar results, but the inactivation rates of Renn and Chesney (1953–1956), who used comparable concentrations of silver, were faster.

TABLE II-23   Concentrations and Contact Times Necessary for Silver to Effect 99.9% Inactivation of *Escherichia coli* in 0.005 *M* Phosphate Buffer[a]

| Contact Time Required for 99.9% Inactivation by Silver as Silver Nitrate, min | | | | | Temperature, °C |
0.01 mg/liter	0.03 mg/liter	0.09 mg/liter	0.27 mg/liter	pH	
1,010	837	156	53	6.3	5
466	214	81	34	7.5	
268	109	58	18	8.7	
831	344	144	32	6.3	15
316	177	63	21	7.5	
216	100	38	13	8.7	
1,210	152	68	20	6.3	25
423	86	32	13	7.5	
203	40	20	8	8.7	

[a] Data from Wuhrmann and Zobrist, 1958.

Both Wuhrmann and Zobrist (1958) and Chambers and Proctor (1960) found that the presence of phosphate (at 60 mg/liter) slowed bacterial inactivation. Because phosphate is typically found at much lower concentrations in drinking water, this observation has little practical significance, but it may account for disparate results in some laboratory studies.

Increasing water hardness slowed bacterial inactivation. According to Wuhrmann and Zobrist, an increase of 3 min was required to achieve 99.9% bacterial inactivation (at 20°C and pH 7.0) for each 10 mg/liter increase in hardness. Likewise, chlorides interfered with the action of silver. At 10 mg/liter, they increased the inactivation time by 25% and at 100 mg/liter, by 70%.

The source of silver seemed to be irrelevant to the inactivation rate because silver either added as silver nitrate or dissolved from metallic silver gave approximately equal results.

In most studies of the disinfection of water with silver, *Escherichia coli* has been the test organism. Wuhrmann and Zobrist also tested a *Salmonella* species and found it to be at least as sensitive as *E. coli*. Yasinskii and Kuznetsova (1973) observed that 90 μg/liter inactivated *Vibrio comma* (1×10^6 cells/ml) in 30 min or 22.5 μg/liter in 60 min.

Fair (1948) and Harrison (1947) suggested that silver salts were ineffective against cysts of *Entamoeba histolytica*, but the data provided in these reports were limited. By contrast, Newton and Jones (1949) observed that electrolytically produced silver in tap water gave greater than 99% cyst inactivation in 1 hr and highly variable residual concentrations that ranged between 17 and 33 mg/liter at pH's of 9.0 to 9.8. When silver nitrate in distilled water at 0.5 mg/liter was used, 4 to 6 hr were required for a 90% to 99% inactivation. At 5 mg/liter, a >99% inactivation occurred in 3 hr, and at 30 mg/liter, a >99% inactivation occurred in 1 to 2 hr.

Chang and Baxter (1955) used 150 mg/liter of silver nitrate (95 mg/liter Ag^+) with contact lines of 1 to 6 min. They concluded that cysticidal activity was only moderate compared to that of iodine. Apparently, there are no data on silver as a virucidal agent in water except for one study by Lund (1963), who decreased poliovirus activity by 2.5 logs in 4 hr with a concentration of approximately 68 mg/liter.

A good general review of silver and its compounds and a more thorough medical examination of their applications was published by Grier (1977), who concluded that there would be a "significant place for silver compounds in the prevention and treatment of at least some bacterial diseases."

Mechanism of Action

Romans (1954) summarized the mechanism of so-called oligodynamic activity: "However, there is much difference of opinion as to the form of the active principle, as to the mechanism of its action, and the value of the results obtained. Some authorities believe that the active form is a positively charged ion, some think it is a complex ion, others a salt and still others think it acts by formation of proteinates or merely as a catalyst. These are only a few of the ideas that have been expressed with formidable experimental support."

Chang (1970) attributed a direct action to silver in the nonreversible formation of silver–sulfhydryl complexes that could not function as hydrogen carriers:

$$2R—SH \rightarrow R—S—S—R \text{ (normal sulfhydryl)} + H_2 \qquad (30)$$

$$R—SH + Ag^+ \rightarrow R—SAg \text{ (inactive silver complex)} + H^+ \qquad (31)$$

He considered silver to be bacteriostatic as well as bactericidal. This would explain the relatively long contact times that are required for antibacterial activity at the concentrations that are normally used.

Zimmerman (1952) demonstrated that low concentrations of silver do not enter the cell but are adsorbed onto the bacterial surface just as silver tends to be adsorbed on other surfaces (Chambers and Proctor, 1960). According to Chang (1970), the adsorbed silver ions must immobilize the dehydrogenation process because bacterial respiration takes place at the cell surface membrane.

Conclusions

As a disinfectant, silver may be applicable to home treatment systems and swimming pools. These applications may be more effective in keeping filters free from bacteria than in actually inactivating organisms that are suspended in the water. This is because of the relatively low rate of solution of silver in water and its low biocidal activities.

Woodward (1963) ably summarized the situation: "The high cost of silver will limit it to specialty uses. The fact that silver does not impart taste, odor, or color to water makes it attractive for use. Its slow bactericidal action, although a disadvantage in some situations, may be an advantage in others, particularly where water is stored for long times before use, as on shipboard. Until some of the uncertainties regarding silver are resolved, it would be prudent to use it as a drinking water disinfectant only in situations where substantial factors of safety can be provided and where the bactericidal effectiveness of the procedure can be monitored."

Silver and its compounds are weak, costly disinfectants that are unsuitable for use in municipal drinking water supplies. To achieve acceptable disinfection in a reasonable time would require concentrations exceeding the MCL of 0.05 mg/liter.

Research Recommendations

Now that adequate chemical analytical techniques are available for measuring low concentrations of silver, it would be desirable to conduct disinfection studies in which both dose and residual are measured accurately. To relate disinfection efficiency to more conventional practices, parallel studies using chlorine should be conducted.

ULTRAVIOLET LIGHT

Electromagnetic radiation, in wavelengths from 240 to 280 nm, is an effective agent for killing bacteria and other microorganisms in water

(Luckiesh and Holladay, 1944). Conveniently, from a practical point of view, from 30% to more than 90% of the energy emitted by a low-pressure mercury arc, which is enclosed in special UV transmitting glass, is emitted at a wavelength of 253.7 nm (Anonymous, 1960; Childs, 1962; Luckiesh and Taylor, 1946).

Two basically different physical arrangements are commonly used for the application of UV light to water. In one, lamps are placed above the solution to be disinfected at the apex or focus of parabolic or elliptical reflectors. For this purpose, aluminum is preferred because of its high reflectance for the germicidal 253.7-nm wavelength (Luckiesh and Taylor, 1946). Although this is an efficient way of applying UV radiation to water, the open nature of the structure can permit contamination. Furthermore, it must operate at atmospheric pressure. Tubular reactors are more common in water treatment because they are sealed and operate under pressure.

To increase intensities and permit higher flow rates, multiple lamp reactors are being designed and put into use. These units generally contain lamps that are positioned parallel to the flow of water through them. A recent patent (Wood, 1974) describes an apparatus using a water film approximately 0.64 cm thick and a flow of liquid that is perpendicular to the lamp in a baffled system. This type of unit is designed for disinfection of fluids with low UV transmittance. For liquids with high transmittance like drinking water, such a design is inefficient, because insufficient depth is available for absorption of UV and a large fraction of the radiant energy is dissipated as heat when the UV is reflected on the walls of the contactor.

In units containing lamps that are surrounded by water, an insulation space must be provided to maintain their efficiency. The maximum efficiency of modern cold cathode lamps is near 40°C, dropping off to a 50% output at 24°C and 65°C. Lamps are normally placed in sleeves that are made of high-silica glass or quartz in order to maximize transmission at the 253.7-nm wavelength. Solarization or opacity can develop in the sleeve as it deteriorates with age. The sleeves must be cleaned regularly for efficient functioning.

Another consideration in the mechanical design of UV contactors is the degree of agitation that is provided and the plug flow characteristics of the contactor. In all disinfection systems that require several orders of magnitude of disinfection, short circuiting or nonplug flow characteristics of contactors, which bypass a part of the flow, limit the efficiency of the process. It was recognized by Cortelyou et al. in 1954 that the degree of agitation in the UV disinfection of water is important in bringing the target microorganism into close proximity to the UV source where the intensity is highest.

Dose

The dose, D, of electromagnetic radiation that is applied to a solution is commonly measured as the intensity of radiant energy input, I_0, at the lamp surface or at some given distance from the lamp (I_0 being expressed as $\mu W/cm^2$), multiplied by the time of exposure, t, in seconds (Luckiesh and Holladay, 1944):

$$D = I_0 \, t \; \mu W \cdot s/cm^2 \qquad (32)$$

Another measurement of dose is chemical actinometry (Calvert and Pitts, 1966). In this method, a photochemical reaction with a known quantum yield is used to measure the intensity (quanta per second) of light that is absorbed by the actinometry solution. Knowing the time of exposure, the volume of solution, and the volume of sample analyzed, the moles of photochemical reaction per unit of time can be related through the quantum yield to the Einsteins or moles of photons per second that are absorbed by the fluid. From the wavelength of radiation, λ, and the area of lamp surface, the average intensity at the lamp surface can be determined.

$$E = hc/\lambda = 1.2 \times 10^7/\lambda \; W \cdot s/Einstein \; nm \qquad (33)$$

Neither of these measurements of energy input, I_0, per unit area of lamp exposed considers the change in intensity through the depth of exposed fluid and the solid angle over which this energy interacts. Recently, attempts have been made to correct the decrease in intensity with depth in studies of wastewater disinfection where this problem is acute (Roeber and Hoot, 1975; Severin, 1978; Venosa et al., 1978). These studies have shown that the usual water quality indices, such as chemical oxygen demand (COD), color, and turbidity, do not adequately predict the loss of intensity through the solution. The direct measurement of UV transmittance has been successful. In spite of these difficulties, Huff et al. (1965) suggested that color at a maximum level of 5 units, iron at 3.7 mg/liter, and turbidity up to 5 units did not decrease treatment efficiency below acceptable limits in a unit with a maximum water depth of approximately 7.5 cm.

Biocidal Dose

The biocidal dose of UV energy consists of the intensity of UV energy that is absorbed at the reactive site within the microbe over the time of interaction. The biocidal dose is then a function of the energy input from the UV source into the solution, dispersion of the energy as a function of distance from the source, the depth of the fluid between the organisms and the source as well as its absorptivity, and, finally, the losses and reflection of UV light within the contactor. All of these factors determine the actual intensity of radiation that is available to the microorganism at any one point within the contactor (Childs, 1962; Luckiesh and Holladay, 1944; Luckiesh *et al.*, 1944).

Quite early in the study of the batericidal action of UV light, Gates (1929) found that the relation between the intensity of incident energy and time required for bacterial destruction were not of equal importance in determining experimental disinfection. However, Hoather (1955) found that when one corrects for the transmitted intensity of radiation, taking into consideration the absorptivity of the water and dispersion as a function of distance from the source, the required time of exposure is inversely proportional to the calculated intensity of radiation penetrating the water for a given degree of inactivation. Finally, Oliver and Cosgrove (1975) used chemical actinometry and a pulsed laser to show that their coliform and streptococcal inactivation in wastewater depended only on the total dose that is delivered and not on the dose rate or intensity of light that impinged on the sample. Thus, the same number of $\mu W \cdot s/cm^2$ provided the same disinfection regardless of the time and intensity that were used to produce that dosage.

Bacterial spores have also been studied with chemical actinometry. For certain stocks, the rate at which the energy was deposited affected the degree of response (Powers *et al.*, 1974). Powers and his colleagues observed that the effect of the dose rate was not due to geometric factors or intensity variations with depth and solution absorptivity. This explains many earlier results. They did find that dependence on dose rate was seen only for some of their stocks of spores, it was not as dramatic with monochromatic-filtered light of a wavelength of 253.7 nm, and it was observed only at very low doses. The explanations usually given for these low-dose effects are photochemical back reactions, enzymatic repair, and photoreactivation mechanisms (Deering and Setlow, 1963; Harm, 1968).

Residual

UV radiation produces no residual. Therefore, monitoring and control of disinfection efficiency are more difficult for UV than for chemical disinfectants.

However, this is not a major problem, because disinfection can be controlled by adjusting the contact time and the UV energy that is transmitted through the solution. The major disadvantage is the lack of a tracer for ensuring the integrity of the distribution system.

Biocidal Activity

UV disinfection follows Chick's Law of kinetics (Luckiesh and Holladay, 1944):

$$-\log N/N_0 = \frac{I \times t}{Q} \tag{34}$$

where N is the number surviving at time t of an original population N_0 that has been exposed to an intensity I. Q is the dose for 1 log survival, one lethal unit exposure, or a lethe.

The variables discussed above interfere with the accurate determination of the average intensity and time of exposure in a practical UV contactor. Consequently, there is considerable disagreement in the literature concerning the absolute magnitude of Q for the microorganisms that have been studied.

Of the Gram-negative bacteria, *Escherichia coli* is consistently more resistant to disinfection by UV than are the *Salmonella* and *Shigella* species that have been studied (Cortelyou *et al.*, 1954; Kawabata and Harada, 1959). The vegetative forms of the Gram-positive bacteria were more resistant than *E. coli*. Kawabata and Harada found *Streptococcus faecalis* nearly 3 times more resistant than *E. coli*, while *Bacillus subtilis* was 4 times more resistant. The spores of *B. subtilis* were 6 times more resistant than *E. coli*.

Luckiesh and Holladay (1944) reported that a dosage of 2,400 $\mu W \cdot s/cm^2$ at a wavelength of 254 nm produced one lethe of disinfection of *E. coli*. Huff *et al.* (1965) studied a two-lamp shipboard disinfection unit with an approximately 75-cm long, 20-cm diam. unbaffled stainless steel cylinder. Their dosages were generally quite high, ranging from 3,000 to 11,000 $\mu W \cdot s/cm^2$ at a maximum water depth of approximately 19 cm. At the lowest dosage, there was a 0.02% to 0.04% survival of *E. coli*, which, assuming Chick's Law, gives a dosage of less than 400 $\mu W \cdot s/cm^2$/lethe. They also found approximately 2 logs

TABLE II-24   Ultraviolet Energy Necessary to Inactivate
Various Organisms[a]

Test Microorganism	Lethal Dose, (μW$\cdot$s/cm^2)
Escherichia coli	360
Staphylococcus aureus	210
Serratia marcescens	290
Sarcina lutea	1,250
Bacillus globiggii spores	1,300
T3 coliphage	160
Poliovirus	780
Vaccinia virus	30
Semliki Forrest virus	470
EMC virus	650

[a] Data from Morris, 1972.

less spore inactivation with the same dose as required for vegetative cells.
They reported more than 4 logs of inactivation of polio-, echo-, and
coxsackievirus with 4,000 μW $\cdot$ s/cm^2. Based on these results, the U.S.
Department of Health, Education, and Welfare issued a policy statement
on April 1, 1966, stating criteria for the acceptability of UV disinfecting
units as a minimum dosage of 16,000 μW $\cdot$ s/cm^2 with a maximum water
depth of approximately 7.5 cm.

Morris (1972) has compared the dose of 254-nm UV energy required
to inactivate a range of microorganisms suspended in droplets of buffer
solution on an aluminum surface. Their results are shown in Table II-24
expressed as μW $\cdot$ s/cm^2/lethe.

Required dosages reported by Morris (1972) are similar in magnitude
to those found by Huff *et al.* (1965). Both Huff's values and those of
Morris (1972) are lower than those of Luckiesh and Holladay (1944),
partly because of the additional dose of UV that was provided by
reflections from the contactor and aluminum surface, which produce an
estimated dosage approximately twice the values given. No studies of the
action of UV light on parasitic helminths and protozoa in the treatment
of drinking water appear to have been reported.

Mechanism of Action

Inactivation by UV light is believed to act through the direct absorption
of UV energy by the microorganism, causing a molecular rearrangement

of one or more of the biochemical components that are essential to the organism's functioning. The major site of UV absorption in microorganisms is the purine and pyrimidine components of the nucleoproteins. Since the relative efficiency of disinfection by UV energy as a function of wavelength follows the absorption spectrum of these chromophore groups and because the first law of photochemistry states that the light that is absorbed by a molecule can produce photochemical change, the mechanism of action of UV probably occurs through the progressive biochemical change that is produced primarily in the nucleoproteins. Witkin (1976) has reviewed both UV mutagenesis and inducible DNA repair. The major specific mechanisms that have been suggested for UV damage involve the reversible formation of pyrimidine hydrates and pyrimidine dimers. Breaks in the bonding structure, known as nicking, also occur. The older literature has been reviewed by Reddish (1957).

The repair of damaged nucleoprotein with light of a wavelength longer than that of the damaging radiation is commonly referred to as photoreactivation (Witkin, 1976). This process, originally identified by Kelner (1949), has been studied extensively. It occurs in the visible wavelength range from 300 to 550 nm (Jagger, 1960; Kelner, 1949). In addition, repair of nucleoproteins that have been damaged by UV radiation can also occur in the dark. The mechanisms of repair of damage to DNA caused by UV radiation are generally thought to involve induced enzymes (Witkin, 1976), but repair has also been observed in inactive systems for which photochemical back reactions have been suggested (Powers *et al.*, 1974).

Conclusions

UV light produces no residual. Therefore, if a residual is desired, another disinfectant must be used. Current technology is limited to the use of UV light in small systems. Requirements for equipment maintenance limits widespread adoption of UV light for drinking water disinfection.

SUMMARY

Tables II-25 and II-26 present significant characteristics of the methods that are considered for disinfection of drinking water.

The biocidal activity of various disinfectants can be compared conveniently through the numerical value of the product (c · t) of the concentration of disinfectant (c) multiplied by the time of exposure (t) that is required to achieve a particular degree of inactivation (e.g., 99%)

under similar conditions of pH, temperature, etc. The lower its c · t product, the more effective the disinfecting action of a particular agent.

Table II-27 displays c · t products for the methods that are regarded as the major possibilities for drinking water disinfection. The c · t products for similar inactivation under the same conditions obtained for other possible agents (ranked less promising by this or other criteria) are up to several orders of magnitude greater than those shown in Table II-27, e.g., 33,000 and 10^6 for inactivation of *E. coli* and poliovirus 1 by hydrogen peroxide, respectively. Therefore, they were not included.

Conclusions

Table II-28 provides the current status of theoretically possible methods for disinfecting drinking water. To derive the conclusions in the table, the specific biocidal activity data summarized in Table II-27 were considered as well as information (or lack of it) on the practical application and reliability of the methods.

Chlorination, ozonization, and the use of chlorine dioxide come closest to meeting the criteria desired. At this time none of the other possibilities considered can substitute for techniques presently used to disinfect drinking water.

The ultimate choice between methods will require weighing the characteristics detailed in this evaluation against the nature of by-products to be expected from the use of the particular method and the potential toxicities of the by-products. Evaluations of these aspects of drinking water disinfection, also carried out by the Safe Drinking Water Committee, are reported in parallel to this study and should be consulted before final conclusions are drawn.

RESEARCH RECOMMENDATIONS

The lack of data, particularly data on pathogens or data that are amenable to comparison, on the biocidal efficacy of various disinfectants needs to be remedied. Particular emphasis should be placed on the methodology for determining biocidal activity and defining those parameters that need to be controlled for the study to yield data for comparative purposes. Disinfection efficacy studies should be conducted with actual pathogens (bacteria, viruses, and cysts of *Giardia lamblia* and *Entamoeba histolytica*) as well as with model systems. Careful control of the character and concentration of the disinfecting species and of the

TABLE II-25   Summary of Major Possible Disinfection Methods for Drinking Water

Disinfection Agent[a]	Technological Status	Efficacy in Demand-Free Systems[b]			Persistence of Residual in Distribution System
		Bacteria	Viruses	Protozoan cysts	
Chlorine[c] As hypochlorous acid (HOCl)	Widespread use in U.S. drinking water	++++	++++	++	Good
As hypochlorite ion (OCl⁻)		++	++	NDR[d]	
Ozone[c]	Widespread use in drinking water outside United States, particularly in France, Switzerland, and the province of Quebec	++++	++++	+++	No residual possible
Chlorine dioxide[c,e]	Widespread use for disinfection (both primary and for distribution system residual) in Europe; limited use in United States to	++++	++++	NDR[d]	Fair to good (but possible health effects)

	counteract taste and odor problems and to disinfect drinking water				
Iodine					
As diatomic iodine (I_2)	No reports of large-scale use in drinking water	++++	+++	+++	Good (but possible health effects)
As hypoiodous acid (HOI)		++++	++++	+	
Bromine	Limited use for disinfection of drinking water	+++f	+++f	+++f	Fair
Chloramines	Limited present use on a large scale in U.S. drinking water	++	+	+	Excellent

[a] The sequence in which these agents are listed does not constitute a ranking.

[b] Ratings: ++++, excellent biocidal activity; +++, good biocidal activity; ++, moderate biocidal activity; +, low biocidal activity; ±, of little or questionable value.

[c] By-product production and disinfectant demand are reduced by removal of organics from raw water prior to disinfection.

[d] Either no data reported or only available data were not free from confounding factors, thus rendering them not amenable to comparison with other data.

[e] MCL 1.0 mg/liter because of health effects (Symons et al., 1977).

[f] Poor in the presence of organic material.

TABLE II-26 Summary of Minor Possible Disinfection Methods for Drinking Water

Disinfection Agent[a]	Technological Status	Efficacy in Demand-Free Systems[b]			Persistence of Residual in Distribution System
		Bacteria	Viruses	Protozoan cysts	
Ferrate	No reports of use in drinking water	++	+++	NDR[c]	Poor
High pH conditions (pH 12-12.5)	No reports of large-scale use in drinking water	+++	+++	NDR[c]	Feasibility restricted since consumption of high pH water not recommended
Hydrogen peroxide	No reports of large-scale use in drinking water	±	±	NDR[c]	Poor
Ionizing radiation	No reports of use in drinking water	++	++	NDR[c]	No residual possible
Potassium permanganate	Limited use for disinfection	±	NDR[c]	NDR[c]	Good, but aesthetically undesirable
Silver[d]	No reports of large-scale use in drinking water	+	NDR[c]	+	Good, but possible health effects
UV light	Use limited to small systems	+++	+++	NDR[c]	No residual possible

[a] The sequence in which these agents are listed does not constitute a ranking.

[b] Ratings: ++++, excellent biocidal activity; +++, good biocidal activity; ++, moderate biocidal activity; +, low biocidal activity; ±, of little or questionable value.

[c] Either no data reported or only available data were not free from confounding factors, thus rendering them not amenable to comparison with other data.

[d] MCL 0.05 mg/liter because of health effects (Symons et al., 1977).

TABLE II-27 Comparative Efficacy of Disinfectants in the Production of 99% Inactivation of Microorganisms in Demand-Free Systems[a]

Disinfection Agent	E. coli pH	Temperature, °C	c·t[b]	Poliovirus 1 pH	Temperature, °C	c·t[b]	Entamoeba histolytica cysts pH	Temperature, °C	c·t[b]
Hypochlorous acid	6.0	5	0.04	6.0	0	1.0	7	30	20
				6.0	5	2.0			
				7.0	0	1.0			
Hypochlorite ion	10.0	5	0.92	10.5	5	10.5		NDR[c]	
Ozone	6.0	11	0.031	7.0	20	0.005	7.5-8.0	19	1.5[d]
	7.0	12	0.002	7.0	25	0.42			
Chlorine dioxide	6.5	20	0.18	7.0	15	1.32		NDR[c]	
	6.5	15	0.38	7.0	25	1.90			
	7.0	25	0.28						
Iodine	6.5	20-25	0.38	7.0	26	30	7.0	30	80
	7.5	20-25	0.40						
Bromine		NDR[c]		7.0	20	0.06	7.0	30	18
Chloramines									
Monochloramine	9.0	15	64	9.0	15	900		NDR[c]	
	9.0	25	40	9.0	25	320			
Dichloramine	4.5	15	5.5	4.5	15	5,000		NDR[c]	

[a] Conditions closest to pH 7.0 and 20°C were selected from studies discussed in the text. Values for other conditions and agents appear in the text along with discussions of the cited studies.

[b] Concentration of disinfectant (mg/liter) times contact time (min).

[c] Either no data reported or only available data were not free from confounding factors, thus rendering them not amenable to comparison with other data.

[d] This value was derived primarily from experiments that were conducted with tap water; however, some parallel studies with distilled water showed essentially no differences in inactivation rates.

TABLE II-28   Status of Possible Methods for Drinking Water Disinfection

Disinfection Agent	Suitability as Inactivating Agent	Limitations	Suitability for Drinking Water Disinfection[a]
Chlorine	Yes	Efficacy decreases with increasing pH; affected by ammonia or organic nitrogen	Yes
Ozone	Yes	On-site generation required; no residual; other disinfectant needed for residual	Yes
Chlorine dioxide	Yes	On-site generation required; interim MCL 1.0 mg/liter	Yes
Iodine	Yes	Biocidal activity sensitive to pH	No
Bromine	Yes	Lack of technological experience; activity may be pH sensitive	No
Chloramines	No	Mediocre bactericide, poor virucide	No[b]
Ferrate	Yes	Moderate bactericide; good virucide; residual unstable; lack of technological experience	No
High pH conditions	No	Poor biocide	No
Hydrogen peroxide	No	Poor biocide	No
Ionizing radiation	Yes	Lack of technological experience	No
Potassium permanganate	No	Poor biocide	No
Silver	No	Poor biocide; MCL 0.05 mg/liter	No
UV light	Yes	Adequate biocide; no residual; use limited by equipment maintenance considerations	No

[a] This evaluation relates solely to the suitability for controlling infectious disease transmission. See conclusions.

[b] Chloramines may have use as a secondary disinfectant in the distribution system in view of their persistence.

degree of aggregation and other characteristics of the test organisms (or cysts) are required in these tests.

Studies should be conducted to define the mechanisms resulting in the different responses to disinfectants of laboratory-acclimated cultures and organisms that have been freshly isolated from natural conditions or that are resistant to specific disinfectants for other reasons. Techniques should be developed to facilitate accurate predictions from laboratory data to disinfectant susceptibilities under operating conditions in treatment plants.

There are no practical assays for many human viruses of known or suspected importance, e.g., hepatitis A virus and rotaviruses. Assay models should be developed for such viruses, and studies should be conducted on their susceptibilities to disinfection. Support is also needed for research that would result in better appraisals of the significance to human health of the presence of viruses in water supplies. Such studies should include investigation of the causative agents that are involved in the large number of illnesses presently characterized as "gastroenteritis of unknown etiology" and of the doses of various enteroviruses that are required to establish infections.

In investigations of factors affecting biocidal activity in full-scale treatment plant operations, priority should be given to studying more thoroughly the effects of turbidity (both organically and inorganically caused) on disinfection.

It should be determined if any data are available from treatment plants on the effectiveness of ozone or chlorine dioxide in disease prevention, where these methods of disinfection are not used sequentially or, in the case of ozone, with subsequent chlorination. If such data, free of complications, are available, they should be compared with the records on the efficacy of chlorination disinfection.

REFERENCES

General Aspects of Disinfection

Bond, W.W., M.S. Favero, and M.R. Korber. 1973. Bacillus sp. ATCC 27380: a spore with extreme resistance to dry heat. Appl. Microbiol. 26:614–616.

Buchanan, R.E., and N.E. Gibbons, eds. 1974. Bergey's Manual of Determinative Bacteriology, 8th ed. Williams & Wilkins, Inc., Baltimore, Md. 1246 pp.

Butterfield, C.T., and E. Wattie. 1946. Influence of pH and temperature on the survival of coliforms and enteric pathogens when exposed to chloramine. Public Health Rep. 61:157–192.

Butterfield, C.T., E. Wattie, S. Megregian, and C.W. Chambers. 1943. Influence of pH and temperature on the survival of coliforms and enteric pathogens when exposed to free chlorine. Public Health Rep. 58:1837–1866.

Carson, L.A., M.S. Favero, W.W. Bond, and N.J. Petersen. 1972. Factors affecting comparative resistance of naturally occurring and subcultured *Pseudomonas aeruginosa* to disinfectants. Appl. Microbiol. 23:863–869.

Cramer, W.N., K. Kawata, and C.W. Krusé. 1976. Chlorination and iodination of poliovirus and f_2. J. Water Pollut. Control Fed. 48:61–76.

Dahling, D., P.V. Scarpino, M. Lucas, G. Berg, and S.L. Chang. 1972. Destruction of viruses and bacteria in water by chlorine. Abstr. Ann. Meet. Am. Soc. Microbiol. Washington, D.C. Abstr. No. E152, p. 26.

Engelbrecht, R.S., B.F. Severin, M.T. Masarik, S. Farooq, and S.H. Lee. 1975. New Microbial Indicators of Disinfection Efficiency. U.S. National Technical Information Service, AD Report 1975, AD-A030547. 88 pp.

Fair, G.M., and J.C. Geyer. 1954. Water Supply and Waste-Water Disposal. John Wiley & Sons, New York. 973 pp.

Favero, M.S. 1961. Comparative chlorine resistance of some bacteria of public health significance. M.S. thesis. Washington State University, Pullman, Wash.

Favero, M.S., and C.H. Drake. 1966. Factors influencing the occurrence of high numbers of iodine-resistant bacteria in iodinated swimming pools. Appl. Microbiol. 14:627–635.

Favero, M.S., C.H. Drake, and G.B. Randall. 1964. Use of staphylococci as indicators of swimming pool pollution. Public Health Rep. 79:61–70.

Favero, M.S., L.A. Carson, W.W. Bond, and N.J. Petersen. 1971. *Pseudomonas aeruginosa*: growth in distilled water from hospitals. Science 173:836-838.

Favero, M.S., N.J. Petersen, L.A. Carson, W.W. Bond, and S.H. Hindman. 1975. Gram-negative water bacteria in hemodialysis systems. Health Lab. Sci. 12:321–334.

Hoehn, R.C., C.W. Randall, R.P. Good, and P.T.B. Shaffer. 1977. Chlorination and water treatment for minimizing trihalomethanes in drinking water. Pp. 519–535 in R.L. Jolley, H. Gorchev, and D.H. Hamilton, Jr., eds. Water Chlorination: Environmental Impact and Health Effects, Vol. 2. Ann Arbor Science Publishers, Inc., Ann Arbor, Mich. 909 pp.

Hsu, Y-C. 1964. Resistance of infectious RNA and transforming DNA to iodine which inactivates f_2 phage and cells. Nature 203:152–153.

Hsu, Y-C., S. Nomura, and C.W. Krusé. 1966. Some bactericidal and virucidal properties of iodine not affecting infectious RNA and DNA. Am. J. Epidemiol. 82:317–328.

Hubbs, S.A., J.S. Zogorski, D.A. Wilding, A.N. Arbuckle, G.D. Allgier, and R.L. Mullins. 1977. Trihalomethane reduction at the Louisville Water Company. Pp. 605–611 in R.L. Jolley, H. Gorchev, and D.H. Hamilton, Jr., eds. Water Chlorination: Environmental Impact and Health Effects, Vol. 2. Ann Arbor Science Publishers, Inc., Ann Arbor, Mich. 909 pp.

Krusé, C.W. 1969. Mode of action of halogens on bacteria and viruses and protozoa in water systems. Final report to the Commission on Environmental Hygiene of the Armed Forces Epidemiological Board, U.S. Army Med. Res. Dev. Command. Contract No. DA-49-193-MD-2314.

Milbauer, R., and N. Grossowicz. 1959. Effect of growth conditions on chlorine sensitivity of *Escherichia coli*. Appl. Microbiol. 7:71–74.

Morris, J.C. 1975. Formation of halogenated organics by chlorination of water supplies. U.S. Environmental Protection Agency, Washington, D.C. Report No. 600/1-75-002. 54 pp.

National Academy of Sciences. 1977. Drinking Water and Health. National Academy of Sciences, Washington, D.C. 939 pp.

Neefe, J.R., J. Stokes, Jr., J.B. Baty, and J.G. Reinhold. 1945. Disinfection of water containing causative agent of infectious (epidemic) hepatitis. J. Am. Med. Assoc. 128:1076–1080.

Shah, P.C., and J. McCamish. 1972. Relative chlorine resistance of poliovirus I and coliphages f_2 and T_2 in water. Appl. Microbiol. 24:658–659.

Stevens, A.A., C.J. Slocum, D.R. Seeger, and G.R. Robeck. 1975. Chlorination of organics in drinking water. Pp. 77–104 in E.R. Jolley, ed. Water Chlorination: Environmental Impact and Health Effects, Vol. 1. Ann Arbor Science Publishers, Inc., Ann Arbor, Mich. 439 pp.

Stringer, R.P., W.N. Cramer, and C.W. Kruse. 1975. Comparison of bromine, chlorine and iodine as disinfectants for amoebic cysts. Pp. 193-209 in J.D. Johnson, ed. Disinfection: Water and Wastewater. Ann Arbor Science Publishers, Inc., Ann Arbor, Mich. 425 pp.

Symons, J.M., J.K. Carswell, R.M. Clark, P. Dorsey, E.E. Geldreich, W.P. Heffernan, J.C. Hoff, O.T. Love, L.J. McCabe, and A.A. Stevens. 1977. Ozone, Chlorine Dioxide, and Chloramines as Alternatives to Chlorine for Disinfection of Drinking Water: State of the Art. Water Supply Research Division, U.S. Environmental Protection Agency, Cincinnati, Ohio. 84 pp.

Wattie, E., and C.T. Butterfield. 1944. Relative resistance of *Escherichia coli* and *Eberthella typhosa* to chlorine and chloramines. Public Health Rep. 59:1661– 1671.

Chlorine and Chloramines

Analytical Reference Service. 1969. Water Chlorine (Residual) No. 1. Report No. 35. Environmental Control Administration, Cincinnati, Ohio. 126 pp.

Analytical Reference Service. 1971. Water Chlorine (Residual) No. 1. Report No. 40. Environmental Control Administration, Cincinnati, Ohio. 97 pp.

Berg, A. 1966. Virus transmission by the water vehicle, III. Removal of viruses by water treatment procedures. Health Lab. Sci. 3:170–181.

Bocharov, D.A. 1970. Content of nucleic acids in bacterial suspension after influence on it of chlorinated and alkaline solutions. Tr. Vses. Nauchno-Issled. Inst. Vet. Sanit. 34:242–252.

Bocharov, D.A., and A.V. Kulikovskii. 1971. Structural and biochemical changes of bacteria after the action of some chlorine-containing preparations, Report 1. Tr. Vses. Nauchno–Issled. Inst. Vet. Sanit. 38:165–170.

Brady, F.J., M.F. Jones, and W.L. Newton. 1943. Effect of chlorination of water on viability of cysts of *Endamoeba histolytica*. War Med. 3:409–419.

Brigano, F.A.D., P.V. Scarpino, S. Cronier, and M.L. Zink. 1978. Effect of particulates on inactivation of enteroviruses in water. Presented at U.S. Environmental Protection Agency Symposium on Wastewater Disinfection. September 18–20, 1978. Cincinnati, Ohio.

Butterfield, C.T. 1948. Bactericidal properties of chloramines and free chlorine in water. Public Health Rep. 63:934–940.

Butterfield, C.T., E. Wattie, S. Megregian, and C.W. Chambers. 1943. Influence of pH and temperature on the survival of coliforms and enteric pathogens when exposed to free chlorine. Public Health Rep. 58:1837–1866.

Chang, S.L. 1944a. Destruction of micro-organisms. J. Am. Water Works Assoc. 36:1192–1207.

Chang, S.L. 1944b. Studies on *Endamoeba histolytica*. III. Destruction of cysts of *Endamoeba histolytica* by a hypochlorite solution, chloramines in tap water and gaseous chlorine in tap water of varying degrees of pollution. War Med. 5:46–55.

Chang, S.L. 1971. Modern concepts of disinfection. J. Sanit. Eng. Div. Am. Soc. Civ. Eng. 97:689–707.

Chang, S.L., and G.M. Fair. 1941. Viability and destruction of the cysts of *Endamoeba histolytica*. J. Am. Water Works Assoc. 33:1705–1715.

Chang, S.L., G. Berg, N.A. Clarke, and P.W. Kabler. 1960. Survival and protection against chlorination of human enteric pathogens in free living nematodes isolated from water supplies. Am. J. Trop. Med. Hyg. 9:136–142.

Clarke, N.A., and S.L. Chang. 1959. Enteric viruses in water. J. Am. Water Works Assoc. 51:1299–1317.

Clarke, N.A., and P.W. Kabler. 1954. Inactivation of purified coxsackie virus in water by chlorine. Am. J. Hyg. 59:119–127.

Clarke, N.A., R.E. Stevenson, and P.W. Kabler. 1956. The inactivation of purified type 3 adenovirus in water by chlorine. Am. J. Hyg. 64:314–319.

Clarke, N.A., G. Berg, P.W. Kabler, and S.L. Chang. 1964. Human enteric viruses in water source, survival and removal and removability. Pp. 523–541 in W.W. Eckenfelder, ed. Advances in Water Pollution Research, Vol. 2, Proceedings of the 1st International Conference on Water Pollution Research, London, September 1962. Macmillan Co., New York.

Dennis, W.H. 1977. The mode of action of chlorine on f_2 bacterial virus during disinfection. Sc.D. thesis. School of Hygiene and Public Health, Johns Hopkins University, Baltimore, Md.

Dorn, J.M. 1974. A comparative study of disinfection of viruses and bacteria by monochloramine. M.S. thesis. University of Cincinnati, Ohio. 67 pp.

Enders, J.F., T.H. Weller, and F.C. Robbins. 1949. Cultivation of the Lansing strain of poliovirus in cultures of various human embryonic tissues. Science 109:85–87.

Engelbrecht, R.S., B.F. Severin, M.T. Masarik, S. Farooq, and S.H. Lee. 1975. New Microbial Indicators of Disinfection Efficiency. U.S. National Technical Information Service, AD Report 1975, AD-A030547. 88 pp.

Engelbrecht, R.S., M.J. Weber, C.A. Schmidt and B.L. Salter. 1978. Virus Sensitivity to Chlorine Disinfection of Water Supplies. EPA 600/2-78-123. U.S. Environmental Protection Agency, Washington, D.C. 44 pp.

Esposito, P. 1974. The Inactivation of Viruses in Water by Dichloramine. M.S. thesis. University of Cincinnati, Ohio. 121 pp.

Esposito, P., P.V. Scarpino, S.L. Chang, and G. Berg. 1974. Destruction by dichloramine of viruses and bacteria in water. Abstr. No. G99. Abstracts of the Annual Meeting, American Society for Microbiology, Washington, D.C.

Fair, G.M., J.C. Morris, S.L. Chang, I. Weil, and R.J. Burden. 1948. The behavior of chlorine as a water disinfectant. J. Am. Water Works Assoc. 40:1051–1061.

Feng, T.H. 1966. Behavior of organic chloramines in disinfection. J. Water Pollut. Control Fed. 38:614-628.

Fetner, R.H. 1962. Chromosome breakage in Vicia faba by monochloramine. Nature 196:1122-1123.

Friberg, L. 1957. Further quantitative studies on the reaction of chlorine with bacteria in water disinfection. 2. Experimental investigations with Cl^{36} and P^{32}. Acta Pathol. Microbiol. Scand. 40:67–80.

Green, D.E., and P.K. Stumpf. 1946. The mode of action of chlorine. J. Am. Water Works Assoc. 38:1301–1305.

Haas, C.N. 1978. Mechanisms of inactivation of new indicators of disinfection efficiency by free available chlorine. Ph.D. thesis. Department of Civil Engineering, University of Illinois at Urbana-Champaign. 158 pp.

Ingols, R.S., H.A. Wyckoff, T.W. Kethley, H.W. Hodgen, E.L. Fincher, J.C. Hildebrand, and J.E. Mandel. 1953. Bactericidal studies of chlorine. Ind. Eng. Chem. 45:996–1000.

Kaminski, J.J., M.M. Huycke, S.H. Selk, N. Bodor, and T. Higuchi. 1976. N-halo derivatives V: Comparative antimicrobial activity of soft N-chloramine systems. J. Pharm. Sci. 65:1737–1742.

Kelly, S., and W.W. Sanderson. 1958. The effect of chlorine in water on enteric viruses. Am. J. Public Health 48:1323–1334.

Kelly, S.M., and W.W. Sanderson. 1960. The effect of chlorine in water on enteric viruses. II. The effect of combined chlorine on poliomyelitis and coxsackie viruses. Am. J. Public Health 50:14–20.

Knox, W.E., P.K. Stumpf, D.E. Green, and V.H. Auerbach. 1948. The inhibition of sulfhydryl enzymes as the basis of the bactericidal action of chlorine. J. Bacteriol. 55:451–458.

Kulikovsky, A., H.S. Pankratz, and H.L. Sadoff. 1975. Ultrastructural and chemical changes in spores of *Bacillus cereus* after action of disinfectants. J. Appl. Bacteriol. 38:39–46.

Laubush, E.J. 1971. Chlorination and other disinfection processes. Pp. 158–224 in Water Quality and Treatment, A Handbook of Public Water Supplies, 3rd ed. Prepared by the American Water Works Association, Inc., McGraw-Hill Book Company, New York.

Liu, O.C., H.R. Seraichekas, E.W. Akin, D.A. Brashear, E.L. Katz, and W.J. Hill, Jr. 1971. Relative resistance of twenty human enteric viruses to free chlorine in Potomac water. Pp. 171–195 in Virus and Water Quality: Occurrence and Control. Proceedings of the 13th Water Quality Conference conducted by the Department of Civil Engineering, University of Illinois at Urbana-Champaign, and the U.S. Environmental Protection Agency, Urbana.

Lothrop, T.L., and O.J. Sproul. 1969. High-level inactivation of viruses in wastewater by chlorination. J. Water Pollut. Control Fed. 41:567–575.

Morris, J.C. 1970. Modern Chemical Methods, Part I, International Courses in Hydraulic and Sanitary Engineering. International Institute of Hydraulics and Environmental Engineering, Delft, Netherlands.

National Academy of Sciences. 1977. Drinking Water and Health. National Academy of Sciences, Washington, D.C. 939 pp.

Nusbaum, I. 1952. Sewage chlorination mechanism. A survey of fundamental factors. Water and Sewage Works 99:295–297.

Olivieri, V.P., T.K. Donovan, and K. Kawata. 1971. Inactivation of virus in sewage. J. Sanit. Eng. Div. Am. Soc. Civ. Eng. 97:661–673.

Olivieri, V.P., C.W. Kruse, Y-C. Hsu, A.C. Griffiths, and K. Kawata. 1975. The comparative mode of action of chlorine, bromine and iodine on f_2 bacterial virus. Pp. 145–162 in J. D. Johnson, ed. Disinfection: Water and Wastewater. Ann Arbor Science Publishers, Ann Arbor, Mich. 425 pp.

Rosenkranz, H.S. 1973. Sodium hypochlorite and sodium perborate: Preferential inhibitors of DNA polymerase-deficient bacteria. Mutat. Res. 21:171–174.

Scarpino, P.V., G. Berg, S.L. Chang, D. Dahling, and M. Lucas. 1972. A comparative study of the inactivation of viruses in water by chlorine. Water Res. 6:959–965.

Scarpino, P.V., M. Lucas, D.R. Dahliing, A. Berg, and S.L. Chang. 1974. Effectiveness of hypochlorous acid and hypochlorite ion in destruction of viruses and bacteria. Pp. 359–

368 in A.J. Rubin, ed. Chemistry of Water Supply, Treatment and Distribution. Ann Arbor Science Publishers, Ann Arbor, Mich.

Shih, K.L., and J. Lederberg. 1976a. Chloramine mutagenesis in *Bacillus subtilis*. Science 192:1141–1143.

Shih, K.L., and J. Lederberg. 1976b. Effects of chloramine on *Bacillus subtilis* deoxyribonucleic acid. J. Bacteriol. 125:934–945.

Siders, D.L., P.V. Scarpino, M. Lucas, G. Berg, and S.L. Chang. 1973. Destruction of viruses and bacteria in water by monochloramine. Abstr. No. E27. Abstracts of the Annual Meeting, American Society for Microbiology, Washington, D.C.

Skvortsova, E.R., and N.S. Lebedeva. Cited in M.N. Bekhtereva and O.A. Krainova. 1973. Changes in the activity of enzyme systems in *Bacillus anthracoides* spores during germination and due to the action of calcium hypochlorite. Mikrobiologiya 44:791–795.

Standard Methods for the Examination of Water and Wastewater, 14th ed. 1976. American Public Health Association, Washington, D.C. 1193 pp.

Stringer, R.P., W.N. Cramer, and C.W. Krusé. 1975. Comparison of bromine, chlorine and iodine as disinfectants for amoebic cysts. Pp. 193–209 in J.D. Johnson, ed. Disinfection: Water and Wastewater. Ann Arbor Science Publishers, Ann Arbor, Mich. 425 pp.

Symons, J.M., J.K. Carswell, R.M. Clarke, P. Dorsey, E.E. Geldreich, W.P. Heffernam, J.C. Hoff, O.T. Love, L.J. McCabe, and A.A. Stevens. 1977. Ozone, Chlorine Dioxide, and Chloramines as Alternatives to Chlorine for Disinfection of Drinking Water: State of the Art. Water Supply Research Division, U.S. Environmental Protection Agency, Cincinnati, Ohio. 84 pp.

Taras, M.J. 1953. Effect of free residual chlorination on nitrogen compounds in water. J. Am. Water Works Assoc. 45:47–61.

Venkobachar, C. 1975. Biochemical model for chlorine disinfection. Ph.D. thesis. Department of Civil Engineering, Indian Institute of Technology at Kanpur.

Venkobachar, C., L. Iyengar, and A.V.S.P. Rao. 1977. Mechanism of disinfection: effect of chlorine on cell membrane functions. Water Res. 11:727–729.

Walton, G. 1969. Water treatment: prevention of waterborne disease. Pp. 21–36 in U. Weise, ed. Influence of Raw Water Characteristics on Treatment, Proceedings 11th Sanitary Engineering Conference, University of Illinois, Urbana.

Weidenkopf, S.J. 1958. Inactivation of Type I poliomyelitis virus with chlorine. Virology 5:56–67.

White, G.C. 1972. Handbook of Chlorination. Von Nostrand Reinhold Company, New York. 744 pp.

Ozone

Broadwater, W.T., R.C. Hoehn, and P.H. King. 1973. Sensitivity of three selected bacterial species to ozone. Appl. Microbiol. 26:391–393.

Burleson, G.R., T.M. Murray, and M. Pollard. 1975. Inactivation of viruses and bacteria by ozone, with and without sonication. Appl. Microbiol. 29:340–344.

Coin, L., C. Hannoun, and C. Gomella. 1964. Ozone inactivation of poliomyelitis virus present in water. (In French) La Presse Medicale 72(38):2153–2156.

Evison, L.M. 1977. Disinfection of water using ozone: comparative studies with enteroviruses, phage and bacteria. Paper presented at the 3rd Congress of the International Ozone Institute, Paris.

Farooq, S. 1976. Kinetics of inactivation of yeasts and acid-fast organisms with ozone. Ph.D. thesis. University of Illinois, Urbana. 134 pp. (Diss. Abstr. Int. 37B:2406B, Nov.–Dec., 1976.)

Farooq, S., E.S.K. Chian, and R.S. Engelbrecht. 1977a. Basic concepts in disinfection with ozone. J. Water Pollut. Control Fed. 49:1818–1831.

Farooq, S., R.S Engelbrecht, and E.S.K. Chian. 1977b. The effect of ozone bubbles on disinfection. Prog. Water Technol. 9:233–247.

Farooq, S., R.S. Engelbrecht, and E.S.K. Chian. 1977c. Influence of temperature and U.V. light on disinfection with ozone. Water Res. 11:737–741.

Katzenelson, E., B. Kett, and H.I. Shuval. 1974. Inactivation kinetics of viruses and bacteria in water by use of ozone. J. Am. Water Works Assoc. 66:725–729.

Keller, J.W., R.A. Morin, and T.J. Schaffernoth. 1974. Ozone disinfection pilot plant studies at Laconia, N.H. J. Am. Water Works Assoc. 66:730–733.

Morris, J.C. 1976. The role of ozone in water treatment. Paper 29–26 in Proceedings of the 96th Annual Conference of the American Water Works Association, Vol. 2. New Orleans, La.

National Academy of Sciences. 1977. Drinking Water and Health. National Academy of Sciences, Washington, D.C. 939 pp.

Newton, W.L., and M.F. Jones. 1949. Effect of ozone in water on cysts of *Endamoeba histolytica*. Am. J. Trop. Med. 29:669–681.

Peleg, M. 1976. The chemistry of ozone in the treatment of water. Water Res. 10:361–365.

Prat, R., C. Nofre, and A. Cier. 1968. Effects of sodium hyperchlorite, ozone, and ionizing radiation on the pyrimidine constituents of *Escherichia coli*. (In French) Annales de L'Institut Pasteur. 114:595–607.

Riesser, V.N., J.R. Perrich, E.B. Silver, and J.R. McCammon. 1977. Possible mechanisms of poliovirus inactivation by ozone. Pp. 186–192 in E.G. Fochtman, R.G. Rice, and M.F. Browning, eds. Forum on Ozone Disinfection. International Ozone Institute, Cleveland, Ohio. 435 pp.

Rosen, A.M. 1972. Ozone generation and its economical application wastewater treatment. Water and Sewage Works 119:114–120.

Ross, W.R., J. van Leeuwen, and W.O.K. Grabow. 1976. Studies on disinfection and chemical oxidation with ozone and chlorine in water reclamation. Pp. 497–513 and discussion, pp. 509–510, in R.G. Rice, P. Pichet, and M.A. Vincent, eds. Proceedings of the Second International Symposium on Ozone Technology, Montreal, Canada, May 11–14, 1975. Jamesville, N.Y. Ozone Press Internationale, Cleveland, Ohio. 725 pp.

Schecter, H. 1973. Spectrophotometric method for determination of ozone in aqueous solutions. Water Res. 7:729–739.

Scott, D.B. McN., and E.C. Lesher. 1963. Effect of ozone on survival and permeability of *Escherichia coli*. J. Bacteriol. 85:567–576.

Singer, P.C., and W.B. Zilli. 1975. Ozonation of ammonia: application to wastewater treatment. Pp. 269–287 in R.G. Rice and M.E. Browning, eds. Proceedings First International Symposium on Ozone for Water and Wastewater Treatment. International Ozone Institute, Waterbury, Conn. 910 pp.

Smith, D.K. 1967. Disinfection and sterilization of polluted water with ozone. P. 52 in Proceedings of 2nd Annual Symposium on Water Research. McMasters University, Hamilton, Ontario.

Sproul, O.J., H.A. Emerson, H.A. Howser, D.M. Boyce, D.S. Walsh, and C.E. Buck. 1978. Effects of particulate matter on virus inactivation by ozone. Presented at the 98th Annual Conference of the American Water Works Association in Atlantic City, N.J. To be published by the American Water Works Association, Denver, Colo.

Standard Methods for the Examination of Water and Wastewater, 14th ed. 1976. American Public Health Association, Washington, D.C. 1193 pp.

Stumm, W. 1958. Ozone as a disinfectant for water and sewage. J. Boston Soc. Civ. Eng. 45:68-79.

U.S. Environmental Protection Agency. 1976. Interim Treatment Guide for the Control of Chloroform and Other Trihalomethanes. Water Supply Research Division, Municipal Environmental Research Laboratory, U.S. Environmental Protection Agency, Cincinnati, Ohio. 251 pp.

Vrochinskii, K.K. 1963. Decontaminating water with ozone. (In Russian) Gig. Sanita. 28(12):3–9. (Chemical Abstracts. 60:1039d. 1964.)

Wuhrmann, K., and Meyrath. 1955. On the bactericidal effects of aqueous ozone solutions. (In German) Schweiz. Z. Path. Bakteriol. 18:1060–1069.

Chlorine Dioxide

Adams, D.B., D.H. Jackson, and J.W. Ogleby. 1966. Determination of trace quantities of chlorine, chlorine dioxide, chlorite and chloramines in water. Proc. Soc. Water Treat. Exam. 15(2):117–150.

Aston, R.N. 1950. Developments in the chlorine dioxide process. J. Am. Water Works Assoc. 42:151–154.

Bedulevich, T.S., M.N. Svetlakova, and N.N. Trakhtman. 1953. Use of chlorine dioxide in purification of water. Gig. Sanit. 10:14–17.

Benarde, M.A., B.M. Israel, V.P. Olivieri, and M.L. Granstrom. 1965. Efficiency of chlorine dioxide as a bactericide. Appl. Microbiol. 13:776–780.

Benarde, M.A., W.B. Snow, and V.P. Olivieri. 1967a. Chlorine dioxide disinfection temperature effects. J. Appl. Bacteriol. 30:159–169.

Benarde, M.A., W.B. Snow, V.P. Olivieri, and B. Davidson. 1967b. Kinetics and mechanism of bacterial disinfection by chlorine dioxide. Appl. Microbiol. 15:257–265.

Cronier, S.D. 1977. Destruction by chlorine dioxide of viruses and bacteria in water. M.Sc. thesis. University of Cincinnati, Ohio. 85 pp.

Davy, H. 1811. On a combination of oxymuriatic gas and oxygene gas. Philos. Trans. R. Soc. London 101:155–162.

Dowling, L.T. 1974. Chlorine dioxide in potable water treatment. Water Treat. Exam. 23:190–204.

Feuss, J.X. 1964. Problems in determination of chlorine dioxide residuals. J. Am. Water Works Assoc. 56:607–615.

Gall, R.J. 1978. Chlorine dioxide, an overview of its preparation and uses. Pp. 356–382 in R.G. Rice and J.A. Cotruvo, eds. Ozone/Chlorine Dioxide Oxidation Products of Organic Materials. Proceedings of a Conference held in Cincinnati, Ohio, November 17–18, 1976. Sponsored by the International Ozone Institute, Inc., and the U.S. Environmental Protection Agency. Ozone Press International, Cleveland, Ohio. 487 pp.

Gordon, G., R.G. Kieffer, and D.H. Rosenblatt. 1972. The chemistry of chlorine dioxide. Pp. 201–286 in S.J. Lippard, ed. Progress in Inorganic Chemistry, Vol. 15, Wiley Interscience, New York.

Granstrom, M.L., and G.F. Lee. 1958. Generation and use of chlorine dioxide in water treatment. J. Am. Water Works Assoc. 50:1453–1466.

Haller, J.F., and S.S. Listek. 1948. Determination of chlorine dioxide and other active chlorine compounds in water. Anal. Chem. 20:639–642.

Hettche, O., and H.W.S. Ehlbeck. 1953. Epidemiology and prophylaxis of poliomyelitis in respect of the role of water in transfer. Arch. Hyg. Bakteriol. 137:440–449.

Hodgen, H.W., and R.S. Ingols. 1954. Direct colorimetric method for the determination of chlorine dioxide in water. Anal. Chem. 26:1224–1226.

Ingols, R.S., and G.M. Ridenour. 1948. Chemical properties of chlorine dioxide in water treatment. J. Am. Water Works Assoc. 40:1207–1227.

Issacsson, U., and G. Wettermark. 1976. The determination of inorganic chlorine compounds by chemiluminescence reactions. Anal. Chim. Acta 83:227–239.

Masschelein, W. 1966. Spectrophotometric determination of chlorine dioxide with acid chrome violet K. Anal. Chem. 38:1839–1841.

Masschelein, W. 1967. Developments in the chemistry of chlorine dioxide and its applications. Chim. Ind. Genie Chim. 97:49–61.

McCarthy, J.A. 1944. Bromine and chlorine dioxide as water disinfectants. J. N. Engl. Water Works Assoc. 58:55–68.

McCarthy, J.A. 1945. Chlorine dioxide for the treatment of water supplies. J. N. Engl. Water Works Assoc. 59:252–264.

Miltner, R.J. 1976. The Effect of Chlorine Dioxide on Trihalomethanes in Drinking Water. M.S. thesis. University of Cincinnati, Ohio. 88 pp.

Moffa, P.E., E.C. Tifft, S.L. Richardson, and J.E. Smith. 1975. Bench-scale High Rate Disinfection of Combined Sewer Overflows with Chlorine and Chlorine Dioxide. U.S. Environmental Protection Agency Report No. EPA-670/2-75-021. Washington, D.C. 193 pp.

Myhrstad, J.A., and J.E. Samdal. 1969. Behavior and determination of chlorine dioxide. J. Am. Water Works Assoc. 61:205–208.

Olivieri, V.P. 1968. Chlorine dioxide and protein synthesis. M.S. thesis. West Virginia University, Morgantown. 63 pp.

Palin, A.T. 1957. The determination of free and combined chlorine in water by the use of diethyl-p-phenylene diamine. J. Am. Water Works Assoc. 49:873.

Palin, A.T. 1960. Colorimetric determination of chlorine dioxide in water. Water and Sewage Works 107:457–478.

Palin, A.T. 1967. Methods for the determination in water of free and combined available chlorine, chlorine dioxide and chlorite, bromine, iodine and ozone using diethyl-p-phenylene diamine (DPD). J. Inst. Water Eng. 21:537–547.

Palin, A.T. 1970. Determining chlorine dioxide and chlorite. J. Am. Water Works Assoc. 62:483–484.

Palin, A.T. 1974. Analytical control of water disinfection with special reference to differential DPD methods for chlorine, chlorine dioxide, bromine, iodine, and ozone. J. Inst. Water Eng. 28:139–154.

Palin, A.T. 1975. Current DPD methods for residual halogen compounds and ozone in water. J. Am. Water Works Assoc. 67:32–33.

Post, M.A., and W.A. Moore. 1959. The determination of chlorine dioxide in treated surface waters. Anal. Chem. 31:1872–1874.

Ridenour, G.M., and E.M. Armbruster. 1949. Bactericidal effects of chlorine dioxide. J. Am. Water Works Assoc. 41:537–550.

Ridenour, G.M., and R.S. Ingols. 1946. Inactivation of poliomyelitis virus by "free" chlorine. Am. J. Public Health 36:639–644.

Ridenour, G.M., and R.S. Ingols. 1947. Bactericidal properties of chlorine dioxide. J. Am. Water Works Assoc. 39:561–567.

Ridenour, G.M., R.S. Ingols, and E.H. Armbruster. 1949. Sporicidal properties of chlorine dioxide. Water and Sewage Works 96:279–283.

Rosenblatt, D.H. 1978. Chlorine dioxide: chemical and physical properties. Pp. 332–343 in R.G. Rice and J.A. Cotruvo, eds. Ozone/Chlorine Dioxide Products of Organic Materials. Proceedings of a Conference held in Cincinnati, Ohio, November 17–19, 1976. Sponsored by the International Ozone Institute, Inc., and the U.S. Environmental Protection Agency. Ozone Press International, Cleveland, Ohio. 487 pp.

Scarpino, P.V., S.D. Cronier, M.L. Zink, F.A.O. Brigano, and J.C. Hoff. 1977. Effect of particulates on disinfection of enterovirus and coliform bacteria in water by chlorine dioxide. Water Quality Technology Conference—Water Quality in the Distribution System. Kansas City, Mo. 19 pp.

Schilling, K. 1956. Chlordioxyd in der Wasseraufbereitung. Wasser 23:95–101.

Standard Methods for the Examination of Water and Wastewater, 14th ed. 1976. American Public Health Association, Washington, D.C. 1193 pp.

Stevens, A.A., D.R. Seeger, and C.J. Slocum. 1978. Products of chlorine dioxide treatment of organic materials in water. Pp. 383–395 in R.G. Rice and J.A. Cotruvo, eds. Ozone/Chlorine Dioxide Products of Organic Materials. Proceedings of a Conference held in Cincinnati, Ohio, November 17–19, 1976. Sponsored by the International Ozone Institute, Inc., and the U.S. Environmental Protection Agency. Ozone Press International, Cleveland, Ohio. 487 pp.

Stevenson, R.G., Jr., L.L. Dailey, and B.J. Ratigan. 1978. The continuous analysis of chlorine dioxide in process solutions. Pp. 23–24 in Preprints of Papers presented at the 175th National Meeting of the Environmental Chemistry Division, American Chemical Society, Anaheim, Calif., March 12–17, 1978.

Sussman, S. 1978. Use of chlorine dioxide in water and wastewater treatment. Pp. 344–355 in R.G. Rice and J.A. Cotruvo, eds. Ozone/Chlorine Dioxide Oxidation Products of Organic Materials. Proceedings of a Conference held in Cincinnati, Ohio, November 17-19, 1976. Sponsored by the International Ozone Institute, Inc., and the U.S. Environmental Protection Agency. Ozone Press International, Cleveland, Ohio. 487 pp.

Symons, J.M., J.K. Carswell, R.M. Clark, P. Dorsey, E.E. Geldreich, W.P. Heffernam, J.C. Hoff, O.T. Love, L.J. McCabe, and A.A. Stevens. 1977. Ozone, Chlorine Dioxide and Chloramines as Alternatives to Chlorine for Disinfection of Drinking Water: State of the Art. Water Supply Research Division, U.S. Environmental Protection Agency, Cincinnati, Ohio. 84 pp.

Synan, J.F., J.D. MacMahon, and G.P. Vincent. 1945. Chlorine dioxide in potable water treatment. Water Eng. 48:285–286.

Trakhtman, N.N. 1946. Chlorine dioxide in water disinfection. Gig. Sanit. 11(10):10–13.

U.S. Environmental Protection Agency. 1978. Interim primary drinking water regulations: control of organic chemical contaminants in drinking water. Fed. Reg. 43(28):5756–5780.

Warriner, T.R. 1967. Inaktwering av Poliovirus med Klordioxid. Institute for Vattenforsorgning och Avlopp, Publikation A67:284–290.

Watt, C., and H. Burgess. 1854. Improvement in the manufacture of paper from wood. U.S. Patent No. 11,343.

Iodine

Allen, T.L., and R.M. Keefer. 1955. The formation of hypoiodous acid and hydrated iodine cation by the hydrolysis of iodine. J. Am. Chem. Soc. 77:2957–2960.

Bell, R.P., and E. Gelles. 1951. The halogen cations in aqueous solution. J. Chem. Soc. Pt. III 2734–2740.

Berg, G., S.L. Chang, and E.K. Harris. 1964. Devitalization of microorganisms by iodine. I. Dynamics of the devitalization of enteroviruses by elemental iodine. Virology 22:469–481.

Black, A.P., J.B. Lackey, and E.W. Lackey. 1959. Effectiveness of iodine for the disinfection of swimming pool water. Am. J. Public Health 49:1060–1068.

Black, A.P., R.N. Kinman, W.C. Thomas, Jr., G. Freund, and E.D. Bird. 1965. Use of iodine for disinfection. J. Am. Water Works Assoc. 57:1401–1421.

Black, A.P., W.C. Thomas, Jr., R.N. Kinman, W.P. Bonner, M.A. Keirn, J.J. Smith, Jr., and A.A. Jabero. 1968. Iodine for the disinfection of water. J. Am. Water Works Assoc. 60:69–83.

Brammer, K.W. 1963. Chemical modification of viral ribonucleic acid. II. Bromination and iodination. Biochim. Biophys. Acta 72:217–229.

Chambers, C.W., P.W. Kabler, G. Malaney, and A. Bryant. 1952. Iodine as a bactericide. Soap Sanit. Chem. 28(10):149–151, 153, 163, 165.

Chang, S.L. 1958. The use of active iodine as a water disinfectant. J. Am. Pharm. Assoc. 47:417–423.

Chang, S.L., and J.C. Morris. 1953. Elemental iodine as a disinfectant for drinking water. Ind. Eng. Chem. 45:1009–1012.

Chang, S.L., and M. Baxter. 1955. Studies on the destruction of cysts of *Endamoeba histolytica*. I. Establishment of the order of reaction in destruction of cysts of *E. histolytica* by elemental iodine and silver nitrate. Am. J. Hyg. 61:121–132.

Chang, S.L., M. Baxter, and L. Eisner. 1955. Studies on the destruction of *Endamoeba histolytica*. II. Dynamics of destruction of cysts of *E. histolytica* in water by tri-iodine ion. Am. J. Hyg. 61:133–141.

Cramer, W.N., K. Kawata, and C.W. Kruse. 1976. Chlorination and iodination of poliovirus and f_2. J. Water Pollut. Control Fed. 48:61–76.

Fraenkel-Conrat, H. 1955. The reaction of tobacco mosaic virus with iodine. J. Biol. Chem. 217:373–381.

Gershenfeld, L. 1977. Iodine. Pp. 196-218 in S.S. Block, ed. Disinfection, Sterilization, and Preservation, 2nd ed. Lea & Febiger, Philadelphia, Pa.

Hsu, Y-C. 1964. Resistance of infectious RNA and transforming DNA to iodine which inactivates f_2 phage and cells. Nature 203:152–153.

Hsu, Y-C., S. Normura, and C.W. Kruse. 1965. Some bactericidal and viricidal properties of iodine not affecting infectious RNA and DNA. Am. J. Epidemiol. 82:317–328.

Hughes, W.L. 1957. The chemistry of iodination. Ann. N.Y. Acad. Sci. 70:3–18.

Kruse, C.W. 1969. Mode of action of halogens on bacteria and viruses and protozoa in water systems. Pp. 1–89 in Final report to the Commission on Environmental Hygiene of the Armed Forces Epidemiological Board, U.S. Army Med. Res. Dev. Command Contract No. DA-49-193-MD-2314.

Li, C.H. 1942. Kinetics and mechanism of 2,6-di-iodotryosine formation. J. Am. Chem. Soc. 64:1147–1152.

Li, C.H. 1944. Kinetics of reactions between iodine and histidine. J. Am. Chem. Soc. 66:225–227.

Longley, K.E. 1964. Some aspects of iodination of bacteriophage f_2. MSE essay. The Johns Hopkins University, Baltimore, Md.

Marks, H.C., and F.B. Strandskov. 1950. Halogens and their mode of action. Ann. N.Y. Acad. Sci. 53:163–171.

O'Connor, J.T., and S.K. Kapoor. 1970. Small quantity field disinfection. J. Am. Water Works Assoc. 62(2):80–84.

Standard Methods for the Examination of Water and Wastewater, 14th ed. 1976. American Public Health Association, Washington, D.C. 1193 pp.

Stringer, R.P. 1970. Amoebic cysticidal properties of halogens in water. Sc.D. thesis. Johns Hopkins University, Baltimore, Md.

Stringer, R., and C.W. Krusé. 1971. Amoebic cysticidal properties of halogens in water. J. Sanit. Eng. Div. Am. Soc. Civ. Eng. 97:801–811.

Stringer, R.P., W.N. Cramer, and C.W. Krusé. 1975. Comparison of bromine, chlorine and iodine as disinfectants for amoebic cysts. Pp. 193–209 in J.D. Johnson, ed. Disinfection: Water and Wastewater. Ann Arbor Science Publishers, Inc., Ann Arbor, Mich. 425 pp.

Wallis, C., A.M. Behbehani, L.H. Lee, and M. Bianchi. 1963. The ineffectiveness of organic iodine (Wescodyne) as a viral disinfectant. Am. J. Hyg. 78:325–329.

Wyss, O., and F.B. Strandskov. 1945. The germicidal action of iodine. Arch. Biochem. 6:261–268.

Bromine

Farkas, L., and M. Lewin. 1950. The dissociation constant of hypobromous acid. J. Am. Chem. Soc. 72:5766–5767.

Farkas-Hinsley, H. 1966. Disinfection. Pp. 554–562 in Z.E. Jolles, ed. Bromine and Its Compounds. Academic Press, New York. 940 pp.

Floyd, R., J.D. Johnson, and D.G. Sharp. 1976. Inactivation by bromine of single poliovirus particles in water. Appl. Environ. Microbiol. 31:298–303.

Floyd, R., D.G. Sharp, and J.D. Johnson. 1978. Inactivation of single poliovirus particles in water by hypobromite ion, molecular bromine, dibromamine, and tribromamine. Environ. Sci. Tech. 12:1031–1035.

Galal-Gorchev, H., and J.C. Morris. 1965. Formation and stability of bromamide, bromimide, and nitrogen tribromide in aqueous solution. Inorg. Chem. 4:899–905.

Henderson, C.T. 1935. Process of antisepticizing water. U.S. Patent No. 1995639.

Inman, G.W., Jr., T.F. LaPointe, and J.D. Johnson. 1976. Kinetics of nitrogen tribromide decomposition in aqueous solution. Inorg. Chem. 15:3037–3042.

Johannesson, J.K. 1958. Anomalous bactericidal action of bromamine. Nature 181:1799–1800.

Johnson, J.D., and R. Overby. 1971. Bromine and bromamine disinfection chemistry. J. Sanit. Eng. Div. Am. Soc. Civ. Eng. 97:617–628.

Kanyaev, N.P., and E.A. Shilov. 1940. Constants of some equilibrium reactions of hypobromous acid. Tr. Ivanov. Khim. Tekhnol. Inst. (USSR) 3:69–73.

Kolthoff, I.M., and R. Belcher. 1957. Volumetric Analysis. Interscience Pub., New York. 714 pp.

Krusé, C.W., Y. Hsu, A.C. Griffiths, and R. Stringer. 1970. Halogen action on bacteria, viruses, and protozoa. Pp. 113–136 in Proceedings of the National Specialty Conference on Disinfection. American Society of Civil Engineers, New York.

Liebhafsky, H.A. 1934. The equilibrium constant of the bromine hydrolysis and its variation with temperature. J. Am. Chem. Soc. 56:1500–1505.

Marks, H.C., and F.B. Strandskov. 1950. Halogens and their mode of action. Ann. N.Y. Acad. Sci. 53:163–171.

Mills, J.F. 1969. The control of microorganisms with polyhalide resins. U.S. Patent No. 3462363.

Mills, J.F. 1975. Interhalogens and halogen mixtures as disinfectants. Pp. 113–143 in J.D. Johnson, ed. Disinfection: Water and Wastewater. Ann Arbor Science Publishers, Inc., Ann Arbor, Mich. 425 pp.

Morris, J.C. 1975. Aspects of the quantitative assessment of germicidal efficiency. Pp. 1–10 in J.D. Johnson, ed. Disinfection: Water and Wastewater. Ann Arbor Science Publishers, Inc., Ann Arbor, Mich. 425 pp.

Olivieri, V.P., C.W. Krusé, Y.C. Hsu, A.C. Griffiths, and K. Kawata. 1975. The comparative mode of action of chlorine, bromine, and iodine on f_2 bacterial virus. Pp. 145–162 in J.D. Johnson, ed. Disinfection: Water and Wastewater. Ann Arbor Science Publishers, Inc., Ann Arbor, Mich. 425 pp.

Sharp, D.G., R. Floyd, and J.D. Johnson. 1975. Nature of the surviving plaque forming unit of reovirus in water containing bromine. Appl. Microbiol. 29:94–101.

Sharp, D.G., R. Floyd, and J.D. Johnson. 1976. Initial fast reaction of bromine on reovirus in turbulent flowing water. Appl. Environ. Microbiol. 31:173–181.

Standard Methods for the Examination of Water and Wastewater, 14th ed. 1976. American Public Health Association, Washington, D.C. 1193 pp.

Stringer, R.P., W.N. Cramer, and C.W. Krusé. 1975. Comparison of bromine, chlorine, and iodine as disinfectants for amoebic cysts. Pp. 193–209 in J.D. Johnson, ed. Disinfection: Water and Wastewater. Ann Arbor Science Publishers, Inc., Ann Arbor, Mich. 425 pp.

Tanner, F.W., and G. Pitner. 1939. Germicidal action of bromine. Proc. Soc. Exp. Biol. Med. 40:143–145.

Taylor, D.G., and J.D. Johnson. 1974. Kinetics of viral inactivation by bromine. Pp. 369–408 in A.J. Rubin, ed. Chemistry of Water Supply, Treatment, and Distribution. Ann Arbor Science Publishers, Inc., Ann Arbor, Mich.

Wyss, O., and J.R. Stockton. 1947. The germicidal action of bromine. Arch. Biochem. 12:267–271.

Ferrate

Audette, R.J., R.J. Quail, and P.J. Smith. 1971. Ferrate (VI) ion, a novel oxidizing agent. Tetrahedron Lett. 3:279–282.

Becarud, N. 1966. Analytical Study of Ferrates. Comm. Energie at France Rapt. No. 2895. 52 pp.

Fremy, E.G. 1841. Studies of the action of alkaline peroxides on metal oxides. (In French) C.R. Acad. Sci. Ser. A 12:23–24.

Gilbert, M.D., T.D. Waite, and C. Hare. 1976. An investigation of the applicability of ferrate ion for disinfection. J. Am. Water Works Assoc. 68:495–497.

Murmann, R.K. 1974. The preparation and oxidative properties of ferrate (FeO_4^{2-}). Studies directed towards its use as a water purifying agent. NTIS publication PB Rept. 238–057. National Technical Information Service, Springfield, Va.

Schreyer, J.M., and L.T. Ockerman. 1951. Stability of the ferrate (VI) ion in aqueous solution. Anal. Chem. 23:1312–1314.

Schreyer, J.M., G.W. Thompson, and L.T. Ockerman. 1950. Ferrate oxidimetry. Oxidation of arsenite with potassium ferrate (VI). Anal. Chem. 22:691–692.

Strong, A.W. 1973. An Exploratory Work on the Oxidation of Ammonia by Potassium Ferrate (VI). M.S thesis. Department of Chemical Engineering [Rept. OWRR-A-031-OHIO(2)] Ohio State University, Columbus. NTIS publication PB-231 873. National Technical Information Service, Springfield, Va.

Wagner, W.F., J.R. Gump, and E.N. Hart. 1952. Factors affecting the stability of aqueous potassium ferrate (VI) solutions. Anal. Chem. 24:1497–1498.

Waite, T.D. 1978a. Management of Wastewater Residuals with Iron (VI) Ferrate. First Annual Report Grant # ENV 76-83897. National Science Foundation: RANN, Washington, D.C. 207 pp.

Waite, T.D. 1978b. Inactivation of *Salmonella* sp., *Shigella* sp., *Streptococcus* sp., and f2 virus by Iron (VI) Ferrate. Paper 33-4 presented at the Annual Meeting of the American Water Works Association, Atlantic City, N.J. 1978 Annual Conference Proceedings. American Water Works Association, Denver, Colo.

Wood, R.H. 1958. The heat, free energy and entropy of the ferrate (VI) ion. J. Am. Chem. Soc. 80:2038–2041.

Zhdanov, Y.A., and O.A. Pustovarova. 1967. Oxidation of alcohols and aldehydes by potassium ferrate. Zh. Onsch. Khim. 37(12):2780.

High pH Conditions

Berg, G., and D. Berman. 1967. Final Report of Progress on Quarterly Contract AMXREC 66-51 and First Quarterly Report on Quartermaster Contract AMXRED 67-54 on Effectiveness of Military Phenolic Dry-Type Disinfectant (MIL-D-51061) Against Viruses. Federal Water Pollution Control Administration, Cincinnati, Ohio.

Boeye, A., and A. Van Elsen. 1967. Alkaline disruption of poliovirus: kinetics and purification of RNA-free particles. Virology 33:335–343.

Donovan, T.K. 1972. Virus inactivation associated with lime precipitation of phosphate from sewage. D.Sc. thesis. Johns Hopkins University, Baltimore, Md.

Maizel, J.V., Jr., B.A. Phillips, and D.F. Summers. 1967. Composition of artificially produced and naturally occurring empty capsids of poliovirus type·1. Virology 32:692–699.

Riehl, M.L., H.H. Weiser, and B.T. Rheins. 1952. Effect of lime-treated water upon survival of bacteria. J. Am. Water Works Assoc. 44:466–470.

Sproul, O.J. 1975. Investigation to Increase the Viricidal Capacity of Disinfectant, Germicidal and Fungicidal Phenolic, Dry Type. Technical Report TR 76-90 FSL, Department of Civil Engineering, University of Maine, Orono. 46 pp.

Sproul, O.J., R.T. Thorup, D.F. Wentworth, and J.S. Atwell. 1970. Salt and virus inactivation by chlorine and high pH. Pp. 385–396 in Proceedings of the National Specialty Conference of Disinfection. American Society of Civil Engineers, New York.

Standard Methods for the Examination of Water and Wastewater, 11th ed., p. 485. 1960. American Public Health Association, Inc., New York.

Van Elsen, A., and A. Boeye. 1966. Disruption of type 1 poliovirus under alkaline conditions: role of pH, temperature and sodium dodecyl sulfate (SDS). Virology 28:481–483.

Wattie, E., and C.W. Chambers. 1943. Relative resistance of coliform organisms and certain enteric pathogens to excess-lime treatment. J. Am. Water Works Assoc. 35:709–720.

Wentworth, D.F., R.T. Thorup, and O.J. Sproul. 1968. Poliovirus inactivation in water softening precipitation processes. J. Am. Water Works Assoc. 60:939–946.

Hydrogen Peroxide

Chadwick, A.F., and G.L.K. Hoh. 1966. Hydrogen peroxide. Pp. 319–417 in Kirk-Othmer Encyclopedia of Chemical Technology, Vol. 11, 2nd ed. Wiley Interscience Publishers, New York.

Gasset, A.R., R.M. Ramer, and D. Katzin. 1975. Hydrogen peroxide sterilization of hydrophilic contact lenses. Arch. Ophthamol. 93:412–415.

Lund, E. 1963. Significance of oxidation in chemical inactivation of poliovirus. Arch. Gesamte Virusforsch. 12:648–660.

Mentel, R., and J. Schmidt. 1973. Investigations on rhinovirus inactivation by hydrogen peroxide. Acta Virol. 17:351–354.

Schumb, W.C., C.N. Satterfield, and R.L. Wentworth. 1955. Stabilization. Pp. 515–547 in Hydrogen Peroxide. Reinhold Publishing Corporation, New York.

Sezgin, M., D. Jenkins, and D.S. Parker. 1978. A unified theory of filamentous activated sludge bulking. J. Water Pollut. Control Fed. 50:362–381.

Snell, F.D., and C.T. Snell. 1949. Colorimetric Methods of Analysis: Including some Turbidimetric and Nephelometric Methods, 3rd ed. D. Van Nostrand Company, New York. 5 Vols.

Spaulding, E.H., K.R. Cundy, and F.J. Turner. 1977. Chemical disinfection of medical and surgical materials. Pp. 654–684 in S.S. Block, ed. Disinfection, Sterilization, and Preservation, 2nd ed. Lea & Febiger, Philadelphia, Pa.

Taki, M., and R. Hashimoto. 1977. Sterilization of biologically treated water. I. Sterilizing effects of chlorine and hydrogen peroxide. Mizu Shori Gijutsu (Jap.) 18(2):149–156.

Toledo, R.T. 1975. Chemical sterilants for aseptic packaging. Food Technol. 29:102, 104, 105, 108, 110, 112.

Toledo, R.T., F.E. Escher, and J.C. Ayres. 1973. Sporicidal properties of hydrogen peroxide against food spoilage organisms. Appl. Microbiol. 26:592–597.

Wardle, M.D., and G.M. Renninger. 1975. Bactericidal effect of hydrogen peroxide on spacecraft isolates. Appl. Microbiol. 30:710–711.

Yoshpe-Purer, Y., and E. Eylan. 1968. Disinfection of water by hydrogen peroxide. Health Lab. Sci. 5:233–238.

Ionizing Radiation

Ballantine, D.S., L.A. Miller, D.F. Bishop, and F.A. Rohrman. 1969. The practicality of using atomic radiation for wastewater treatment. J. Water Pollut. Control. Fed. 41:445–458.

Brannan, J.P., D.M. Garst, and S. Langley. 1975. Inactivation of Ascaris lumbricoides eggs by heat, radiation, and thermoradiation. Sandia Laboratories Report Sand. 75–0163. Albuquerque, N.Mex. 26 pp.

Compton, D.M.J., W.L. Whittemore, and S.J. Black. 1970. An evaluation of the applicability of ionizing radiation to the treatment of municipal waste waters and sewage sludge. Trans. Am. Nucl. Soc. 13:71–72.

Dunn, C.G. 1953. Treatment of water and sewage by ionizing radiations. Sewage Ind. Wastes 25:1277–1281.

Eliassen, R., and J.G. Trump. 1973. High Energy Electron Treatment of Wastewater and Sludge. Paper presented at 45th Annual Meeting of the California Water Pollution Control Association, San Diego.

Lea, D.E. 1955. Actions of Radiations on Living Cells, 2nd ed. Cambridge University Press, London.

Lowe, H.N., Jr., W.J. Lacy, B.F. Surkiewicz, and R.F. Jaeger. 1956. Destruction of microorganisms in water, sewage, and sewage sludge by ionizing radiations. J. Am. Water Works Assoc. 48:1363–1372.

Massachusetts Institute of Technology. 1977. High Energy Electron Radiation of Wastewater Liquid Residuals. Report to U.S. National Science Foundation. NSF Grant ENV 74 13016, Dec. 31, 1977. National Science Foundation, Washington, D.C.

Ridenour, G.M., and E.H. Armbruster. 1956. Effect of high-level gamma radiation on disinfection of water and sewage. J. Am. Water Works Assoc. 48:671–676.

Silverman, G.F., and A.J. Sinskey. 1977. Sterilization by ionizing radiation. Pp. 542–567 in S.S. Block, ed. Disinfection, Sterilization, and Preservation, 2nd ed. Lea & Febiger, Philadelphia, Pa.

Wright, K.A., and J.G. Trump. 1956. High energy electrons for the irradiation of blood derivatives. Pp. 230–239 in Proc. 6th Congress of the International Society of Blood Transfusion. Supplement to Acta Haematologica, 1956.

Potassium Permanganate

American Water Works Association. 1971. Water Quality and Treatment: A Handbook of Public Water Supplies, 3rd ed. McGraw-Hill Book Company, New York. 654 pp.

Cleasby, J.L., E.R. Baumann, and C.D. Black. 1964. Effectiveness of potassium permanganate for disinfection. J. Am. Water Works Assoc. 56:466–474.

Derbyshire, J.B., and S. Arkell. 1971. Activity of some chemical disinfectants against Talfan virus and porcine adenovirus type 2. Br. Vet. J. 127(3):137–142.

Eskarous, J.K., and H.M. Habib. 1972. Effect of potassium permanganate and toluquinone on mosaic symptoms and necrosis caused by tomato streak virus on tobacco. Adv. Front. Plant Sci. 29:125–169.

Fitzgerald, G.P. 1964. Laboratory evaluation of potassium permanganate as an algicide for water reservoirs. Southwest Water Works J. 45(10):16–17.

Heuston, K.H. 1972. Tablets for the sterilization of water. Ger. Offen. 2:303, 364.

Hughes, C.G., and D.R.L. Steindl. 1955. Ratoon stunting disease of sugar cane. Bur. Sugar Exp. Stn., Brisbane, Tech. Commun. No. 2:1–54.

Kemp, H.T., R.G. Fuller, and R.S. Davidson. 1966. Potassium permanganate as an algicide. J. Am. Water Works Assoc. 58:255–263.

Lund, E. 1963. Oxidative inactivation of poliovirus at different temperatures. Arch. Ges. Virusforsch. 13:375–386.

Lund, E. 1966. Oxidative inactivation of adenovirus. Arch. Ges. Virusforsch. 19:32–37.

Peretts, L.G., O.V. Bychkovskaia, M.A. Bazhedomova, N.S. Babina, and N.S. Semenova. 1960. Effect of potassium permanganate on poliomyelitus virus. Probl. Virol. 5:441–447.

Schultz, E.W., and F. Robinson. 1942. The in vitro resistance of poliomyelitus virus to chemical agents. J. Infect. Dis. 70:193–200.

Seidel, K. 1973. Purification of swimming pool water. Ger. Offen. 2:141, 620.

Shull, K.E. 1962. Operating experiences at Philadelphia suburban treatment plants. J. Am. Water Works Assoc. 54:1232–1240.

Spicher, R.G., and R.T. Skrinde. 1963. Potassium permanganate oxidation of organic contaminants in water supplies. J. Am. Water Works Assoc. 55:1174–1194.

Standard Methods for the Examination of Water and Wastewater, 14th ed. 1976. American Public Health Association, Washington, D.C. 1193 pp.

Wagner, R.R. 1951. Studies on the inactivation of influenza virus. Comparison of the effects of p-benzoquinone and various inorganic oxidizing agents. Yale J. Biol. Med. 23:288–298.

Welch, W.A. 1963. Potassium permanganate in water treatment. J. Am. Water Works Assoc. 55:735–741.

Silver

Chambers, C.W., and C.M. Proctor. 1960. The Bacteriological and Chemical Behavior of Silver in Low Concentrations. Robert A. Taft Sanitary Engineering Center, Tech. Rep. W60-4, U.S. Department of Health, Education, and Welfare. 18 pp.

Chang, S.L., and M. Baxter. 1955. Studies on destruction of cysts of Entamoeba histolytica. I. Establishment of the order of reaction in destruction of cysts of E. histolytica by elemental iodine and silver nitrate. Am. J. Hyg. 61:121–132.

Chang, S.L. 1970. Modern concept of disinfection. Pp. 635–681 in Proceedings of the National Specialty Conference on Disinfection. American Society of Civil Engineers, New York.

Davies, R.L. 1976. Improved circulation systems use silver to maintain pool water. Swimming Pool Weekly and Swimming Pool Age, Data and Reference Annual 50.

Fair, G.M. 1948. Water disinfection and allied subjects. Pp. 520–531 in E.C. Andrus, D.W. Bronk, G.A. Garden, Jr., C.S. Keefer, J.S. Lockwood, J.T. Wearn, and M.C. Winternitz, eds. Advances in Military Medicine, Vol. 2. Little, Brown and Company, Boston, Mass.

Grier, N. 1977. Silver and its compounds. Pp. 395–407 in S.S. Block, ed. Disinfection, Sterilization, and Preservation, 2nd ed. Lea & Febiger, Philadelphia, Pa.

Harrison, C.J. 1947. Purification of tea-estate water supplies. Indian Tea Association, Tockai Experimental Station, Memo 18. 10 pp.

Just, J., and A. Szniolis. 1936. Germicidal properties of silver in water. J. Am. Water Works Assoc. 28:492–506.

Lund, E. 1963. Significance of oxidation in chemical inactivation of poliovirus. Arch. Ges. Virusforsch. 12:648–660.

Newton, W.L., and M.F. Jones. 1949. Effectiveness of silver ions against cysts of Entamoeba histolytica. J. Am. Water Works Assoc. 41:1027–1034.

Rattonetti, A. 1974. Determination of soluble cadmium, lead, silver, and indium in rainwater and stream water with the use of flameless atomic absorption. Anal. Chem. 46:739–742.

Renn, C.E., and W.E. Chesney. 1953–1956. Reports to Salem-Brosius, Inc., on Research on Hyla System of Water Disinfection.

Romans, I.B. 1954. Oligodynamic metals. Pp. 388–428 in G.F. Reddish, ed. Antiseptics, Disinfectants, Germicides, and Chemical and Physical Sterilization. Lea & Febiger, Philadelphia, Pa.

Seidel, K. 1973. Purification of swimming pool water. Ger. Offen. 2:141, 620.

Standard Methods for the Examination of Water and Wastewater, 14th ed. 1976. American Public Health Association, Washington, D.C. 1193 pp.

U.S. Environmental Protection Agency. 1974. Methods for Chemical Analysis of Water and Wastes. EPA-625/6-74-003. U.S. Environmental Protection Agency, Washington, D.C.

U.S. Environmental Protection Agency. 1975. Interim primary drinking water regulations. Fed. Reg. 40(51):11989–11998.

Woodward, R.L. 1963. Review of the bactericidal effectiveness of silver. J. Am. Water Works Assoc. 55:881–886.

Wuhrmann, K., and F. Zobrist. 1958. Bactericidal effect of silver in water. Schweiz. Z. Hydrol. 20:218–254.

Yasinskii, A.V., and V.F. Kuznetsova. 1973. Disinfection of water containing vibrios by silver ions. Aktual. Vopr. Sanit. Mikrobiol. 112–113.

Zimmermann, W. 1952. Oligodynamic silver action. I. The action mechanism Z. Hyз. Infektionskr. 135:403–413.

Ultraviolet Light

Anonymous. 1960. Germicidal Lamps and Applications. General Electric Bulletin LS-179. 15 pp.

Calvert, J.G., and J.N. Pitts, Jr. 1966. Photochemistry. John Wiley, New York. 890 pp.

Childs, C.B. 1962. Low-pressure mercury arc for ultraviolet calibration. Appl. Opt. 1:711–716.

Cortelyou, J.R., M.A. McWhinnie, M.S. Riddiford, and J.E. Semrad. 1954. Effects of ultraviolet irradiation on large populations of certain water-borne bacteria in motion. I. The development of adequate agitation to provide an effective exposure period. Appl. Microbiol. 2:227–235.

Deering, R.A., and R.B. Setlow. 1963. Effects of ultraviolet light on thymidine dinucleotide and polynucleotide. Biochim. Biophys. Acta 68:526–534.

Gates, F.L. 1929. A study of the bactericidal action of ultraviolet light. II. The effect of various environmental factors and conditions. J. Gen. Physiol. 13:249–260.

Harm, W. 1968. Effects of dose fractionation on ultraviolet survival of *Escherichia coli*. Photochem. Photobiol. 7:73–86.

Hoather, R.C. 1955. The penetration of ultra-violet radiation and its effects in waters. J. Inst. Water Eng. 9:191–207.

Huff, C.B., H.F. Smith, W.D. Boring, and N.A. Clarke. 1965. Study of ultraviolet disinfection of water and factors in treatment efficiency. Public Health Rep. 80:695–705.

Jagger, J. 1960. Photoreactivation. Radiat. Res. Suppl. 2:75–90.

Kawabata, T., and T. Harada. 1959. J. Illumination Society 36:89.

Kelner, A. 1949. Photoreactivation of ultraviolet-irradiated *Escherichia coli*, with special reference to the dose-reduction principle and to ultraviolet-induced mutation. J. Bacteriol. 58:511–522.

Luckiesh, M., and A.H. Taylor. 1946. Transmittance and reflectance of germicidal (2537) energy. J. Opt. Soc. Am. 36:227–234.

Luckiesh, M., A.H. Taylor, and G.P. Kerr. 1944. Germicidal energy. Gen. Electr. Rev. 47(9):7–9.

Luckiesh, M., and L.L. Holladay. 1944. Disinfecting water by means of germicidal lamps. Gen. Electr. Rev. 47(4):45–50.

Morris, E.J. 1972. The practical use of ultraviolet radiation for disinfection purposes. Med. Lab. Technol. 29:41–47.

Oliver, B.G., and E.G. Cosgrove. 1975. The disinfection of sewage treatment plant effluents using ultraviolet light. Can. J. Chem. Eng. 53:170–174.

Powers, E.L., M. Cross, and C.J. Varga. 1974. A dose-rate effect in the ultraviolet inactivation of bacterial spores. Photochem. Photobiol. 19:273–276.

Reddish, G.G., ed. 1957. Antiseptics, Disinfectants, Fungicides and Chemical and Physical Sterilization, 2nd ed. Lea & Febiger, Philadelphia, Pa. 975 pp.

Roeber, J.A., and F.M. Hoot. 1975. Ultraviolet Disinfection of Activated Sludge Effluent Discharging to Shellfish Waters. EPA 600/2-75/060 Municipal Environmental Research Laboratory Office of Research and Development, U.S. Environmental Protection Agency, Cincinnati, Ohio. 85 pp.

Severin, B.F. 1978. Disinfection of Municipal Wastewater Effluents With Ultraviolet Light. Paper presented to Annual Meeting, Water Pollution Control Federation, Anaheim, Calif.

Venosa, A.D., H.W. Wolf, and A.C. Petrasek. 1978. Ultraviolet disinfection of municipal effluents. Pp. 675–684 in R. Jolley, H. Gorchev, and D. H. Hamilton, Jr., eds. Water Chlorination: Environmental Impact and Health Effects, Vol. 2. Ann Arbor Science Publishers, Ann Arbor, Mich. 909 pp.

Witkin, E.M. 1976. Ultraviolet mutagenesis and inducible DNA repair in *Escherichia coli.* Bacteriol. Rev. 40:869–907.

Wood, M.D. 1974. Apparatus method for purifying fluids. U.S. Patent No. 3,837,800. September 24. (Chem. Abs. 85:4749v.)

ERRATUM

On page iv, under the "Subcommittee on Chemistry of Disinfectants and Products," please insert

GEORGE R. HELZ, University of Maryland, College Park.

Drinking Water and Health
Volume 2
ISBN 0-309-02931-7

III

The Chemistry of Disinfectants in Water: Reactions and Products

A major objective of this review of disinfectant chemistry is the identification of likely by-products that might be formed through the use of specific disinfectants. The review is part of a comprehensive study of the possible health effects of contaminants in drinking water. The prediction of possible products, which is attempted herein, is intended to be a guide to those contaminants that might require removal or toxicological evaluation; however, neither of these two aspects of the overall study is discussed in this chapter.

While there is some current research on using combinations of disinfectants sequentially, the chemical consequences and benefits of this strategy are not yet clear. This subject has been omitted from the report. Similarly the subcommittee did not review the chemical side benefits of disinfection, such as removal of cyanides, phenols, and, possibly, many other compounds, although these side benefits may be of considerable importance.

Although there is now a rapidly growing body of scientific literature on chlorine by-products in drinking waters, comparable information for other disinfectants is very scarce. The subcommittee believed that reviewing chlorine by-products in detail, while saying little about other disinfectants, could suggest (probably erroneously) that these alternate disinfectants are free of the difficulties that are encountered with chlorine. In an attempt to circumvent this problem, the subcommittee found it necessary to broaden its information base by reviewing not only data on potable water, but also studies on nonpotable water, such as treated sewage effluents, and on synthetic model solutions, the data from which might be applicable to potable waters. These studies on nonpotable water shed light on the chemistry of disinfectants in drinking waters, although it is obvious that many compounds produced in treated sewage or in artificial laboratory experiments may never be found in drinking waters. To avoid confusion, a clear distinction has been drawn throughout this chapter between information acquired from actual drinking waters and information derived from other sources.

A great deal of research on the chemistry of disinfectants is now in progress. An attempt was made to ensure that this chapter was current by contacting many scientists who are working in this field in the United States and abroad. However, in an active field such as this, any review can become rapidly outdated.

The chapter begins with a preliminary discussion of the character of the natural organic substances from which by-products of organic disinfectants are thought to originate. Subsequent sections describe the chemistry of chlorine, chloramines, halogens (Br_2 and I_2), chlorine dioxide, and, finally, ozone.

PRECURSOR COMPOUNDS AND THE HALOFORM REACTION

Since 1975, many investigators have assumed that the ubiquitous appearance of chloroform ($CHCl_3$) and other THM's (trihalomethanes, or haloforms) in chlorinated water can be explained by the mechanisms involved in the "haloform reaction" and that the principal precursors of THM's that are found in natural waters are humic substances. As discussed subsequently in the section pertaining to chlorine chemistry, the haloform reaction will proceed only if specific functional groups are present in the available pool of organic compounds. It is likely that the haloform reaction does occur when natural waters are chlorinated and that humic substances provide the necessary functional groups, but it is not certain that either of these postulates is true. For that reason, both topics—the haloform reaction and humic substances—merit further discussion.

The Haloform Reaction

The terms "trihalomethanes" and "haloforms" are synonymous, but the term "haloform reaction" is often misused in discussions of THM formation in natural waters. In recent literature, it has been used to mean any reaction between aqueous solutions of organic compounds and hypohalous acids that results in THM formation, but it actually has a classic chemical definition that is more restrictive. In the future, the expanded meaning may be preferred, but at present the term "haloform reaction" is inappropriate from a strict chemical interpretation, unless one is sure that the THM's are formed by reactions between hypohalous acids and compounds containing acetyl groups or substituents that can be converted to acetyl groups.

The classic haloform reaction, which is actually a series of well-defined reactions, has been known since the 1800's (Fuson and Bull, 1934). The earliest studies were conducted with nonaqueous solvents, high concentrations of organic compounds, and chlorine gas, but research since 1974 has focused more on defining the reactions that yield THM's under conditions that are closer to those more commonly encountered during the treatment of drinking water supplies.

Compounds, or classes of compounds, with the general formula CH_3CHOHR or CH_3COR, which includes ethanol, acetaldehyde, methyl ketones, and secondary alcohols, can participate in the haloform reaction. So may olefinic substances with the general structure $CH_3CH = CR_1R_2$, which will be oxidized by hypochlorous acid (HOCl) first to secondary alcohols and then to methyl ketones. The site of attack by chlorine is the carbon adjacent to the one bearing oxygen, and this attack, wherein the hydrogen atoms are successively replaced by chlorine, is preceded by a dissociation of one hydrogen (as H^+) to produce a carbanion ($-CH_2^-$) that can react with Cl(I), from hypochlorous acid. Chlorine substitution continues until all hydrogen atoms on the same carbon have been replaced. The final step involves a hydrolytic cleavage of the trihalogenated carbon (the trichlorinated carbon, in this example) to form the THM, which in this example would be chloroform (Morris, 1975).

While it is well known that compounds containing acetyl groups are reactants in the haloform reaction, methyl ketone (acetone, CH_3COCH_3) itself is not a likely precursor during water treatment. According to Morris and Baum (1978), who cited a study by Bell and Lidwell (1940), the half-life for chloroform formation from acetone at pH 7 and room temperature is nearly a year. Stevens *et al.* (1978) also discounted acetone as a precursor of THM because of the slow reaction rate. The rate-limiting step in the haloform reaction is the ionization that produces carbanions, and, apparently, simple ketones are not representative of those which react quickly to produce chloroform under conditions in water treatment plants. Studies with model compounds, which are discussed in the section pertaining to chlorine chemistry, have shown that other types of compounds, including other ketones, may react more rapidly than the simple ketones.

Humic Substances

As was mentioned previously, it is an attractive assumption that naturally occurring humic substances, which are derived from the structural components of living and decaying plants and/or soil dissolution and runoff, provide the most ubiquitous source of haloform precursors in natural water systems. Only limited information is available concerning the structure of these complex natural products, and it is not yet known whether all the *major* structural features have been identified, if any structural differences exist among the humic substances in waters from different geographic areas, and if these substances are closely or distantly related to soil humic and marine humic materials.

The term "humic acid" is generic and refers to that fraction of soil organic material that is soluble in alkaline solutions but insoluble in acid and ethyl alcohol (Christman and Oglesby, 1971). The fraction that is soluble in acid is commonly labelled "fulvic acid," and that material precipitated by acid but soluble in ethyl alcohol is "hymatomelanic acid." Soils vary widely in their relative compositions of these acids, but aquatic organic material behaves operationally as fulvic acid (Black and Christman, 1963), which typically contains more oxygen and less nitrogen than the humic acid fraction in both soil and aquatic organic matter. Marine organic matter (including sedimentary material) is derived largely from marine organisms and contains more sulfur than its fresh water equivalent (Nissenbaum and Kaplan, 1972; Stuermer and Harvey, 1978). Christman and Oglesby (1971), Steelink (1977), Schnitzer and Kahn (1972), and Dubach *et al.* (1964) have reported the presence of carboxyl, phenolic and alcoholic hydroxyl, carboxyl, and methoxyl functional groups in humic material. It would appear that the more oxygenated fulvic acid fraction has a greater carboxyl acidity than the humic acid fraction.

Whittaker and Likens (1973) estimated that 90% of the terrestrial biospheric carbon (standing biomass) is tied up in woody tissue. Lignin is a dominant (20%–40%) chemical entity in woody tissue. Because of its refractory nature, it is probably a principal precursor of soil humus, although a myriad of other natural products unquestionably contribute to the complex pool of soil organic matter. Lignin itself is a mixed polymer of guaiacyl (I), syringyl (II), and *p*-hydroxyphenylpropane (III) aromatic moieties:

I II III

No other substitution patterns are known in nature and no other length of alkyl side chain has been found in lignin from any source. Oxidative degradation of lignin produces, therefore, only three aromatic substitution patterns (I, II, and III), although the relative amounts of each vary among the gymnosperms, angiosperms, and the grasses. Intermonomeric linkages in the lignin macromolecule are of both carbon-to-carbon and ether linkage types. The largest single contributor is believed to be the β-4' ether configuration. Side-chain carbon atoms may be in various states of oxygenation or unsaturation, and may contain methyl ketone, allyl, and secondary alcohol configurations.

Significant changes occur in the humification process as reflected by comparative functional group data for lignin and soil humic acid (Table III-1).

This process, which is oxidative in nature, may strongly affect the characteristics of aquatic humic material. Microbial mediation is apparent when there is a marked decrease in methoxyl groups and increases in phenolic hydroxyl and carboxyl acidity.

TABLE III-1 Comparative Functional Group Analysis of Soil Humic Acid and Spruce Lignin[a]

	Group Content, mM/g	
Functional Group	Lignin	Soil Humic Acid
Methoxyl	5.1	0.2
Total hydroxyl	6.2	5.1
Phenolic hydroxyl	1.6	2.9
Alcoholic hydroxyl	4.6	2.2
Carbonyl	1.0	5.5
Carboxyl	Trace	86.0

[a] From Christman and Oglesby, 1971.

The contribution of woody tissues to marine humus is not apparent from the results of degradative experiments on marine fulvic acids, which are considered to be autochthonous materials. Degradation of both soil humic acid and aquatic humic material reflects a partial lignitic origin (Table III-2), although a variety of other aromatic patterns (m-dihydroxy) and aliphatic chain lengths (C_2—C_{17}) must result from other natural product sources. The data in Table III-2 indicate key areas of inadequacy in our knowlege of the chemical nature of aquatic humic substances. It is not possible to model natural aquatic humic material with a desirable degree of chemical accuracy, and it certainly is not possible to state that THM's, which appear in chlorinated water containing humic substances, are derived by the classic haloform reaction.

The ultimate concern for public health protection is, of course, the fact that THM's are formed during the chlorination of drinking water sources. Consequently, a discussion of chemical mechanisms may appear to be rather academic. However, a precise understanding of the mechanisms by which the THM's are formed may prove to be truly beneficial by helping water utility personnel avoid the conditions during treatment that promote the appearance of high concentrations of these compounds in finished water. Studies with model compounds under well-defined laboratory conditions have been useful in elucidating these mechanisms and reaction conditions. Examples are given in the section pertaining to chlorine chemistry.

CHLORINE

Chlorine has been the principal disinfectant of community water supplies for several decades. Until recently, its use had never been questioned seriously because the health benefits derived from it were so obvious. Although an occasional taste-and-odor problem in finished water was attributable to the reaction of chlorine with some substance in the raw water, the events were usually intermittent, short-lived, and presumably did not affect the public health. However, in 1974, Rook (1974) in the Netherlands and Bellar et al. (1974) in the United States reported that chlorine reacts with organic precursors that are found in many source waters to produce a potential carcinogen, chloroform ($CHCl_3$).

In December 1974, Congress passed the Safe Drinking Water Act (PL 93-523), and in early 1975, the U.S. Environmental Protection Agency (EPA) began an 80-city water supply survey—the National Organics Reconnaissance Survey (NORS)—to determine the extent of the problem (Symons *et al.*, 1975). As part of NORS, finished waters from five cities (Miami, Florida; Seattle, Washington; Ottumwa, Iowa; Philadelphia, Pennsylvania; and Cincinnati, Ohio), which represented the major types of water sources in the United States, were analyzed as thoroughly as possible for all volatile organic compounds, i.e., those that can be stripped from solution by purging with an inert gas (Coleman *et al.*, 1976). Seventy-two compounds were identified, 53% of them containing one or more halogens. A later study, the EPA National Organic Monitoring Survey (NOMS), included analyses of samples that had been taken from the water supplies of 113 cities (Brass *et al.*, 1977) on four occasions over an 18-month period during 1976 and 1977. The source waters of a few cities were examined, but most of the effort was directed toward an analysis of finished waters for chloroform and 20 other volatile organic compounds. In addition to the 21 compounds that were orginally selected, five others appeared frequently and were reported.

Since 1974, there have been numerous other surveys similar to NORS and NOMS, but they have been more restricted in scope. In addition, research activity has been intensified to isolate and identify the precursors, products, and mechanisms that are associated with the presence of potentially toxic organic compounds in both water and wastewater. In December 1976, the EPA published a list of 1,259 compounds that had been identified in a variety of waters (including industrial effluents) in Europe and in the United States (Shackelford and Keith, 1976). The agency is currently compiling a comprehensive register of all data concerning the identification of organic pollutants in water.

Properties of Aqueous Chlorine

Various aspects of chlorine chemistry have been reviewed by Jolley *et al.* (1978), Miller *et al.* (1978), Morris (1975, 1978), and Rosenblatt (1975). A synopsis of the basic principles will provide some understanding of the various forms that chlorine can assume in water and the reactions that it can undergo with certain types of compounds.

REACTIVE FORMS OF CHLORINE IN WATER

"Aqueous chlorine" is a misleading term because the active form of chlorine that is present in treated water and wastewater is not the gaseous chlorine molecule (Cl_2) but, rather, a hydrolysis product, hypochlorous acid (HOCl), which is formed from the reaction between the chlorine molecule and water:

$$Cl_2 + H_2O \rightleftharpoons HOCl + H^+ + Cl^- \tag{1}$$

TABLE III-2 Chemical Degradation Products of Humic Substances

Technique	Marine Humus[a]	Soil Humus[b]	Freshwater Humus[c]
Acid hydrolysis	(FA) nine amino acids (Gagosian and Stuermer, 1977) (FA) 20% organic soluble (not identified)	20 amino acids (Kahn and Sowden, 1972), peptides, sugars, phenolic carboxylic acids (trace)[d]	No amino acids (Gjessing, 1976)
Alkaline hydrolysis	No data	(HA) 11% aliphatic (C_{16}-C_{18}) fatty acids 7% phenolic acids (principally quaiacyl and syringyl) 2% polycarboxylic aromatic acids (Neyroud and Schnitzer, 1975)	(HA) phenols, phenolic acids (including quaiacyl and syringyl), aliphatic acids (C_{13}-C_{17}), and citric acid (Christman, 1978a)
Oxidation	Conversion to carbon dioxide and water noted with strong oxidants. (Limited experimental data) (Stuermer and Harvey, 1978)	Alkaline cupric oxide: (HA) vanillin, p-hydroxybenz-aldehyde, syringaldehyde, p-hydroxybenzoic acid, vanillic acid, 3,5-dihydroxybenzoic acid, m-hydroxybenzoic acid (Green and Steelink, 1962) Alkaline potassium permanganate: aliphatic monocarboxylic acids (C_2-C_6) and dicarboxylic acids	Alkaline cupric oxide: (HA) vanillin p-hydroxybenzaldehyde, syringaldehyde, p-hydroxybenzoic acid, vanillic acid, 3,5-dihydroxybenzoic acid (Christman and Ghassemi, 1966) Alkaline potassium permanganate: aliphatic monocarboxylic acids (C_7-C_{15}) and dicarboxylic acids

Reductive degradation	High-pressure hydrogenation: n-alkanes (C_{12}-C_{26}, predominance of even carbon no.), alkyl benzenes (four homologous series, with side chains of C_{10}, C_{11}, and C_{12} predominant)	Zinc dust distillation: polynuclear aromatic hydrocarbons (low yields) (Schnitzer and Kahn, 1972) Sodium-amalgam: p-hydroxybenz-aldehyde, vanillic acid, syringic acid, protocatechuic acid, quaiacyl and syringyl propionic acids, resorcinol, phloroglucinol, pyrogallol methylphloroglucinol, 2,6- and 2,4-dihydroxytoluene, and 3,5-dihydroxybenzoic acid (Burgess et al., 1964)	(C_2-C_8), phenolic acids, and benzene polycarboxylic acids (including methoxy-substituted analogs) (Schnitzer and Kahn, 1972)	No data	(C_1-C_{15}), phenolic acids, and benzene polycarboxylic acids (including methoxy-substituted analogs) (Christman, 1978b)

[a] FA/HA (Fulvic acid/humic acid) >1.0 (Gagosian and Stuermer, 1977); HA + FA <5% DOC (dissolved organic carbon); autochthonous (Stuermer and Harvey, 1978).

[b] FA/HA variable.

[c] FA/HA 1.0 (Black and Christman, 1963); % DOC variable; allochthomous (Shapiro, 1957).

[d] From total soil organic matter; acid hydrolysis has little effect on HA per se.

Hypochlorous acid, a weak acid, can ionize as follows:

$$HOCl \rightleftharpoons H^+ + OCl^- \tag{2}$$

The degree of ionization depends primarily on the pH and temperature of the water. The concentration of hypochlorous acid and the hypochlorite ion (OCl^-) are approximately equal at pH 7.5 and 25°C.

Another form of chlorine, the hypochloronium acidium ion (H_2OCl^+), is known to exist (Miller *et al.*, 1978; Rosenblatt, 1975), but its concentration would be extremely low in water at pH's between 5 and 9. Still another form of chlorine, the chloronium (or chlorinium) ion (Cl^+), has been proposed as an important reactant in aqueous solutions of organic compounds (Carlson and Caple, 1978), although its existence is disputed (Rosenblatt, 1975). Nevertheless, Morris (1978) pointed out that "the reactant behavior of HOCl with organic carbon and amino nitrogen is as an electrophilic agent in which the chlorine atom takes on partially the characteristics of Cl^+ and combines with an electron pair in the substrate." Finally, Carlson and Caple (1978) mentioned that another form of chlorine, the chlorine radical ($Cl\cdot$), may react in the light to produce chlorine-substituted organic compounds when the parent chlorine molecule is not lost by any other significant reaction pathway. Rosenblatt (1975), citing others, described this form as "probably the most selective chlorinating species of all."

Free chlorine species (HOCl, OCl^-, Cl_2, H_2OCl^+, Cl^+) will oxidize both the bromide ion (Br^-) and iodide ion (I^-) to hypobromous and hypoiodous acids (HOBr and HOI). This reaction, as will be discussed later, is postulated to account for the presence of bromine- and iodine-substituted organic compounds, particularly the mixed-halide haloforms, in waters that had been disinfected by chlorination.

REACTIONS OF HYPOCHLOROUS ACID WITH ORGANIC COMPOUNDS

Chlorine reacts in solutions of organic compounds by one or more of three basic mechanisms (Jolley *et al.*, 1978; Miller *et al.*, 1978; Morris, 1975; Morris, 1978), namely, addition, during which chlorine atoms are added to a compound; oxidation; and substitution, during which chlorine atoms are substituted for some other atom that is present in the organic reactant. All three of these reactions involve hypochlorous acid as an electrophile.

Only addition and substitution reactions produce chlorinated organic compounds. Oxidation reactions account for most of the "chlorine demand" of natural waters and waste treatment effluents (Jolley et al., 1978; Morris, 1975), but the end products are not chlorinated organic compounds. That is not to say that those products cannot be harmful. Miller et al. (1978) have mentioned that epoxides can be produced from carbon-chlorinated compounds at pH values that are common in water treatment plants (e.g., pH 9.5–10.5) where softening is practiced. To illustrate, they describe the reaction between ethylene (C_2H_4) and hypochlorous acid, which yields ethylene chlorohydrin ($ClCH_2CH_2OH$) as an intermediate. This hydrolyzes to form the epoxide, ethylene oxide (C_2H_4O). Carlson and Caple (1978) mentioned one such reaction, in which a mixture of chlorohydrins resulted from the reaction of oleic acid [$CH_3(CH_2)_7CH=CH(CH_2)_7COOH$] with hypochlorous acid. Presumably, these would be converted to epoxides if the pH were to be increased. Carlson and Caple also showed how a ubiquitous natural compound, α-terpineol [$CH_3C_6H_4C(CH_3)_2OH$], could form epoxides when reacted with hypochlorous acid. These reactions illustrate how chlorination may result in the development of nonchlorinated products, e.g., the epoxides, which may pose health risks. In instances such as those just discussed, a chlorinated intermediate, which itself should be evaluated toxicologically, is involved.

Chlorine By-Products Found in Drinking Water and Selected Nonpotable Waters

The most frequently mentioned products of aqueous reactions between chlorine and selected types of organic compounds are discussed in this section. Special attention is given to the trihalomethanes (THM's) because of the current interest in them as potentially hazardous by-products of chlorination in municipal water treatment facilities. The specific reactions by which THM's are produced in chlorinated natural waters are not well understood because the chemical structures of the precursor organic compounds, which are thought to be primarily humic substances, are highly varied and extremely complex. A summary of the relevant facts concerning these ubiquitous, natural organic substances is presented in the section on precursors. The term "haloform reaction" is often mentioned as the mechanism by which THM's are produced when natural waters are chlorinated. This has not been validated definitively in actual water treatment systems. However, the reaction will be discussed in conjunction with THM formation in natural waters because it is one possible mechanism that has been described thoroughly in the literature.

Other products of chlorination that are discussed below include the chlorinated phenols, which have been of concern primarily because they impart offensive tastes to drinking water, and compounds that have been isolated during carefully controlled experiments involving analyses of both chlorinated and unchlorinated samples of freshwater and its analogs. Data derived from in-plant studies are difficult to interpret because raw waters are seldom uniform in composition over time, especially surface waters and raw sewages. Thus, there is always some unavoidable uncertainty as to whether compounds that have been isolated from finished waters were produced by chlorination of precursor organic compounds in the influent or whether they were present before the influent entered the plant. Despite the uncertainty, some published in-plant studies are described in this section. Those related to THM formation are especially noteworthy. Abundant laboratory evidence shows that the high concentrations of THM's that have been observed in many finished drinking waters are produced by reactions between chlorine and precursor organic compounds that are commonly found in natural waters.

TRIHALOMETHANES

The current interest in THM's was prompted by the reports of Rook (1974) and Bellar et al. (1974), which linked the presence of chloroform and other trihalogenated derivatives of methane (CH_4) in finished drinking water to the chlorination of raw waters during treatment. Rook (1974) demonstrated that THM's were produced by the chlorination of aqueous extracts of peat, and he postulated that the precursors were the humic substances. The presence of THM's in laboratory-chlorinated waters that had been taken from a lake in a "peaty region" helped confirm Rook's hypothesis. Later laboratory studies involving the chlorination of aqueous solutions of humic substances (e.g., Babcock and Singer, 1977; Hoehn et al., 1978; Stevens et al., 1976) further confirmed Rook's hypothesis. Bellar et al. (1974) reported that THM concentrations in Ohio River water increased as it was being treated and chlorinated at several points in the Cincinnati, Ohio, waterworks. Rook (1974) reported similar observations for treated water from the Rhine and Meuse rivers at the Berenplaat treatment plant in the Netherlands.

The prevalence of THM's in U.S. municipal water supplies was demonstrated by the NORS survey in 1975 and the NOMS survey in 1976. According to Symons et al. (1975), the total THM (TTHM) concentrations in the 80-city survey (NORS) were log-normally distributed, while chloroform appeared in the highest concentrations (median, 21 μg/liter), followed by bromodichloromethane ($CHCl_2Br$) (median, 6 μg/liter) and lesser concentrations of chlorodibromomethane ($CHBr_2Cl$) and tribromomethane ($CHBr_3$). The distributions are shown in Figure III-1. Brass *et al.* (1977) reported median concentrations of chloroform and bromodichloromethane of 27 and 10 μg/liter, respectively, in the 113 supplies that were surveyed during the first phase of NOMS. During that phase, sampling and handling procedures were identical to those used during NORS. The THM concentrations in the raw water sources, which included rivers, groundwaters, and lakes, were much lower. Hoehn *et al.* (1977) and Hoehn and Randall (1977) reported results of an extensive 2-yr THM monitoring program at a water treatment plant and at the distribution system of a northern Virginia water supply that was supplied by a reservoir. Mean finished-water THM concentrations varied seasonally and were from 1 to 2 orders of magnitude greater than those found in the source water. Average chloroform concentrations in finished drinking water were from 5 to 10 times greater than the median reported for NORS and NOMS, but concentrations of bromodichloromethane were comparable.

As was mentioned earlier, it is difficult to determine whether many organic compounds that are recovered from finished waters during in-plant studies actually were formed during the treatment process, especially when analyses of intermittently collected "grab" samples provide the data base. The uncertainty factor is greater when compounds are seldom recovered from finished water and when they are occasionally detected in untreated water at concentrations that are similar to those found in treated water. In these instances, the origin of a substance that has been isolated from finished water would be determined more accurately by a comparative analysis of samples from both influent and effluent water that has been collected and composited for a period at least equal to the hydraulic detention time within the plant. In the in-plant surveys, the attribution of THM's to chlorination is more certain, although grab samples were used, primarily because THM's have often been found in finished waters in much higher concentrations than in the untreated influent waters.

Mention has already been made of the fact that mixed-halide THM's have been identified on numerous occasions, the most common ones being the bromochloromethanes, $CHCl_2Br$ and $CHClBr_2$. These, and occasionally iodine-containing, mixed-halide THM's, have been report-

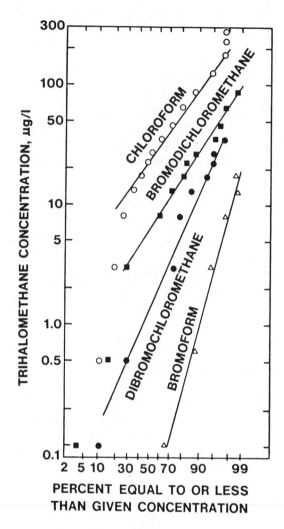

FIGURE III-1   Frequency distribution of trihalomethane data (NORS). From Stevens *et al.*, 1978.

ed but in much lower concentrations than chloroform. The mechanisms that are involved in the formation of these compounds during chlorination are discussed in the bromine–iodine section of this chapter. Fluorinated isomers are not expected to be produced by these mechanisms (Kleopfer, 1976).

The production of chlorinated THM's in concentrations that are typical of those reportedly recovered from finished drinking waters is dependent upon the initial presence of free chlorine. Thus, unnitrified, chlorinated sewage effluents that contain no free chlorine usually contain low ($<$10 μg/liter) THM concentrations (Stevens et al., 1978) unless industrial wastes containing THM's are discharged into the sewers. The reason for this phenomenon is that free chlorine species react extremely rapidly with ammonia (NH_3) (Morris, 1967), which is present in sewage in concentrations of parts per million. Under those conditions, the concentration of free chlorine is extremely low (Jolley et al., 1976).

NONHALOFORM PRODUCTS OF THM REACTIONS

While it is not certain that the classic haloform reaction is solely responsible for the appearance of THM's in chlorinated drinking water, it illustrates the fact that organic compounds other than THM's are formed as a natural consequence of reactions involving carbanions that lead to THM formation. Some of these compounds are chlorinated intermediates, while others are terminal products that are formed simultaneously with the THM's. For example, if the classic haloform reaction (involving a ketone) is operative, a carboxylic acid is formed during the final hydrolysis step, which results in the production of a THM:

$$R—C—CCl_3 + H_2O \rightarrow R—C—OH + CHCl_3 \tag{3}$$

Nonhalogenated products, which may contain aromatic or alicyclic structures (e.g., benzene rings or cyclic hydrocarbons, respectively), should not be ignored when assessing potential health risks that are associated with water chlorination.

Another fact to consider is that if the free THM were not produced (e.g., by hydrolysis, in the haloform reaction), some chlorinated intermediate containing a chlorinated methyl group might be present. Suffet et al. (1976) have reported finding 1,1,1-trichloroacetone (Cl_3CCOCH_3) in two different potable water supplies near Philadelphia. One water treatment plant is on the Delaware River; the other is on the

Schuylkill River. The 1976 EPA Survey (Shackelford and Keith, 1976) reported no instances of trichloroacetone in rivers, lakes, or groundwaters. Trichloroacetone is readily hydrolyzed at a pH above 5 (Suffet *et al.*, 1978, private communication). Suffet *et al.* (1976) utilized two different on-line composite isolation methods with dechlorination and adjustment to pH 4 to stabilize the compound. They isolated it with a XAD-2 resin and continuous liquid–liquid extractor. This compound is a likely intermediate in the haloform reaction, especially when acetone (C_3H_6O) is present in the river water. The haloform reaction for acetone is extremely slow (Bell and Lidwell, 1940; Morris and Baum, 1978). Trichloroacetone hydrolysis is much quicker. To be observed, the compound must be extracted immediately or the pH must be lowered to ≤ 4 to stabilize it.

Morris and Baum (1978) reported that trichloroacetate (CCl_3COO^-) and hexachloroacetone (CCl_3COCCl_3) are possible intermediates of the classic haloform reaction, but they argued that substantial quantities of other chlorinated organic compounds, except chloroform, should not be formed. Obviously, the formation of chlorinated intermediates other than these could occur by mechanisms other than the haloform reaction.

Pfaender *et al.* (1978) presented corroborating evidence that trichlorinated intermediates do occur in chlorinated waters. They detected more chloroform in water samples that had been analyzed by direct aqueous injections (DAI) of samples into a gas chromatograph than by a conventional technique that involves stripping the volatile THM's from solution with an inert purge gas. They attributed the higher recoveries to thermal decomposition of nonvolatile, chlorinated intermediate compounds that had been introduced into the analytical instrument by DAI but which remained in solution during the analysis involving the purge technique. They did not identify any of the intermediates but did show that chloral (CCl_3CHO), a previously suspected intermediate, was stable under the conditions of the anlaysis by DAI and could not account for the observed increases in chloroform concentration.

Carbon tetrachloride (CCl_4) is not produced during the haloform reaction, nor should it be produced by any other mechanism involving electrophilic substitution of chlorine on a carbanion. Shackelford and Keith (1976) reported its presence in finished drinking water on numerous occasions when it had not been detected in the untreated water. The most likely source of carbon tetrachloride in these instances is the chlorine itself. Carbon tetrachloride and hexachloroethane (C_2Cl_6) have been identified as contaminants of the chlorine-manufacturing process (Laubusch, 1959). Hexachlorobenzene (C_6Cl_6) has also been identified as a contaminant (Blankenship, 1978).

REACTIONS INVOLVING PHENOLIC SUBSTANCES

The primary concern with phenolic compounds in drinking water supplies has been the offensive tastes that result from their reaction with hypochlorous acid. The presence of the hydroxyl group on the benzene ring activates the ring and permits chlorine to substitute readily. Multiple substitutions can lead to rupture of the parent ring (Burttschell et al., 1959). Morris (1975) has provided a good overview of the available literature of the subject, including that related to the products that have been observed after rupture of the ring. Lee and Morris (1962) and Lee (1967) have described in detail the kinetics of phenol chlorination and have recommended controls for the taste and odor problem that is caused by chlorophenols.

Phenolic substances that are present in natural waters are highly varied. Reactions produced in the laboratory with the simple phenols may not occur when the more complex phenols are present. Therefore, conclusions that are derived from these laboratory studies should be extended with caution to systems that contain the more complex and diverse forms of phenols that exist in nature.

REACTION PRODUCTS FROM CHLORINATED SURFACE WATERS AND
SEWAGE EFFLUENTS

Because of the difficulties of interpreting in-plant studies involving analyses of influent and effluent grab samples, most of the investigations discussed below are limited to those involving analyses of pairs of influent water or sewage samples that differed only in that one of each pair was chlorinated in the laboratory. Despite the uncertainties that are associated with data from influent– effluent analyses, a few investigations involving in-plant studies have been reviewed, either because the compounds that were detected in the chlorinated effluents were seldom, if ever, detected in untreated waters or because the study involved a broad survey of many treatment facilities.

PRODUCTS FROM CHLORINATED SURFACE WATERS

Jolley et al. (1978) chlorinated surface sources that were used to cool water at two Tennessee electric power-generating facilities, one in Kingston (Watts Bar Lake) and the other near Memphis (Mississippi River). Radioisotopic ^{36}Cl in $HO^{36}Cl$ was applied in dosages of 2.1 mg/liter at Kingston and 3.4 mg/liter at Memphis and was allowed to react for 75 and 15 min, respectively. The waters were concentrated by vacuum distillation, and compounds were separated for analysis with a scintillation counter by high-pressure liquid chromatography (HPLC). Chlorination yields (as Cl) of chloroorganic constituents that were separated by HPLC were 0.5% at Kingston and 3.0% at Memphis. A variety of compounds was recovered. The influent water was not analyzed because the presence of the [36]Cl isotope in the molecules indicated that the product was derived from the chlorination. There was no attempt to confirm the identity of the reported compounds by gas chromatography/mass spectrometry analysis.

Among the chlorinated compounds that were recovered in concentrations ranging from a few tenths of a part per billion (ppb) to as high as 20 ppb were a nucleoside, three purines, a pyrimidine, seven aromatic acids, and five phenolics. The Mississippi River sample from Memphis contained the highest concentrations (0.7 to 20.0 ppb), because it contained less ammonia—hence more free chlorine to serve as the active oxidizing agent. The analytical methods recovered only nonvolatile, or slightly volatile, compounds and did not permit detection of large polymeric substances such as humic acids or nucleic acids. The pyrimidine, 5-chlorouracil, which was present at concentrations of 0.6 and 7.0 ppb in the two samples, has captured attention because it could be incorporated into cellular genetic material (Gehrs and Southworth, 1978; Jolley et al., 1978). Gehrs and Southworth (1978) commented that one of the chlorophenols, 4-chlororesorcinol [ClC_6H_3-1,3-$(OH)_2$], was potentially toxic, but they made no mention of the possible impacts of the other chloroderivatives that were recovered.

In a study of chlorinated (2.0 mg/liter, 68-hr contact time) and unchlorinated waters from Lake Zurich, Giger et al. (1976) recovered several α-chloroketones and a variety of THM's that contained chlorine, bromine, and iodine, all of which were absent in the unchlorinated control sample. The ketones included 2,2-dichlorobutanone (CH_3CCl_2-$COCH_3$), 2,2-dichloropentan-3-one ($CH_3CCl_2COC_2H_5$), 1,1,1-trichloroacetone (also recovered by Suffet et al., 1976), and 3,3-dichlorohexan-4-one ($C_2H_5CCl_2COC_2H_5$). In addition, they detected minor quantities of chlorinated alkylated benzene compounds. The α-ketones and THM's were identified by mass spectrometry.

Brass et al. (1977) mentioned that two sets of raw and finished waters from an unidentified city were analyzed for volatile organics during NOMS Phase III. They observed that aromatic compounds (unspecified) were found in finished water but not in the raw water samples. Further work was anticipated. A later publication concerning NOMS-III (Munch et al., 1977) lists the relative recoveries of 25 various organic compounds from the raw and finished waters at 11 locations. Compounds other than THM's, which were recovered more often in finished waters than in raw, included benzene (C_6H_6) (4 versus 0), chlorobenzene (C_6H_5Cl) (3 versus 1), ethylbenzene ($C_6H_5C_2H_5$) (3 versus 0), dichloromethane (CH_2Cl_2) (3 versus 0), toluene ($C_6H_5CH_3$) (3 versus 1), and a xylene isomer [$C_6H_4(CH_3)_2$] (4 versus 1). (Compounds where the difference in recoveries was only 1 are not listed.) The ranges of concentrations that were observed when the compounds were quantified included: 0.58–6.10 μg/liter for chlorobenzene, 0.1–1.5 μg/liter for benzene, 0.42–0.57 μg/liter for ethylbenzene, and 0.48–19.00 μg/liter for toluene. The means were 2.7, 0.88, 0.50, and 6.9 μg/liter, respectively.

PRODUCTS FROM CHLORINATED SEWAGE EFFLUENTS

Jolley (1975) chlorinated primary- and secondary-treated sewage effluents with various forms of ^{36}Cl-tagged chlorine compounds to determine which chlorination products could be found. Chlorine was dispensed as a gas at dosages and contact times that were similar to those expected in actual plant operations. Additional experiments were performed in the laboratory, wherein a ^{36}Cl-tagged hypochlorite solution was used as the chlorinating agent. Of the 44 compounds that were recovered, 17 mentioned previously as having been recovered from cooling waters were identified in the sewage effluents. Less than 1% of the chlorine could be accounted for within organic compounds. Most of it was in the form of chloride ion (Cl^-), indicating that most of the chlorine that is applied to sewage serves as an oxidant. There are many difficulties inherent in the separation and identification of compounds in waters that are heavily laden with organic and inorganic contaminants. It may be that more chloroorganics were present than could be recovered. However, this possibility does not alter the basic conclusion that most of the chlorine is simply reduced to chloride ion during the oxidation of sewage constituents. Nevertheless, the oxidized organic compounds have importance from an environmental perspective whether or not they contain chlorine.

Garrison *et al.* (1976) identified extractable volatile organics in lime-clarified, tertiary-treated sewage from the Blue Plains pilot plant near Washington, D.C. Chlorination was effected by sodium hypochlorite (NaOCl), which was added to achieve breakpoint and a final, free residual of 3–5 mg/liter. The final pH was between 7.0 and 7.5. Samples were extracted and fractionated by standard analytical procedures, then concentrated and methylated before analysis. The most pronounced effect of the chlorination was evidenced by the appearance of chlorocyclohexane ($C_6H_{11}Cl$) and tetra-, penta-, and hexachloroethanes ($C_2H_2Cl_4$; C_2HCl_5; C_2Cl_6) in the effluent. None of the compounds was quantified.

These compounds are unusual constituents of chlorinated waters. The pentachloroethane is not an ordinary commercial material and, therefore, would probably not have an industrial origin. Commenting on his previous work (Garrison et al., 1976), Garrison (1978) provided some insight concerning the appearance of these compounds. Studies at the EPA Laboratory in Athens, Georgia, have shown that cyclohexene (C_6H_{12}) is a common contaminant of methylene chloride (CH_2Cl_2), which is used as the extracting solvent. If the aqueous system being extracted contained residual chlorine, the cyclohexene could be converted to 1,2-dichlorocyclohexane by the addition of chlorine to the double bond. During the original study, the solvent may have contained other alkene impurities that could have reacted with chlorine to form the tetra-, penta-, and hexachloroethanes, but that possibility was not explored. If those impurities had existed, they would have been masked during analysis by the methylene chloride peak on the gas chromatogram, since they are highly volatile substances. No "blanks" (control tests) were analyzed because the possible problem was not recognized. Moreover, both raw and treated sewages were being analyzed and the differences in composition were of prime interest. However, Garrison (1978) emphasized that these chlorinated aliphatic compounds, although unusual, have been identified in studies subsequent to the one reported in the 1976 publication.

Glaze et al. (1976, 1978) and Glaze and Henderson (1975) reported the appearance of 38 compounds that were generated by superchlorination (2,000 mg/liter) of sewage effluent that had received secondary treatment. Most of the chlorinated compounds that were identified were aromatic derivatives. Many of them involved aromatics with no activating substituent groups. Among those that appeared were the chloroderivatives of benzene, toluene, and benzyl alcohol (C_6H_5-CH_2OH) and the nonaromatic derivatives such as chlorocyclohexane (reported also by Garrison et al., 1976), a chloroalkyl acetate, and three chlorinated acetone derivatives (tri-, penta-, and hexachloroacetone). The acetone derivatives may be precursors of chloroform (see also Suffet et al., 1976). According to the authors, they may have been produced by an acid-catalyzed reaction between acetone and chlorine.

Glaze and Henderson (1975) and Glaze et al. (1976, 1978) also reported that an increase in the concentration of chlorine-containing compounds, as estimated by the total organic chlorine (TOCl) concentration in nonpurgeable compounds, was observed in the sewage as the chlorine dose was increased from 25 to 2,000 mg/liter. The TOCl concentration increased from 80 to 906 μg/liter, but decreased to 164 μg/liter when the chlorine dose was increased to 3,000 mg/liter, thereby demonstrating the destruction of chloroorganic compounds that were formed at lower chlorine dosages. The chlorine that was bound in organic compounds accounted for less than 0.05% of the applied chlorine. The chlorine dosages far exceeded expected concentrations in routine sewage treatment plant operations. However, there are commercially available treatment units in which sewage and industrial waste sludges can be oxidized by superchlorination within the range of the high dosages used by Glaze *et al.* Superchlorination would probably be required to reduce the concentrations of chloroorganic compounds that increase when chlorine dosages are increased. Fuchs and Kuhn (1976) demonstrated a marked increase in concentrations of chlorinated organic compounds at a water treatment plant when Rhine River water was chlorinated to breakpoint. Activated carbon treatment reduced these concentrations, the removal ranging from 28% to 69% of the influent TOCl concentrations. Superchlorination was not attempted.

Sievers *et al.* (1978) found increased levels of aromatic hydrocarbons—such as toluene, xylenes, and styrene ($C_6H_5CH=CH_2$)—in chlorinated, secondary-treated wastewaters from the Metro-Denver sewage plant in District No. 1. Excess chlorine additions under laboratory conditions resulted in the formation of species of chlorotoluene ($ClC_6H_4CH_3$) and chloroxylene [$ClC_8CH_3(CH_3)_2$]. No industrial discharges enter the system. Therefore, the authors believe that the precursors were not of industrial origin. Concentrations of these aromatics ranged from 0.1 to 2.0 ppb.

In the EPA survey (Shackelford and Keith, 1976), toluene was found in finished drinking waters on several occasions, although it has been detected also in river water. Garrison (1978) reported that recent studies by the EPA laboratories in Las Vegas, Nevada, show toluene to be present at concentrations up to 2 μg/liter in pristine mountain streams in the Great Smoky Mountains National Park. The EPA investigators attributed this to automobile exhausts.

The EPA survey document also reported the frequent detection in finished drinking waters of the xylenes (ortho, meta, and para isomers) and, less frequently, styrene. These compounds were present in various raw water sources as well. Sievers *et al.* (1978) believed the precursors to be nonvolatile but did not postulate what they might be. According to them, toluene, styrene, and xylenes have been identified in 20 U.S. drinking water supplies and in certain Canadian supplies.

Chlorination of Model Compounds

Several recent publications have described the results of laboratory experiments involving chlorination of model compounds in aqueous solutions. The products have been reported, and, in some instances, mechanisms were proposed. A select number of those publications are reported below.

REACTIONS RESULTING IN THM FORMATION

Rook (1976) presented evidence that diketones, which have been described as degradation products of fulvic acids (one component of humic substances), do produce chloroform more rapidly than simple ketones. He chlorinated 1,3-cyclohexanedione [$C_6H_8(=O)_2$], 5,5-dimethylcyclo-1,3-hexanedione [$(CH_3)_2C_6H_6(+O)_2$] (dimedone), and 1,3-indandione [$C_9H_5(=O)_2$] at concentrations (>200 mg/liter Cl_2) that were high in comparison to dosages used in water treatment plants at pH 7.5 and 11.0 at 10°C. He obtained yields of chloroform ranging from 50% to 100% of the theoretical yields (0.5–1.0 mol of chloroform per mole of precursor) in 4 hr.

In a later publication, Rook (1977) reported that the yields of chloroform from a variety of hydroxylated compounds were quite high. Those producing the highest yields with relative low chlorine dosages were metadihydroxy compounds such as 1,3-benzenediol (resorcinol) [$C_6H_4(OH)_2$], 1,3-dihydroxynaphthalene [$C_{10}H_6(OH)_2$], and 3,5-dihydroxybenzoic acid [$HOOCC_6H_3(OH)_2$]. Resorcinol is known to be a degradation product of fulvic acids (Christman and Ghassemi, 1966). The hydroxyl groups are strongly "activating." Consequently, the carbon positioned between the two hydroxyl groups is activated from both sides, thereby becoming a strong carbanion, which is readily attacked by chlorine.

Rook (1977) pointed out that chloroform may be just one of many by-products of reactions between chlorine and these types of compounds. He mentioned that substitution, oxidative ring fissions, or even ring contractions and other fragmentations may occur. Christman *et al.* (1978a) also chlorinated resorcinol under laboratory conditions and found that the carbon between the hydroxyl substituents was removed from the structure, thereby producing a 1,2-diketocyclopentenedione (3-chloro-5,5-dichlorocyclopent-3-ene-1,2-dione). They also identified mono-, di-, and trichlorinated resorcinols that had been produced by simple substitution reactions. Additional work by Christman and co-workers is described below.

Morris and Baum (1978) chlorinated a variety of compounds that could produce reactive carbanions in solutions at pH 7 and 11. Several of the compounds contained the pyrrole ring, which exhibits active carbanion formation and is a component of many natural compounds such as the plant pigments chlorophyll and xanthophyll. The pyrrole ring is also present in tryptophane, proline (both amino acids), and indole (a component of certain protein putrefaction products). They also studied a class of compounds that are described as "acetogenins," which also contain β-ketonic groups in structures that are common to natural pigments.

Other compounds that Morris and Baum investigated as possible haloform precursors were vanillin (4-hydroxy-3-methoxybenzaldehyde and syringaldehyde (4-hydroxy-3,5,dimethoxylbenzaldehyde), both alkaline degradation products of woody materials. Neither compound has the 1,3-dihydroxy configuration that reacts rapidly to produce THM's. In some of the studies, the reactions with chlorine were permitted to proceed in near-neutral solutions for several hours. Then the pH was increased to between 9 and 11. While THM's were produced at the lower pH, greater concentrations were found when the pH was increased. Their major conclusion was that naturally occurring compounds, from which THM's can be produced, are capable of forming chlorinated intermediates as well at neutral pH as at high pH, and that only the final hydrolysis, which results in higher concentrations of THM's, is enhanced by elevated pH. They suggested that the hygienic quality of drinking water might best be monitored by measuring TOCl concentrations.

Christman *et al.* (1978b) have reacted several phenolic humic model compounds with hypochlorous acid in dilute aqueous solution. These models were selected on the basis of results from oxidative degradation of aquatic humic material. Their data (Table III-3) suggest that aromatic substitution patterns that are typical of lignin and soil humic acid (1,3,5- and 1,3,4,5-) produce less chloroform than the basic *m*-dihydroxy model (resorcinol). The decrease is particularly marked when hydroxy is absent or methylated. The yield data from the substituted cinnamic acid (3-phenyl-2-propenoic acid, $C_9H_8O_2$) indicate that the propyl side chain may be involved in the production of chloroform.

The yield of chloroform from resorcinol (Table III-3) compares favorably with the data of Rook (1977). In addition, the configuration of the cyclopentene intermediate suggests that Rook's hypothesis concerning the location of the chloroform-producing carbon is correct.

TABLE III-3   Comparative Chloroform Yields for Some Humic Model Compounds[a]

Compound	Chloroform Yield, Moles of Chloroform/ Mole of Compound	Chlorine Demand, Moles of Chlorine/ Mole of Compound
1,3-dihydroxybenzene (resorcinol)	0.91 (30 min)	6.60
3,5-dihydroxybenzoic acid	0.5 (40 min)	7.06
3,5-dimethoxybenzoic acid	0.009 (40 min)	3.00
3,5-dihyroxytoluene (orcinol)	0.914 (30 min)	6.26
3,5-dimethoxy-4-hydroxybenzoic acid (syringic acid)	0.005 (40 min)	5.18
3,5-dimethoxy-4-hydroxycinnamic acid	0.0228 (40 min)	6.09
(3,5-dimethoxy-4-hydroxyphenyl) propionic acid	0.0959 (221 min)	7.79
3-methoxy-4-hydroxy hydrocinnamic acid	0.0149 (183 min)	5.55
3-methoxy-4-hydroxy cinnamic acid	0.184 (250 min)	8.44

[a] From Christman et al., 1978b.

REACTIONS PRODUCING COMPOUNDS OTHER THAN THM'S

The previous section emphasized model compound studies that were designed primarily to elucidate the mechanisms of THM formation. This section contains a review of published data from investigators who were principally interested in chlorination products other than THM's.

Carlson *et al.* (1975) and Carlson and Caple (1978) addressed the problems of predicting the extent of chlorine incorporation into aromatic substances. They chlorinated aqueous solutions of a variety of compounds whose parent structure was the benzene ring but which contained a variety of substituent groups. Included in their studies were phenol (C_6H_5OH), anisole ($C_6H_5OCH_3$), acetanilide ($CH_3CONHC_6H_5$), toluene ($C_6H_5CH_3$), benzyl alcohol ($C_6H_5CH_2OH$), benzonitrile (C_6H_5CN), nitrobenzene ($C_6H_5NO_2$), chlorobenzene (C_6H_5Cl), methyl benzoate ($C_6H_5COOCH_3$), and benzene (C_6H_6) in concentrations of $9.5 \pm 0.6 \times 10^{-4}$ M. Chlorine (7.0×10^{-4} M) was added and allowed to react at 25°C for 20 min. Experiments were conducted at pH 3, 7, and 10. They also studied biphenyl ($C_6H_5C_6H_5$), the parent compound of polychlorinated biphenyls (PCB's).

As expected their results showed that phenol was the only aromatic compound with one substituent that reacted readily at pH's that are common to water treatment (e.g., pH 7 and 10). Others, like anisole and acetanilide, reacted to some degree, but only at pH 3. The substituent groups in anisole and acetanilide ($-O-CH_3$ and $-NH-CO-CH_3$, respectively) are not highly reactive with hydrochlorous acid at near-neutral pH's that are encountered in water treatment. Biphenyl reactions with chlorine under conditions that are normally found at water treatment plants were not significant. Either extremely long reacting times (days), high dosages of chlorine (>100 mg/liter), or low pH's were required to obtain relatively small yields of the chlorinated biphenyls, but one or more of these conditions might prevail where superchlorination is practiced.

Inference of Possible Chlorination By-Products

INFERENCES REGARDING POLYNUCLEAR AROMATIC HYDROCARBONS

Polynuclear (or polycyclic) aromatic hydrocarbons (PAH's) are commonly found in water (Andelman and Snodgrass, 1974; Harrison *et al.*, 1975), and many are known to be potent toxins, mutagens, and teratogens (Blumer and Youngblood, 1975; Hase and Hites, 1976). Blumer and Youngblood (1975) concluded that PAH's that are found in recent sediments originate primarily from particulates that are produced by forest fires. But Hase and Hites (1976) presented data that they interpreted as evidence that PAH's in water are produced principally from urban air pollutants from man-induced combustion processes. Oyler *et al.* (1978) cited reports indicating that PAH concentrations can be reduced by aqueous chlorination reactions, resulting in the production of chlorinated napthalenes, a chlorobenzopyrene, and a benzopyrene quinone.

Oyler *et al.* (1978) also reported laboratory data indicating that PAH's are susceptible to conversion to "second-order" products in the presence of hypochlorite under conditions that are typical of those in water during disinfection. Specific data concerning chlorine doses were not given. Compounds that were recovered and quantified included anthraquinone (9,10-anthracenedione, $C_{14}H_8O_2$), and monochloro derivatives of fluorene ($C_{13}H_{10}$), phenanthrene ($C_{14}H_{10}$), 1-methylphenanthrene ($C_{14}H_9$-CH_3), and 1-methylnaphthalene ($C_{10}H_7CH_3$). Several PAH's and their derivatives have been detected in finished drinking water (Shackelford and Keith, 1976). Therefore, one should not ignore the possibility that reaction products, similar to those that Oyler and his co-workers identified, can be formed during water chlorination.

INFERENCES REGARDING REACTIONS WITH BIOGENIC SUBSTANCES

Surface waters receive, through runoff, a variety of allochthonous materials other than humic substance that may be important reactants with chlorine during disinfection. The compounds number in the thousands, but few have been studied in detail. In addition to organic compounds that might be washed in, surface waters contain many compounds that are produced by actively growing (or decaying) algae and higher plants. Here, too, there is a myriad of possibilities. Most likely, it will not be practical to isolate, identify, and evaluate the potential toxicity of more than a few. Vallentyne (1957) has written a comprehensive review of the natural aquatic organic compounds.

Morris and Baum (1978) found that THM was produced from chlorophyll. Hoehn *et al.* (1978) observed a seasonal variation in finished-water THM concentrations during a 2-yr study of a northern Virginia water supply. Their data suggested that the high THM concentrations that were observed during the summer months may have been related, at least in part, to the chlorophyll-a concentrations in the reservoir water near the raw water intakes of treatment plants.

Thompson (1978) and Barnes (1978) demonstrated that haloform yields from chlorinated extracellular products (ECP's) of actively growing algae were higher than those that have been reported for chlorinated humic substances. They showed that the THM yields of the organic compounds that dissolved in the culture medium were greater than those from either the living or decaying algal cells. Algal ECP's often account for a large fraction ($\leq 30\%$–35%) of the carbon that was fixed during photosynthesis. This can result in a variety of compounds, including organic acids, especially glycolic ($HOCH_2COOH$), oxalic ($HOOCCOOH$), glyceric [$HOCH_2CH(OH)COOH$], and others; nitrogenous compounds, such as free amino acids and small peptides, which are produced in abundance by bluegreen algae (the cause of many nuisance conditions in reservoirs); carbohydrates, primarily as polysaccharides of reasonably high molecular weight, which are associated with sheaths and capsules; lipids, especially those with C_{16} and C_{18} fatty acids; and a variety of nucleic acids, vitamins, and "volatile substances," including 2-furaldehyde ($C_4H_3O \cdot CHO$), acetaldehyde (CH_3CHO), acetone (CH_3COCH_3), valeraldehyde [$CH_3(CH_2)_3CHO$], heptanal [$CH_3(CH_2)_5$-CHO], and an odor constituent "geosmin" (1,10-dimethyl-*trans*-9-deca-hol). Barnes presented a comprehensive review of the literature pertaining to the organic compounds that have been identified as algal ECP.

Other biologically derived compounds that are ubiquitous in water are the terpenes and related compounds, which are produced in abundance by terrestrial plants, especially conifers. The chlorinated derivatives of α-terpineol, which were reported by Carlson and Caple (1978) and discussed above, are another example of natural organic compounds, which in the past have virtually been ignored in chlorination studies. Chlorination produces a variety of other compounds whose toxicities have not been evaluated.

INFERENCES REGARDING TRICHLOROACETALDEHYDE

Keith *et al.* (1976) reported that trichloroacetaldehyde (CCl_3CHO, chloral) was found in the carbon–chloroform extracts (CCE) from 6 of the 10 city water supplies that were selected for detailed organics analysis during NORS. Two of the cities in which chloral was found (New York and Seattle) secure their water from uncontaminated upland water supplies. Keith *et al.* concluded that although chloral is an industrial product, its appearance in the CCE from these two water supplies is strong evidence that the compound was produced in some manner by chlorination. Chloral in water forms chloral hydrate [$CCl_3CH(OH)_2$], which is a highly toxic hypnotic drug. It is highly soluble; therefore, it is not recoverable by the analytical methods that were routinely used during NORS, which involve purging volatile compounds from solution by an inert gas.

Bellar *et al.* (1974) postulated that both chloral and chloral hydrate would be formed as intermediates in the formation of chloroform by the chlorination of ethanol in aqueous solutions. Keith *et al.* (1976) did not propose this sequence of reactions as an explanation for the appearance of chloral in any of the city water supplies. They did corroborate data from earlier reports that showed that chloral hydrate decomposes to chloroform slowly. In test solutions, only about 2% of the compound hydrolyzed to form chloroform in 24 hr.

As mentioned previously, Pfaender *et al.* (1978) demonstrated that direct aqueous injection of chloral hydrate into a heated gas chromatograph did not appreciably increase the recovery of chloroform. Therefore, while chloral does not appear to be a readily available source of chloroform in drinking water, its demonstrated presence and inferred relationship to chlorination indicate the need for further evaluation from a toxicological viewpoint.

CHLORAMINES

Combining ammonia (NH_3) with chlorine (Cl_2) to form chloramines for the treatment of drinking water has been called combined residual chlorination, chloramination, or the chloramine process. Objectives of this water treatment are to provide disinfecting residual that is more persistent than free chlorine in distribution systems and to reduce the unpleasant tastes and odors that are associated with the formation of chlorophenolic compounds (Symons *et al.*, 1977). Thus, this process utilizes the formation of monochloramine (NH_2Cl) as indicated in the following reaction:

$$NH_3 + HOCl \rightarrow NH_2Cl + H_2O \qquad (4)$$

The production of monochloramine is optimized by a pH range of 7 to 8 and a chlorine-to-ammonia ratio of 5:1 (by weight) or less (Symons *et al.*, 1977). White (1972) states that the preferred ratio is 3:1 (by weight).

At higher chlorine-to-ammonia ratios or at lower pH values, dichloramine ($NHCl_2$) and trichloramine (NCl_3), also called nitrogen trichloride, are formed according to the following reactions:

$$NH_2Cl + HOCl \rightarrow NHCl_2 + H_2O \qquad (5)$$

$$NHCl_2 + HOCl \rightarrow NCl_3 + H_2O \qquad (6)$$

These and organic chloramines are produced during the chlorination of water containing ammonia or organic amines. Their presence may contribute to taste and odor problems in the finished water (Symons *et al.*, 1977).

Ammonia may be added to the water before (preammoniation) or after (postammoniation) addition of chlorine. Preammoniation can prevent the formation of tastes and odors that are caused by reaction of chlorine with phenols and other substances. According to White (1972), postammoniation is the most often used ammonia–chlorine water treatment process.

The *Inventory of Municipal Water Supplies* (U.S. Public Health Service, 1963) indicated that only 308 of the 11,590 water treatment plants surveyed used an ammonia–chlorine process (Symons *et al.*, 1977).

Properties of Chloramines

Hypochlorous acid (HOCl) reacts rapidly with ammonia to form monochloramine, dichloramine, or nitrogen trichloride as shown in Reactions 4 through 6, respectively. The reaction products are dependent upon the pH, the relative concentrations of hypochlorous acid and ammonia, the reaction time, and the temperature (Morris, 1978).

Usually monochloramine is the only chloramine that is observed when pH values are greater than 8 and when the molar ratio of hypochlorous acid to ammonia is 1:1 or less. At pH values less than 3, only nitrogen trichloride is ordinarily detected (Morris, 1978).

Drago (1957) described the general chemistry of monochloramine, and Theilacker and Wegner (1964) and Kovacic *et al.* (1970) reported its organic reactions in some detail. Most of these organic reactions occurred in nonaqueous media. Although extremely useful for organic syntheses, these experiments have only limited value for predicting effects from drinking water treatment.

Monochloramine has been the principal subject of several reviews. Its properties and chemistry have been described by Metcalf (1942), Colton and Jones (1955), Jander (1955a), Drago (1957), Theilacker and Wegner (1964), Czech *et al.* (1961), Gmelin (1969), and Kovacic *et al.* (1970). Monochloramine is a colorless, water-soluble liquid with a freezing point of -66°C. It may decompose violently above that temperature (Kirk-Othmer, 1964, p. 914).

Relatively little is known about dichloramine. Chapin (1929) determined that its odor, volatility from aqueous solution, and relative solubility in various solvents are intermediate between those of monochloramine and nitrogen trichloride. He also found that dichloramine liberates iodine from acidified potassium iodide (KI) solution as do the other chloramines. Dichloramine solutions are reported to be unstable (Corbett *et al.*, 1953; Palin, 1950). Recently, Gray and Margerum (1978) reported that aqueous dichloramine solutions are more stable than previously thought and, thus, may be more significant in the water treatment process.

Nitrogen trichloride is a bright yellow liquid with a strong irritating odor and lachrymatory fumes. Its melting point is below -40°C; its boiling point is 70°C. It is extremely explosive and, therefore, dangerous,

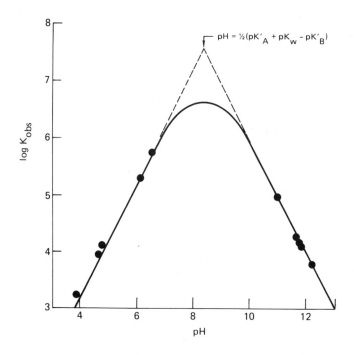

FIGURE III-2 Variation in rate of chloramine formation with pH. Calculated with log K_n Z 8.48. From Morris, 1978.

TABLE III-4   Specific Rates for Chloramine Formation at 20°C[a]

Chloramine	$k, M^{-1} s^{-1}$
Monochloramine[b]	5.6×10^6
Dichloramine[c]	2.7×10^2

[a] From Saguinsin and Morris, 1975.
[b] Assuming reaction between neutral molecules.
[c] For reactions not catalyzed by acid.

except at very low concentrations. Its solubility in water is limited (Kirk-Othmer, 1964, p. 916). In aqueous solutions it decomposes slowly to ammonia and hypochlorous acid (Remick, 1942). Corbett et al. (1953) observed that aqueous solutions of nitrogen trichloride are stabilized by small amounts of acid. The compound is an effective chlorinating agent, particularly in nonaqueous media (Dowell and Bray, 1917; Houben and Weyl, 1962; Jander, 1955b; Kovacic et al., 1970).

Monochloramine is the principal chloramine that is encountered under the usual conditions of water treatment. The rate of its formation, shown in Reaction 4, is extremely rapid at the concentrations and conditions of water treatment. At the pH range of most water supplies, the reaction is usually 90% complete in approximately 1 min. As shown in Figure III-2, the reaction rate is maximum at pH 8.5 (Morris, 1978; Weil and Morris, 1949).

The specific rate of formation of dichloramine is much slower than that for monochloramine except at pH values less than 5.5 (Morris, 1978) (see Table III-4). Because dichloramine forms much more slowly than monochloramine at near-neutral pH values, dichloramine does not constitute a large percentage of the available chlorine unless the waters are quite acid or when the molar ratio of chlorine to ammonia is greater than 1. The relative proportion of dichloramine and monochloramine for equimolar chlorine and ammonia and for 25% excess ammonia from pH 4–9 are shown in Figure III-3 (Morris, 1978). Dichloramine is much less stable than monochloramine or nitrogen trichloride. The decomposition of dichloramine is simplified in Reaction 7. The actual reaction is more complicated: more chlorine is reduced and some nitrate is formed (Morris, 1978).

$$2NHCl_2 + H_2O \rightarrow N_2 + HOCl + 3H^+ + 3Cl^- \tag{7}$$

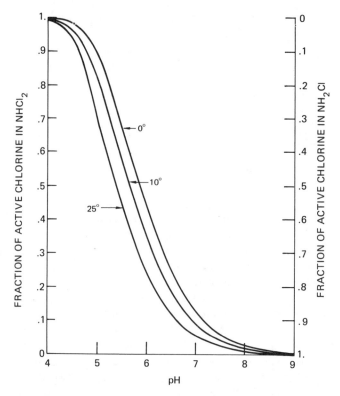

FIGURE III-3 Proportions of monochloramine (NH₂Cl) and dichloramine (NHCl₂) formed in water chlorination with equimolar concentrations of chlorine and ammonia (Morris, personal communication).

In acid solutions (pH 4 or less) or in solutions where chlorine concentrations far exceed those of ammonia, nitrogen trichloride is formed. Because nitrogen trichloride is formed from dichloramine, the reaction occurs only under conditions in which the dichloramine is reasonably stable. Thus, nitrogen trichloride is the only chloramine at pH values less than 3. At chlorine-to-ammonia molar ratios greater than 2, nitrogen trichloride occurs in diminishing proportions up to pH values of 7.5. Above pH 7.5, no nitrogen trichloride is found regardless of the ratio of chlorine to ammonia (Morris, 1978).

When chlorine is added to waters containing ammonia, the "breakpoint" phenomenon becomes significant in the pH range of 6 to 9. At chlorine-to-ammonia molar ratios of 0 up to 1, monochloramine is formed, thereby creating the "peak" shown in Figure II-3 (Chap. II). At values greater than 1, dichloramine is formed. Being unstable, it decomposes, usually as indicated in Reaction 7. Thus, with the addition of chlorine the apparent chlorine residual decreases from a chlorine-to-ammonia molar ratio of 1 up to approximately 1.65, at which the breakpoint occurs, i.e., after the ammonia has been converted principally to nitrogen (N_2) and some nitrate (see Figure II-3 in Chap. II). Chlorine that is added after the breakpoint exists as free chlorine, i.e., hypochlorous acid and the hypochlorite ion (OCl^-) (Morris, 1978; Wei, 1972; Wei and Morris, 1974).

Chloramine By-Products Found in Drinking Water and Selected Nonpotable Waters

Very few chemical studies of drinking water have been designed to identify the products resulting from the reaction of chloramines with organic or inorganic constituents of the water supplies.

Monochloramine is less effective as a chlorinating agent than hypochlorous acid by a factor of approximately 10^4 (Morris, 1967). Presumably, many of the reaction products of chlorination of water will be formed from chloramination because of the hydrolysis of chloramines to hypochlorous acid; however, the products should occur in lower concentrations because of the low equilibrium concentrations of the acid. According to Margerum and Gray (1978) the hydrolysis of monochloramine,

$$NH_2Cl + H_2O \rightarrow HOCl + NH_3 \tag{8}$$

has a reaction half-time of 10 hr. The equilibrium constant is $K = 6.7 \times 10^{-12}$.

Margerum and Gray (1978) indicate that the formation of hydroxylamine (NH_2OH),

$$NH_2Cl + OH^- \rightarrow NH_2OH + Cl^- \tag{9}$$

at pH 8 has a reaction half-time of 350 yr. Therefore, it probably does not occur in water treatment.

Stevens et al. (1978) determined that trihalomethane (THM) formation was minimized when chloramines (mostly monochloramine) were used to treat raw water. Chlorine was added at 5.5 mg/liter to raw water and to raw water spiked with 20 mg/liter ammonium chloride (NH_4Cl) (ammonia nitrogen, 5.2 mg/liter) (see Figure III-4). Thus, during

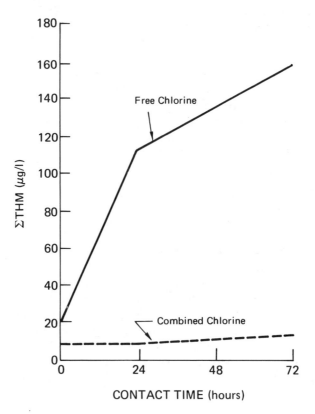

FIGURE III-4   Comparison of THM formation with free
and combined chlorine in Ohio River water, at pH 7.0 and
25°C. (Chlorine dosage 5.5 mg/liter: free chlorine values
represent raw water, combined chlorine values represent raw
water spiked with 20 mg/liter ammonium chloride.) Based on
Stevens *et al.*, 1978; Symons *et al.*, 1975.

chlorination of water where the ammonia breakpoint is not achieved,
THM production may not be great (Stevens *et al.*, 1978).

Rickabaugh and Kinman (1978) determined that chloramination of
Ohio River water with monochloramine at 10 mg/liter, pH 7 to 9, and
25°C resulted in 90.7% to 99.9% less production of THM as compared
with THM production from chlorination with 10 mg/liter chlorine as
hypochlorous and hypochlorite ion.

In the 1975 National Organics Reconnaissance Survey (NORS), 10 of
the 80 water supplies sampled had been disinfected with chloramines.
The concentration of THM's in the finished water of these utilities

ranged from 1 to 81 μg/liter with an average of 19 μg/liter. The THM concentrations in treatment plants using breakpoint chlorination ranged from 1 to 472 μg/liter, averaging 72 μg/liter (Symons *et al.*, 1977).

Chloramination of Model Compounds

N-Chloroorganic compounds, such as *N*-chloroglycine [H(Cl)-NCH$_2$COOH] and chlorophenols, may be by-products of the chloramine water treatment process.

According to Margerum and Gray (1978), monochloramine is a chlorinating agent for *N*-compounds in aqueous solutions. For example, with 10^{-4} *M* glycine the following reaction takes place:

$$NH_2Cl + H_2NCH_2COOH \rightarrow H(Cl)NCH_2COOH + NH_3 \qquad (10)$$

The rate constant (K) for this reaction is 1.5 $M^{-1}s^{-1}$ at pH 5 to 9, making it or similar reactions probable in aqueous systems. This report also corroborates the observation of Ellis and Soper (1954) that monochloramine undergoes chlorine-exchange reactions with primary and secondary aliphatic amines.

Although initially no chlorophenols are formed when low concentrations (milligram-per-liter range) of monochloramine and phenol are mixed, they appear after a reaction time of several days (Burttschell *et al.*, 1959).

Inferences of Possible Chloramine Reaction By-Products

Reaction products from aqueous chloramine reactions are presented in Table III-5. The types of reaction are quite varied. They include addition, chlorine substitution, oxidation, amination, and free radical reactions. The majority of these reactions involve either highly acidic or highly alkaline solutions. Thus, deducing or inferring the presence of such reaction by-products in the chloramine water treatment process is a highly speculative activity. This is particularly true if the substrate is present in the water supply only in trace or very low concentrations. Much of the considerable reported research concerning chloramine reactions used organic solvents, such as ether. Because reactions in organic solvents have limited value in predicting by-products of the chloramine water treatment process, they were not included in Table III-5.

Reactions of chloramides, such as chloramine-T (p-CH$_3$C$_6$-H$_4$SO$_2$NCl$^-$Na$^+$) have been studied extensively. Selected recent papers have been referenced in Table III-6. If present at all, such chloramides

TABLE III-5   Aqueous Chloramine Reactions with Organic Compounds: Summary of Reaction Products

Substrate	Products	Reaction Conditions	Reference
Olefins R–CH=CH–R' + NH₂Cl	β-chloramines $$R-\overset{\underset{\displaystyle H}{|}}{\underset{\underset{\displaystyle Cl}{|}}{C}}-\overset{\underset{\displaystyle H}{|}}{\underset{\underset{\displaystyle NH_2}{|}}{C}}-R$$	0.5 M chloramine, 4 M H₂SO₄, 20°C	Neale, 1964
Acetylenes R–C≡C–H + NH₂Cl	β-chloroaldehydes $$R-\overset{\underset{\displaystyle H}{|}}{\underset{\underset{\displaystyle Cl}{|}}{C}}-\overset{\displaystyle O}{\overset{\|}{C}}-H$$	0.5 M chloramine, 4 M H₂SO₄, 20°C	Neale, 1964
o-Hydroxyacetophenone (structure: benzene ring with O=C–CH₃ and OH)	2-Acetamidophenol (structure: benzene ring with N–C–CH₃ (H, O) and OH)	0.5 M monochloramine, pH ∼ 13, 0°C	Crochet and Kovacic, 1973
Anisaldehyde CH₃–O– (benzene ring) –C=O (H)	Anisalchlorimine CH₃–O– (benzene ring) –C=N–Cl (H) Anisonitrile CH₃–O– (benzene ring) –C≡N	Monochloramine, 0°C	Hauser and Hauser, 1930

175

o-Chlorobenzaldehyde	o-Chlorobenzalchlorimine	Monochloramine, 0°C	Hauser and Hauser, 1930
H C=O with Cl-phenyl	H C=NCl with Cl-phenyl; o-Chlorobenzonitrile C≡N with Cl-phenyl		
Formaldehyde H_2CO	N-trichlorotrimethyl-enetriamine $(CH_2NCl)_3$	0.5 M monochloramine, 15°C	Cross et al., 1910; Lindsay and Soper, 1946
Phenol[a]	p-Aminophenol (H_2N—phenyl—OH); 4,4'-Dihydroxydiphenylamine (HO—phenyl—N(H)—phenyl—OH); Iminoquinone (O=phenyl=N–H); and also quinone chlorimide and indophenol blue.	Monochloramine, neutral pH	Raschig, 1907; Harwood and Kuhn, 1970; Standard Methods, 1975

TABLE III-5 (continued)

Substrate	Products	Reaction Conditions	Reference
Phenol ⟨benzene ring⟩–OH	Chlorophenols ⟨benzene ring⟩ with OH and Cl	Monochloramine at ppm conc., Several days	Burtschell et al., 1959
Thiol groups R–SH	Sulfides R–S–S–R	Monochloramine and dichloramine	Srivastava and Bose, 1975a,b
Thiols R–SH	Sulfenamides R–S–NH$_2$	Monochloramine, pH 12	Sisler et al., 1970
Cysteine HS–CH$_2$–C(NH$_2$)(H)–COOH	Cystine HOOC–C(NH$_2$)(H)–CH$_2$–S–S–CH$_2$–C(NH$_2$)(H)–COOH	Monochloramine 0.5-1.5 ppm, pH 8	Ingols et al., 1953
Tyrosine HO–⟨benzene ring⟩–CH$_2$–C(NH$_2$)(H)–COOH	N-Chlorotyrosine HO–⟨benzene ring⟩–CH$_2$–C(H)(N(H)(Cl))–COOH	Monochloramine 0.5-1.5 ppm, pH 8	Ingols et al., 1953

Substrate	Structure	Product	Conditions	Reference
Alanine	$CH_3-\underset{\underset{H}{\mid}}{\overset{\overset{NH_2}{\mid}}{C}}-COOH$	N-Chloroalanine $CH_3-\underset{\underset{H}{\mid}}{\overset{\overset{H-N-Cl}{\mid}}{C}}-COOH$	Monochloramine 0.5-1.5 ppm, pH 8	Ingols et al., 1953
Glycylglycylglycine	$NH_2-CH_2-C(O)-N(H)-CH_2-C(O)-N(H)-CH_2-COOH$	Terminal N-chloro-compound, N-chloroglycylglycylglycine $Cl-N(H)-CH_2-C(O)-N(H)-CH_2-C(O)-N(H)-CH_2-COOH$	Monochloramine 0.5-1.5 ppm, pH 8	Ingols et al., 1953
DNA		Unidentified	Monochloramine	Shih and Lederberg, 1976a, 1976b
Iodide		Iodine and hypoiodous acid	Monochloramine	Kinman and Layton, 1976; Standard Methods, 1975
Activated carbon		N_2 and NO_3^-, Organics unidentified	Monochloramine, pH 7.4 Dichloramine, pH 7.4	Bauer and Snoeyink, 1973; Stasiuk, 1974

[a]This reaction may be time dependent and may not occur with preformed monochloramine.

TABLE III-6 Aqueous Chloramide Reactions with Organic Compounds: Summary of Reaction Products

Substrate	Products	Reaction Conditions	Reference
Allyl alcohol $CH_2=CH-CH_2OH$	Acrolein $CH_2=CH-CHO$	Chloramine-T, pH ∼ 1	Mahadevappa and Naidu, 1973
Benzyl alcohol CH_2OH (phenyl)	Benzaldehyde $HC=O$ (phenyl)	0.02 M Chloramine-T, pH 1-2, acetic acid and perchloric acid, 25°C	Banerji, 1977
n-Butanol $CH_3CH_2CH_2CH_2OH$	n-Butanal $CH_3CH_2CH_2CHO$	Chloramine-T, pH 4-5.5, 45-60°C	Mushran et al., 1974a
Iso-butanol $(CH_3)_2CHCH_2OH$	Iso-butanal $(CH_3)_2CHCHO$	Chloramine-T, pH 4-5.5, 45-60°C	Mushran et al., 1974a
Iso-pentanol $(CH_3)_2CH_2CH_2CH_2OH$	Iso-pentanal $(CH_3)_2CH_2CH_2CHO$	Chloramine-T, pH 4-5.5, 45-60°C	Mushran et al., 1974a
Crotyl alcohol $CH_3CH=CHCH_2OH$	Crotyl aldehyde $CH_3CH=CHCHO$	0.1 N Chloramine-T, pH 1-7, 25°C	Naidu and Mahadevappa, 1976
Cyclohexanol (structure)	Cyclohexanone (structure)	Chloramine-T, pH 5, 50°C	Kumar et al., 1976a

Propan-2-ol $CH_3CH(OH)CH_3$	Not identified	Chloramine-T, pH $\sim$ 1	Natarajan and Thiagarajan, 1975
Xylose, arabinose, Mannose, galactose	Aldonic acids	Chloramine-T, highly alkaline, 45°C	Agrawal and Mushran, 1973
D(-)Ribose	Aldonic acid	Chloramine-T, pH $\sim$ 13, 32.5°C	Mushran et al., 1974b
D(+)Sorbose	Xylonic acid, Formaldehyde	0.002 M Chloramine-T, pH $\sim$ 13, 50°C	Sanehi et al., 1975
Hydroquinone, hydrazine, cinnamic acid, and ascorbic acid	Not identified	Dichloramine-T	Nair and Nair, 1973
Acetophenone	Phenyl glyoxal	Chloramine-T, ethanol, pH $\sim$ 13, 55°C	Kumar et al., 1975
p-Chloro-, p-bromo-, and p-nitroanilines	Substituted N-Chloroanilines	Chloramine-T, pH 7.4, 50°C	Trieff and Ramanujam, 1977

TABLE III-6 (continued)

Substrate	Products	Reaction Conditions	Reference
Aniline and substituted anilines NH_2—(ring)—R	N-chloroanilines $NHCl$—(ring)—R	Chloramine-T, 50% ethanol, pH 7.4, 25-20°C	Trieff and Ramanujam, 1977
Glutathione $HOOCC(NH_2)HCH_2CH_2C(=O)-NH$ $HSCH_2CHCNHCH_2COOH$ ($=O$)	Glutathione disulfide $R'-C(=O)-NH$ $\|$ $S-CH_2CHR^2$ $\|$ $S-CH_2CHR^2$ $\|$ $R'-C-NH$ ($=O$)	0.1 N Chloramine-T, pH 1.4 or 0.N Dichloramine-T, 25°C	Mahadevappa and Gowda, 1975
Thiols (e.g., cysteine) See Table 5.	Disulfides (e.g., cystine) See Table 5.	Chloramine-T, pH $\sim$ 1	Gowda et al., 1975
Valine, leucine, and phenylalanine e.g., valine $(CH_3)_2CHCCOOH$ (with NH_2 and H)	Nitriles e.g., 3 methylproprionitrile $(CH_3)_2CHCN$	0.1 N Chloramine-T, pH 5	Mahadevappa and Naidu, 1976

Phenylalanine and serine	Nitriles	Chloramine-T, pH 11-12, 40-45°C	Kumar et al., 1976b
e.g., Serine $HOCH_2-\underset{\underset{H}{\overset{NH_2}{\vert}}}{C}-COOH$	e.g., hydroxyacetonitrite $HOCH_2CN$		
Hydroxyproline	Pyrrole	Chloramine-T	Mani and Radhakrishnan, 1976
m- or p-Cresol	Chlorinated cresol	Chloramine-T, pH 1-10, max. rate pH 4.5	Antelo et al., 1974

would occur in the water treatment process only at very low concentrations. However, similar reaction products would be anticipated from chloramine reactions. The reaction summaries in Table III-6 include several substrates, e.g., carbohydrates that might be present in water supplies. They indicate that reaction by-products such as aldonic acids could occur in the chloramine water treatment process.

BROMINE AND IODINE

The use of chlorine for disinfection of public water supplies has proved so successful that there has been little impetus to test alternative halogens. In the late 1930's, bromine was used briefly at Irvington, California, but was abandoned because it was difficult to handle, it produced undesirable tastes, and a residual could not be maintained in the distribution system (White, 1972, p. 712). During the 1920's, iodine was added to the water supplies at Rochester, New York, and Sault Sainte Marie, Michigan. One reason for its use in these cases was goiter prevention, but this motivation disappeared with the advent of iodized table salt (Laubusch, 1971). A long-term study of physiological effects of iodinated drinking water was conducted in Florida prisons (Black et al., 1968; Freund et al., 1966).

Both bromine and iodine have been used in swimming pool disinfection. In addition, iodine that is administered in Globaline tablets, whose active ingredient is tetraglycine hydroperiodide, $2[(NH_2CH_2COOH)_4HI] \cdot 2\frac{1}{2} I_2$, has been adopted by the military to disinfect individual water supplies. Unfortunately, none of these applications has provided data on trace by-products. Therefore, an assessment of the potential of bromine and iodine to produce hazardous substances at the trace level must be based on less direct evidence.

Properties of Bromine and Iodine

Bromine and iodine may be introduced into water in several ways: in pure elemental form (Br_2 liquid or I_2 solid), as interhalogen compounds such as bromine chloride (BrCl) (Mills, 1975), or they may be released from various organic substrates (Goodenough et al., 1969; Morris et al., 1953). They may also be generated within the water by oxidizing bromide or iodide with an agent such as chlorine. Once the halogen has been introduced into water, it reacts rapidly. Consequently, its ultimate chemical form is controlled mainly by the composition and temperature of the water rather than by the nature of the halogen source.

Various aspects of bromine chemistry have been discussed recently by Johnson and Overby (1971), LaPointe *et al.* (1975), and Sugam (1977). In pure water containing no amino-nitrogen, the predominant form of bromine at near-neutral pH is hypobromous acid (HOBr). Above pH 8.6 at 25°C, this gives way to the hypobromite ion (OBr⁻). At pH values below 6, hypobromous acid will convert to Br_2, Br_3^-, bromine chloride, or other halide complexes. The exact nature of the predominant species and the exact pH of the transition is controlled by the halide composition of the water (Sugam, 1977). However, at the pH and halide levels of drinking waters, halide complexes are not abundant. In the presence of ammonia or organic amines, bromamines are formed. Unlike the analogous chloramines, the inorganic bromamines are labile and interconvert rapidly so that the species distribution is controlled by chemical equilibrium (Johnson and Overby, 1971). The bromamines decompose readily into primarily nitrogen gas and bromide (LaPointe *et al.*, 1975). At temperatures above approximately 70°C, alkaline hypo-bromite solutions decompose rapidly to yield the thermodynamically more stable anions bromate (BrO_3^-) and bromide (Br^-). At ordinary temperatures and at near-neutral pH, this reaction is very slow (Engel *et al.*, 1954); however, Macalady *et al.* (1977) have shown that the rate is appreciable in seawater under bright sunlight.

Iodine chemistry in drinking water has been discussed in detail by Chang (1958). Iodine differs from chlorine and bromine in several notable ways. Iodoamines are unstable and do not form to any appreciable extent in aqueous solutions. Hypoiodite (OI⁻), which becomes a predominant species only at very high pH, is not of practical importance because of the tendency of hypoiodous acid (HOI) to decompose rapidly to iodate (IO_3^-) plus iodide (I⁻) above pH 9.

$$3OH^- + 3HOI \rightarrow IO_3^- + 2I^- + 3H_2 \tag{11}$$

This decomposition is much faster than the analogous bromine reaction and results in a loss of most of the disinfecting capacity of the iodine. Unlike oxyanions of chlorine and bromine, iodate is thermodynamically stable in oxygenated water. Once formed, it is likely to be persistent. Also in contrast to both bromine and chlorine, the diatomic form of iodine (I_2) is fairly stable in aqueous solutions and can be the predominant species in neutral-to-acidic solutions. The exact pH at which hypoiodous acid predominance gives way to iodine depends upon the iodide concentration. If iodide is greater than approximately 10^{-3} *M*, then iodine is replaced by I_3^- as the predominant species in neutral-to-acidic solutions.

TABLE III-7   Comparison of Bond Energies and
Relative Hydrolysis Rates for Methyl Halides

Carbon-Halogen	Bond Energy[a] kcal/mol	Relative Hydrolysis Rate[b]
Methyl fluoride	105.4	0.04
Methyl chloride	78.5	1
Methyl bromide	65.9	28
Methyl iodide	57.4	16

[a] Pauling, 1960.
[b] Moelwyn-Hughes, 1971.

Although the predominant chemical form of a halogen under specified conditions of dose, pH, ionic strength of the halide concentration, and temperature can usually be predicted precisely, it may not be the active chemical species in disinfection or in the formation of organic by-products. The long-standing debate over the role of transient species, e.g., Cl^+, Br^+, H_2OBr^+, H_2OI^+, etc., in aromatic substitution reactions (Berliner, 1966; Gilow and Ridd, 1973; Swain and Crist, 1972) illustrates the difficulties, and, commonly, the ambiguities, that are associated with attempts to identify the active species.

With respect to their persistence in distribution systems, alkyl bromides and iodides are somewhat more labile than alkyl chlorides. The data in Table III-7 indicate that carbon–bromine and carbon–iodine bonds are somewhat weaker than carbon–chlorine bonds and are considerably weaker than the carbon–fluoride bond. The relative hydrolysis rates for methyl bromide (CH_3Br) and methyl iodide (CH_3I) are correspondingly greater than for methyl chloride (CH_3Cl) and methyl fluoride (CH_3F). Actual hydrolysis rates for trihalomethanes (THM's) and other disinfection by-products in distribution systems have not yet been determined. Although the bromo and iodo compounds hydrolyze relatively faster than the chloro compounds, absolute rates may be too slow for these reactions to have practical significance.

Bromine and Iodine By-Products Found in Drinking Water or Selected Nonpotable Waters

EXPERIENCE WITH DRINKING WATER SUPPLIES

Since neither bromine nor iodine are used to disinfect major public water supplies, it is only possible to establish the tendency of these disinfectants to produce hazardous by-products in the laboratory. However, it is possible to gain some insight into the problem by examining data for chlorinated water supplies. In these, traces of bromine and iodine are commonly produced by oxidation of very small amounts of bromide and iodide in the raw water. This phenomenon was first reported by Rook (1974), who discovered chloroform ($CHCl_3$), bromodichloromethane ($CHCl_2Br$), dibromochloromethane ($CHClBr_2$), and bromoform ($CHBr_3$) in chlorinated drinking water in Rotterdam. He showed that the ratio of ΣBr to ΣCl in the THM's was in excess of the Br(I) to Cl(I) ratio in the water, even if quantitative oxidation of the trace bromide was assumed. This indicated that the THM formation kinetics favored bromine selectively.

Rook's observations have been confirmed in many water treatment systems throughout the world. Abundant documentation substantiates that THM's are produced mostly by the chlorination process and are quite rare in the raw water (e.g., see Bellar et al., 1974; Environmental Health Directorate, Canada, 1977; Henderson et al., 1976). In addition to the four bromo–chloro haloforms, dichloroiodomethane ($CHCl_2I$) is sometimes observed. In the National Organic Monitoring Survey (NOMS) of the Environmental Protection Agency, this compound was found in 85 of 111 supplies during Phase II of the survey and in 50 of 105 supplies during Phase III, but it was not quantified. Iodine-containing THM's are probably underrepresented in the data on water supplies because the isolation techniques that are used in analysis are usually not very suitable for these relatively nonvolatile compounds. Nevertheless, the total organically bound iodine that can be produced by chlorinating drinking waters will be severely limited by the iodide in the raw water. Typical iodide concentrations in river waters are below 10 μg/liter (Livingstone, 1963; Turekian, 1971).

Shackelford and Keith (1976) listed 20 organic compounds containing bromine and iodine and the number of reports of their presence in water supplies (Table III-8). These compounds were not necessarily produced by disinfection. Indeed, this would be unlikely in many cases. However, the list is very instructive because of the clear analytical bias that it displays. All of the compounds are nonpolar, and most have relatively low molecular weight and high volatility. Undoubtedly, many compounds are overlooked because of limitations in the analytical methods that are used most frequently. For example, in view of the ease with which they form, it is surprising that there have been no reports of bromophenols in drinking water. The NOMS study produced evidence that 2,4-dichlorophenol [$C_6H_3(Cl)_2OH$] is produced by chlorination of drinking waters. It seems likely that some bromophenols would also have been produced, but this remains to be established.

TABLE III-8   Organobromides and Iodides Reported to be Found in Finished Drinking Water[a]

Parent Compound, Derivative	Parent Compound, Derivative
Acetylene, bromo	Methane, bromochloro
Benzene, bromo	Methane, bromochloroiodo
Benzene, bromochloro	Methane, bromodichloro
Benzene, dibromo	Methane, chlorodibromo
Butane, bromo	Methane, dibromo
Butane, dibromochloro	Methane, dibromodichloro
Butane, dibromodichloro	Methane, dichloroiodo
Ether, bromophenyl, phenyl	Methane, iodo
Ethylene, bromotrichloro	Methane, tribromo
Methane, bromo	Propane, 2-bromomethyl

[a] Data from Shackelford and Keith, 1976.

These studies of chlorinated water supplies show that large amounts of THM's would probably result if bromine or iodine replaced chlorine as the principal disinfectant, since THM's containing bromine and iodine are produced from traces of oxidized bromine and iodine.

LABORATORY STUDIES WITH POTABLE WATERS

The conclusion in the previous paragraph is also supported by several laboratory studies of river waters. Bunn *et al.* (1975) treated Missouri River water both with chlorine, in the form of calcium hypochlorite [$Ca(OCl)_2$], and with mixtures of chlorine and halide salts. This is analogous to the treatment of some swimming pools to which bromide or iodide salts are added and then oxidized with chlorine. The results of Bunn *et al.* reveal that the addition of potassium fluoride (KF) or potassium chloride (KCl) has little effect on the composition of the THM products (Table III-9). But in the presence of potassium bromide (KBr) or potassium iodide (KI), appreciable amounts of these halogens are incorporated into the THM products.

Similar experiments were performed by Rickabaugh (1977) and Rickabaugh and Kinman (1978). They treated Ohio River waters with hypochlorous acid (HOCl), hypochlorous acid plus iodide, monochloramine (NH_2Cl), monochloramine plus iodide, and iodine at pH's between 7.5 and 9.0. In addition to the usual four chlorine- and bromine-

TABLE III-9   Effect of Added Potassium Halide on THM Formation in Missouri River Water[a]

Halide Added	THM's, μg/liter			
	Chloroform	Bromodichloromethane	Dibromochloromethane	Bromoform
None	172	20	1	<1
1 ppm fluoride	158	17	1	<1
1 ppm chloride	166	18	1	<1
1 ppm bromide	21	35	30	50
1 ppm iodide[b]	67	15	1	<1

[a] Data from Bunn et al., 1975. Dose: 7 ppm chlorine from calcium hypochlorite.
[b] Substantial amounts of dichloroiodomethane, chlorodiiodomethane ($CHClI_2$), and triiodomethane (CHI_3) were found but not quantified.

containing THM's, they found dichloroiodomethane and bromochloroiodomethane (CHBrClI) when iodine was present. On a molar basis, the total yield of THM's increased with pH. Ten mg/liter of iodine produced 5 to 10 times less total THM than 10 mg/liter of hypochlorous acid. Treatment with monochloramine or monochloramine plus iodide produced even smaller amounts. It would be unwise to generalize too much from these data, since the doses were not comparable on a molar basis. Moreover, little is known about the relative halogen demands under the different treatment conditions. Nevertheless, they suggest that iodine may be a less potent generator of THM's than chlorine.

EXPERIENCE WITH NONPOTABLE WATERS

Kuehl et al. (1978) studied brominated organic compounds in the tissues of fathead minnows that had been exposed to sewage effluent treated with bromine chloride. The compounds that they found and their estimated concentrations are given in Table III-10. These compounds were identified by mass spectrometry. None of the compounds were found in control fish, which were exposed to effluent that had not been treated with bromine chloride. An obvious interpretation is that these compounds were synthesized by reaction of the bromine chloride with organic compounds in the effluent. The authors caution that they cannot rule out the possibility that the enhanced bromide levels in the exposed

TABLE III-10   Brominated Compounds in Fish
Exposed to Secondary Effluent Treated with Bromine
Chloride at Grandville, Michigan[a]

Compound	Estimated Concentration, ng/g
Bromoindole[b]	100-200
Dibromoindole[b]	10-50
Tribromoindole	10-50
Tetrabromoindole	10-50
Dibromomethylindole[b]	10-50
Tribromomethylindole	10-50
Tetrabromomethylindole	. 10-50
Dibromomethylbenzthiazole	5-25
Dibromophenol	10-50
Tribromophenol[b]	50-100
Chlorodibromophenol	5-25
Dichlorobromophenol	5-25
Dibromomethylphenol	5-25
Dibromoanisole	10-50
Tribromoanisole[b]	50-100

[a] Data from Kuehl et al., 1978.
[b] Compounds also found in fish at the treatment plant in Wyoming, Michigan.

fish caused biosynthesis of brominated compounds. Unfortunately, the effluent water was not analyzed.

Bean et al. (1978) examined the compounds that were recovered from XAD-2 resin through which chlorinated seawater had been passed. The bromide content of untreated seawater is about 65 mg/liter, well in excess of chlorine doses that are typically used for disinfection. Thus, in chlorinated seawater, bromide oxidizes rapidly, forming mainly brominated organic by-products (Helz and Hsu, 1978). Using gas chromatography and mass spectrometry, Bean et al. found several halogenated compounds including bromoform, bromoacetal [$BrCH_2CH(OC_2H_5)_2$], and various brominated aromatic compounds. Since the seawater was not dechlorinated prior to its passage through the resin, it is not clear which compounds were formed in the seawater and which were formed in the resin by reaction with bromine in the seawater. The authors concluded that, except for bromoform, the concentration of nonpolar halogenated compounds that were generated by chlorination of relatively pristine seawater appears to be very low, i.e., in the nanogram per liter range.

Bromination of Model Compounds

Rook *et al.* (1978) reported a series of experiments in which they compared the reactivity of chlorine and bromine to peat extracts and to several hydroxybenzene and methoxybenzene model compounds. When these two halogens were applied to peat extracts at the same molar level, the bromine tests produced about twice the molar yield of THM's in a 4-hr period. This was coupled with a much faster oxidant decay rate in the bromine tests. Experiments with the model compounds showed that both oxidants were more reactive at high pH. Chlorine reacted readily with both 1,3-dihydroxybenzene $[C_6H_4(OH)_2]$ and 1,3-dimethoxybenzene $[C_6H_4(CH_3O)_2]$. There was very little chlorine substitution with the 1,3-dimethoxybenzene since the reaction was mainly oxidative. In contrast, there was efficient substitution in both organic substrates when bromine was used. Since organic matter in natural waters is believed to include material containing hydroxybenzene and methoxybenzene structures, these experiments support the notion that bromine may be more effective than chlorine in generating haloorganic compounds.

Discussion and Conclusions

The unsatisfactory state of knowledge concerning potentially hazardous substances that might be generated in drinking water through disinfection with bromine or iodine results from the absence of data from operational water treatment systems. However, the evidence suggests that the behavior of these halogens will be qualitatively similar to chlorine. At the very least, the production of THM's can be anticipated. Traces of halogenated phenols and nitrogen heterocycles also seem likely. Some tenuous evidence suggests that the total THM yield would be greater for bromine than for chlorine, but less for iodine than for chlorine. Factors such as cost, adequacy of supply, and adverse physiological effects of constant exposure to iodide and its disinfectant efficacy are pertinent concerns when considering iodine as a replacement for chlorine in public water supply disinfection.

CHLORINE DIOXIDE

Chlorine dioxide (ClO_2) is an orange-yellow gas with a liquefaction temperature of 9.7°C at atmospheric pressure. It is explosive in either its gaseous or pure liquid state (Robson, 1964). Accordingly, it is usually prepared in solution at the place and time of use.

Properties of Aqueous Chlorine Dioxide

According to Henry's law, the coefficient for aqueous solubility of chlorine dioxide is 1.0 mol/liter/atm at 25°C and 3.1 mol at 0°C (Gordon et al., 1972). Dilute gas mixtures with less than 0.1 atm partial pressure of chlorine dioxide and dilute aqueous solutions are not explosive; they may be handled with ordinary precautions. However, even dilute aqueous solutions are somewhat unstable, particularly in light, tending to decompose through reactions that will be described later. Fresh solutions must be prepared daily and must be protected from light to be suitable as reproducible stock or test solutions.

Two principal methods are used for the preparation of aqueous solutions of chlorine dioxide for water treatment (Gall, 1978; Masschelein, 1967, 1969). The first, which is used in the United States almost exclusively, is the reaction of sodium chlorite ($NaClO_2$) and chlorine (Cl_2) in acidic aqueous solution, primarily by the following equation:

$$HOCl + 2ClO_2^- + H^+ \rightarrow 2ClO_2 + Cl^- + H_2O \qquad (12)$$

Reaction 12 is not entirely stoichiometric. Side reactions producing chlorate (ClO_3^-) consume some extra chlorine, so that an excess over the proportion that is indicated by the equation is required to utilize the chlorite (ClO_2^-) fully. For stoichiometric reaction, according to Reaction 12, 0.39 part of chlorine as Cl_2 is required for each part of sodium chlorite. In practice, 0.5 to 1.0 part of chlorine per part of technical sodium chlorite (80%) is commonly used (Dowling, 1974; Gall , 1978; Symons et al., 1977). The solution resulting after completion of Reaction 12 then contains excess aqueous chlorine and some chlorate along with the chlorine dioxide.

According to Masschelein (1969), optimal yields of chlorine dioxide (90% to 95% of the theoretical yield based on sodium chlorite) are obtained by mixing a strong sodium chlorite solution (300 g/liter) with aqueous chlorine solution containing 2 to 3 g/liter of Cl_2. The mixed solution is then usually passed through a reactor that is packed with inert turbulence-promoting material to give a contact time of 1 to several minutes for reaction. The resulting solution, containing 3 to 5 g/liter of chlorine dioxide, may be dosed directly into the water being treated or may be diluted to about 1 g/liter for short-term intermediate storage before dosing. The other method of preparing chlorine dioxide for use in water treatment is acidification of strong sodium chlorite solution, usually with hydrochloric acid (HCl). The major reaction is:

$$5ClO_2^- + 4H^+ \rightarrow 4ClO_2 + Cl^- + 2H_2O \qquad (13)$$

Side reactions leading to the formation of chlorate and even elemental chlorine also occur in this system, as in the other (Gordon et al., 1972; Taylor, et al., 1940). The side reactions are minimized when hydrochloric acid is used at a 1 to 2 molar concentration and mixed in excess with a strong sodium chlorite solution (Beuerman, 1965; Kieffer and Gordon, 1968; Masschelein, 1969; Toussaint, 1972).

According to Reaction 13, 0.322 part of hydrochloric acid is required per part of sodium chlorite for stoichiometric reaction. In practice, approximately equal parts, representing a threefold excess of hydrochloric acid, have been used. After a few minutes of contact to allow reaction to proceed to completion, the concentrated mixture may be dosed directly or given intermediate storage, as in the previous method.

The latter method, sometimes with an acid other than hydrochloric acid, has often been preferred for laboratory preparation of chlorine dioxide solutions as a means of avoiding the presence of excess aqueous chlorine (Dowling, 1974; Granstrom and Lee, 1957, 1958). Since chlorine or hypochlorous acid (HOCl) may be a product of decomposition of chlorous acid ($HClO_2$) under some conditions, however, the method does not assure freedom from contamination by aqueous chlorine unless special precautionary techniques are followed (Feuss, 1964; Miltner, 1977). Failure to observe such precautions casts doubts on a number of reported findings of chlorinated products from the reaction of aqueous chlorine dioxide with organic matter.

For industrial use, especially in the pulp and paper industry, where much greater amounts are used than in water treatment, chlorine dioxide is prepared by reduction of sodium chlorate ($NaClO_3$) with agents such as sulfur dioxide (SO_2), methanol (CH_3OH), or chloride (Cl^-), generally in several molar sulfuric acid (H_2SO_4) solutions (Gall, 1978; Sussman and Rauh, 1978). These processes are more economical than those based on sodium chlorite for the manufacture of large quantities of chlorine dioxide. However, they are more complex in operation, the formed chlorine dioxide must be swept from the reaction mixture with a gas stream and redissolved in water, contamination with chlorine usually occurs, and disposal of by-product wastes can be a problem. Nonetheless, adaptation of some of these processes to conditions of water treatment is being attempted (Gall, 1978), and practical methods may develop if demand for chlorine dioxide disinfection increases sufficiently.

The principal side reactions occurring during the preparation of chlorine dioxide solutions are:

$$4HClO_2 \rightarrow 2ClO_2 + ClO_3^{\ -} + Cl^- + 2H^+ + H_2O \qquad (14)$$

and

$$HClO_2 + HOCl \rightarrow 2H^+ + ClO_3^{\ -} + Cl^- \qquad (15)$$

These lead to the formation of chlorate as a significant by-product. Accordingly, the health effects of chlorate must be considered in connection with the treatment of water with chlorine dioxide. Gordon *et al.* (1972) have discussed these and other reactions that may occur in solutions containing chlorine dioxide, chlorite, and aqueous chlorine. They pointed out that many of the observed reactions appear to proceed through a transitory, common intermediate, Cl_2O_2, with a suggested structure:

$$
\begin{array}{c}
O \\
\parallel \\
Cl-Cl \\
\diagdown\!\!\diagdown \\
O
\end{array}
$$

This intermediate may undergo several reactions, including the following:

$$2Cl_2O_2 \rightarrow Cl_2 + 2ClO_2 \qquad (16)$$

This reaction is invoked to account for the appearance of aqueous chlorine in the acid solutions of chlorine dioxide that are used to bleach pulp (Lindgren and Ericsson, 1969; Lindgren and Nilsson, 1972). It may also account for the reported presence of hypochlorous acid or chlorine in reaction mixtures that are used for the preparation of supposedly "chlorine-free" chlorine dioxide (Kieffer and Gordon, 1968; Rosenblatt, 1975, 1978). On the other hand, many of these reports may simply reflect the inadequacy of most analytical methods for discriminating accurately between chlorine dioxide and free aqueous chlorine. Gordon *et al.* (1972)

concluded that the reactions of chlorite plus acid do give chlorine dioxide solutions that are free of chlorine. Chlorine dioxide is reasonably stable in neutral or mildly acid aqueous solutions at concentrations of several milligrams per liter or less, provided the solutions are shielded from light (Bowen and Cheung, 1932; Gordon et al., 1972). However, in alkaline solutions, it disproportionates according to the reaction:

$$2ClO_2 + 2OH^- \rightarrow H_2O + ClO_2^- + ClO_3^- \tag{17}$$

whose rate has been measured extensively (Gordon, 1964). Another decomposition reaction:

$$6ClO_2 + 3H_2O \rightarrow 6H^+ + 5ClO_3^- + Cl^- \tag{18}$$

occurs with measurable speed only in quite acid solution (Bray, 1906). As noted earlier, photochemical breakdown takes place readily. The initial reaction appears to be:

$$ClO_2 \overset{h\nu}{\rightarrow} ClO + O \tag{19}$$

but the complete mechanism of the photochemical reaction in solution is unknown. Hydrogen peroxide (H_2O_2), chlorite, chlorate, Cl_2O_3, oxygen (O_2), and chlorine have all been reported as intermediates or products (Gordon et al., 1972). Presumably, the chlorine dioxide will not persist in open basins or reservoirs, although it can remain for days in clean distribution systems. Residual persistence is discussed more fully in Chapter II.

Chlorine dioxide is a strong oxidizing agent. The normal pathway of action in mildly acid, neutral, and alkaline solutions is:

$$ClO_2(aq) + e^- \rightarrow ClO_2^- \tag{20}$$

for which the standard potential is $E° = 0.954$ V at 25°C. Reduction to chloride also occurs, but only in acid solutions, so that the reaction is of little interest for the usual conditions of water treatment.

INORGANIC REACTANTS.

Iodide (I^-), arsenite (AsO_3^-), and bisulfite (HSO_3^-) are some of the inorganic reductants that are oxidized by chlorine dioxide between pH 5 and 9. The chlorine dioxide is reduced to chlorite (Reaction 19). Manganous ions are also oxidized readily to manganic hydroxides, a reaction that is often used to precipitate manganese as hydroxide in water treatment (Sussman and Rauh, 1978; Symons *et al.*, 1977). Oxidation of ammonia (NH_3) in aqueous solution is not known to occur, but may not have been looked for adequately.

Chlorine Dioxide By-Products Found in Drinking Water and Selected Nonpotable Waters

The subcommittee found only one study of compounds that are generated in raw water as a result of treatment with chlorine dioxide. Stevens *et al.* (1978) reported several C_2 to C_8 aliphatic aldehydes, but no THM's as products of the treatment of Ohio River water with chlorine dioxide.

Chlorine Dioxide Reactions with Model Organic Compounds

There have been extensive investigations of reactions of chlorine dioxide with organic compounds, particularly phenols and amines. Results of these studies have been reviewed in detail in several articles and monographs (Gordon *et al.*, 1972; Masschelein, 1969; Miller *et al.*, 1978; Stevens *et al.*, 1978). Unfortunately, most of the studies were conducted in acidic solutions in which concentrations of chlorine dioxide and organic substrate were much greater than those encountered during water treatment. Consequently, the extent to which the findings are applicable to the pH values and concentrations of organic compounds that are found in drinking water sources is not clear. In addition, most reviewers did not specify the ranges of pH and concentrations to which their statements apply, thereby making it difficult to distinguish the conclusions that pertain to highly dilute, nearly neutral aqueous solutions.

Since chlorine dioxide reduces to chlorite when it acts as an oxidant in the nearly neutral pH range, it functions as a one-electron acceptor. The immediate oxidation product must have an odd number of electrons to conform to the general definition of a free radical. Except for the studies of Lindgren with lignin simulators (Lindgren and Ericsson, 1969; Lindgren and Nilsson, 1972) and of Rosenblatt on reactions with tertiary amines (Gordon *et al.*, 1972; Rosenblatt, 1978), this aspect of the reaction of chlorine dioxide with organic materials has seldom been considered in defining reaction pathways and products. Yet, the reactivity of chlorine dioxide with organic material often differs greatly from that of other oxidants because of this one-electron transfer. Despite this, some investigators have stated that products resulting from treatment of organic material in natural waters with chlorine dioxide are generally similar to those found after ozonization (Buydens, 1970; Miller et al., 1978).

In a broad sense, chlorine dioxide is most reactive with tertiary amines and phenols (Masschelein, 1969; Rosenblatt, 1978); it is moderately reactive with olefins (Gordon et al., 1972); and its reactivity with alcohols and aldehydes, yielding the corresponding carboxylic acids, appears greater than that of ozone and aqueous chlorine (Masschelein, 1969; White et al., 1942). It is less reactive with secondary amines than with tertiary ones, and it is very unreactive toward primary amines (Gordon et al., 1972). As noted earlier, its reaction with ammonia is unknown (Miller et al., 1978). Chlorine dioxide is unreactive toward saturated aliphatic hydrocarbons and aliphatic side chains, but the latter may be split from aromatic rings or other functional groups. Saturated carboxylic acids, carbonyl compounds, and amino acids are usually inert with chlorine dioxide (Kennaugh, 1957; Sarkar, 1935).

Chlorine dioxide has sometimes been called a "pure" oxidant, which refers to its failure to form chlorinated derivatives. This is certainly incorrect, for numerous chlorinated aromatic compounds (Masschelein, 1969; Miller et al., 1978; Paluch et al., 1965) and some chlorinated aliphatic substances (Lindgren et al., 1965) have been obtained from aqueous oxidations by chlorine dioxide. However, no THM's have been detected as reaction products of chlorine dioxide with organic materials, although investigators have looked for them carefully (Miller et al., 1978; Vilagenes et al., 1977).

One complication is encountered when considering the reactions of chlorine dioxide with organic materials: the normal reaction product of chlorine dioxide, chlorite, may also be a reactive agent in some circumstances. A nucleophilic reagent (Rosenblatt, 1975), chlorite has been proposed as a possible source of some of the chlorinated products that are found after reaction of aromatic compounds with chlorine dioxide (Lindgren and Nilsson, 1972). Chlorite also reacts with aldehydes in neutral or mildly acidic aqueous solution yielding chlorine dioxide in accord with the following overall equation (White et al., 1942):

$$RCHO + 3ClO_2^- + H^+ \rightarrow RCO_2^- + 2ClO_2 + Cl^- + H_2O \qquad (21)$$

This reaction has been used, for example, in the colorimetric estimation of sugars (Jeanes and Isbell, 1941; Spinks and Porter, 1934). According to Lindgren and co-workers (Lindgren and Ericsson, 1969; Lindgren and Nilsson, 1972), Reaction 21 may involve formation of hypochlorous acid as an initial product, which then reacts on other chlorite to regenerate chlorine dioxide in a chain reaction or reacts to chlorinate or oxidize other organic substrates. Formation of hypochlorous acid as a product in the oxidation of phenols by chlorine dioxide has also been postulated by Lindgren (Lindgren and Ericsson, 1969). His ideas are based on studies at pH 1 to 5 and millimolar or greater concentrations. The extent of these types of reactions for conditions of water treatment is not known.

Reactions of chlorine dioxide with phenol and substituted phenols have been studied by many investigators. An extensive list of references is given by Gordon et al. (1972). Probably the most detailed investigations that are applicable to conditions of water treatment have been those of Glabisz (1968) and Paluch (1964). See Gordon et al. (1972) for other citations. The major products of the reactions are quinones and chlorinated quinones, in which the initial ring structure is retained, and carboxylic acids such as oxalic (HOOCCOOH), fumaric (trans-HOOCCH = CHCOOH), and maleic acids (cis-HOOCCH = CHCOOH), which result from rupture of the aromatic ring.

Phenol has been found to give 1,4-benzoquinone, 2-chloro-1,4-benzoquinone, 2,5-dichloro-1,4-benzoquinone, and the previously listed products of ring rupture (Masschelein, 1969). The chlorine-substituted products have been found to increase with decreasing ratio of chlorine dioxide to phenol, while ring rupture increases with increasing excess of chlorine dioxide over phenol.

Substituted phenols are also oxidized to p-quinones. Para substituents are often stripped away in the process, as is the case with p-nitrophenol, p-chlorophenol, and p-hydroxybenzaldehyde (Miller et al., 1978; Symons et al., 1977). According to Glabisz (1968), p-alkylphenols and o- or m-dihydric phenols are more subject to ring cleavage than are other types of phenols.

There is some evidence that formation of chlorophenols precedes oxidation to chlorinated quinones (Glabisz, 1967). In his work with a limited concentration of chlorine dioxide that was mixed with 0.67 millimolar phenol, Spanggord found 2-chlorophenol, 4-chlorophenol, 2,6-dichlorophenol, 2,4-dichlorophenol, 2,4,6-trichlorophenol, 2-chloro-2,4-dihydroxybenzene, resorcinol [C_6H_4 1,3⁻$(OH)_2$], and fumaric acid as products (Miller et al., 1978). Also, at the Water Supply Research Laboratory of the Environmental Protection Agency in Cincinnati, chlorophenols were observed as reaction products at a chlorine dioxide to phenol molar ratio of 0.8, but not at 3:1 or 14:1 (Miller et al., 1978). Interestingly, hydroquinone [C_6H_4 1,4⁻$(OH)_2$] was observed at all molar ratios. Some formation of polyquinones was also indicated.

Some other types of aromatic organic compounds are much less reactive than the phenols. For example, it has been reported that benzoic acid (C_6H_5COOH), benzenesulfonic acid ($C_6H_5SO_3H$) (Schmidt and

Braunsdorf, 1922), and cinnamic acid ($C_6H_5CH=CHCOOH$) (Sarkar, 1935) do not react with chlorine dioxide. Benzylic acid [(C_6H_5)$_2$-C(OH)COOH] reacts only slowly (Paluch *et al.*, 1965). Dinitrophenols and trinitrophenols have also been found to be inert (Paluch, 1964). According to Gordon *et al.* (1972), anilines should react in much the same manner as do phenols. Reactions with amines have been studied extensively, particularly by Rosenblatt and co-workers (Gordon *et al.*, 1972; Rosenblatt, 1978). Tertiary aliphatic amines are very reactive, undergoing a free-radical, oxidative dealkylation yielding aldehydes and secondary amines as products. The typical reaction with triethylamine [(C_2H_5)$_3$N] has the overall equation:

$$(C_2H_5)_3N + 2ClO_2 + H_2O$$
$$\rightarrow (C_2H_5)_2NH + CH_3CHO + 2H^+ + 2ClO_2^- \quad (22)$$

Secondary amines react through a similar pathway, but more slowly. Most primary amines react only slightly (Rosenblatt, 1978). Benzylamines undergo a hydrogen-abstraction reaction, and β-substituted amines may exhibit oxidative fragmentation as a result of α,β-scission.

Most amino acids are not reactive under conditions that prevail during water treatment (Kennaugh, 1957). In mildly acid solutions, tryptophan (2-amino-3-indoleproprionic acid) is oxidized to indoxyl, isatin, and indigo red, the acetic acid side chain being concurrently removed (Fujii and Ukita, 1957; Schmidt and Braunsdorf, 1922). Tyrosine [*p*-HOC$_6$H$_4$CH$_2$CH(NH$_2$)COOH] gives dopaquinone and dopachrome at pH 4.5 (Hodgden and Ingols, 1954). Histidine [2-amino-4(5)-imidazole proprionic acid] is also somewhat reactive (Schmidt and Braunsdorf, 1922).

Additional reactions of nitrogenous materials are described in considerable detail by Gordon *et al.* (1972). Most of the compounds that are covered are not known as common pollutants in water supplies. Consequently, their findings are not clearly relevant to water treatment with chlorine dioxide.

Studies with other materials have been sparse and have been confined mostly to acid conditions, pH 1 to 4, and to the concentrations between 10^{-3} and 10^{-1} M, which are characteristic of pulp and paper bleaching. However, some of these studies have shown that a number of organic structures are quite unreactive with chlorine dioxide even under these conditions. Observed reactions are often attributed to hypochlorous acid or Cl$_2$ that are formed in other processes.

In contrast to ozone (O$_3$), chlorine dioxide is not highly reactive toward the olefinic double bond. The oleic chain of methyl oleate

$[CH_3(CH_2)_7CH=CH(CH_2)_7COOCH_3]$ (Leopold and Mutton, 1959; Lindgren and Svahn, 1966) or triolein (glyceryl trioleate) (Leopold and Mutton, 1959) reacts, even in acidic solution over several days, primarily by oxidation at a position α or β to the double bond or by scission at the α-β link. Cyclohexene (1,2,3,4-tetrahydrobenzene, C_6H_{10}) does undergo ring opening at the double bond, but also gives cyclohex-1-ene-3-one and 3-chlorocyclohexene as major initial products (Lindgren et al., 1965). With excess ClO_2, ring splitting occurs when dicarboxylic acids form. Moreover, Schmidt and Braunsdorf (1922) found fumaric, maleic, and crotonic ($CH_3CH=CHCOOH$) acids to be unreactive with chlorine dioxide.

Similarly, although primary alcohols may be oxidized to carboxylic acids or ketones in relatively concentrated acidic solutions, much less reactivity is apparent in dilute, nearly neutral aqueous media. For example, glucose at pH 2 oxidizes at the $-CH_2OH$ group, without opening of the furananose or pyranose ring (Flis et al., 1955), but Somsen (1960) found no reaction with ethanol or 2,3-butandiol [CH_3-CH(OH)CH(OH)CH$_3$] at pH 7, even at 80°C.

Aldehyde groups are more reactive. For example, Somsen (1960) found that acetaldehyde (CH_3CHO), butyraldehyde (CH_3CH_2-CH_2CHO), and acetoin [$CH_3CH(OH)COCH_3$] are oxidized to the corresponding carboxylic acids at pH 7. Otto and Paluch (1965) reported that an aqueous dispersion of benzaldehyde (C_6H_5CHO) reacts violently with chlorine dioxide. On the other hand, Stevens et al. (1978) reported that several C_2 to C_8 aliphatic aldehydes were products of the treatment of Ohio River water with chlorine dioxide.

The situation is complicated further by the reaction of chlorite ion with aldehydes to produce chlorine dioxide with concurrent oxidation of the aldehyde to carboxylic acid or carbon dioxide (Lindgren and Nilsson, 1972; White et al., 1942). Reaction takes place in neutral or slightly acidic solution:

$$H^+ + RCHO + 3ClO_2 \rightarrow 2ClO_2 + RCO_2^- + Cl^- + H_2O \qquad (23)$$

Formaldehyde (HCHO), in particular, reacts very readily, but acetaldehyde, benzaldehyde, and reducing sugars are also known to react.

Hydrocarbons and simple carboxylic acids are generally inert towards dilute aqueous chlorine dioxide (Stevens et al., 1978). However, Reichert (1968a,b) has shown that the polynuclear aromatic hydrocarbon, 3,4-benzpyrene ($C_{20}H_{12}$), reacts to give quinones and chlorinated derivatives. Reactions of polycyclic aromatic hydrocarbons have been described by Thielmann (1972).

Humates and fulvates react with chlorine dioxide (Buydens, 1970; Fuchs and Leopold, 1927), as its use for the bleaching of colored waters attests, but the nature of the reactions is not known. Phenolic materials are reported to be released from the humic matrix under certain conditions (Buydens, 1970). Some investigators have conducted studies with model building units for lignin and humic acid; however, they have used acidic, high-concentration solutions. For example, vanillin [4-$(HO)C_6H_3$—3—$(OCH_3)CHO$] at pH 4 or less suffers ring rupture to give β-formylmuconic acid methyl ester (Sarkanen et al., 1962), while vanillyl alcohol [4—$(HO)C_6H_3$—3—$(OCH_3)OH$] at a final pH of 1 forms chlorinated benzoquinones (Dence et al., 1962). Under similar conditions, veratryl alcohol [3,4-$(OCH_3)_2C_6H_3OH$] produces 4,5-dichloroveratrole [4,5—$Cl_2C_6H_4(OH_3)_2$] (Dence and Sarkanen, 1960). However, the pertinence of these findings to water treatment conditions is questionable, in view of the pH at which these reactions were observed.

Discussion

Much remains to be learned about the nature of the organic products that are formed in water supplies during oxidative treatment with chlorine dioxide. Clearly, chlorine dioxide, like other aqueous chemical oxidants, is selective in its attack on organic materials, so that only a small fraction, if any, is oxidized completely to carbon dioxide and water. The specific reactants and reaction products that are formed have been determined for only a few substances and, even then, in a very limited way.

Both oxygenated and chlorinated products may be formed, the latter being found most prominently in connection with the reactions of phenolic substances. Other products that might affect health are quinones and 1,2-epoxy compounds.

Formation of chlorinated products and quinones is greatest when the concentration of chlorine dioxide was limited in comparison with reactive organic matter. When the ratio of chlorine dioxide to organic carbon is large, e.g., 20:1 or more by weight, then many aromatic rings are broken and the principal products are carboxylic acids, ketones, and, possibly, aldehydes.

Unfortunately, economic considerations and concerns about possible toxicities of chlorine dioxide, chlorite, and chlorate will probably limit the use of chlorine dioxide in water treatment to concentrations that do not greatly exceed those of the organic carbon. Consequently, conditions that are conducive to the production of intermediate oxidation products are likely to be realized in practice. Therefore, the hygienic effects of these partial oxidation products— the quinones, chlorinated quinones, and epoxy compounds— need considering before any widespread usage of chlorine dioxide is undertaken.

On the other hand, chlorine dioxide is not known to produce THM's under any conditions (Love et al., 1976; Mallevialle, 1976). It even seems not to be active in oxidizing bromide to bromine or hypobromite, with possible subsequent formation of brominated organic compounds (Vilagenes et al., 1977). Its nonreactivity with ammonia is also an important and advantageous factor in the practical use of chlorine dioxide.

Research Recommendations

Primary targets for research are the potential toxicities and carcinogenicities of chlorine dioxide, chlorite, and chlorate.

Secondly, there is a need for much greater knowledge of the organic products that are formed during the treatment of humates and fulvates with chlorine dioxide and of the hygienic properties of those products, both individually and collectively.

Finally, additional research is needed on the reaction pathways and products for the interaction of specific aquatic pollutants with chlorine dioxide under conditions approximating those anticipated during the preparation of drinking water.

OZONE

Although ozone (O_3) has been used as a disinfectant of water for over eight decades (Lawrence and Cappelli, 1977), relatively little is known about its chemistry as an oxidizing agent of organic and inorganic solutes in aqueous solution. On the other hand, ozone reactions in nonaqueous systems have been studied thoroughly, mainly because of the widespread use of ozone as a degradative tool in the elucidation of organic structure (Murray, 1968). While it is probably true that much of this knowledge may be transferred to aqueous systems, particularly at low pH values (Hoigne and Bader, 1975), few definitive mechanistic studies have been conducted to confirm this view. Thus, a discussion of the chemistry of ozone by-products that are formed during water treatment is severely limited by a lack of specifically designed studies and by the poor definition of the organic materials involved.

This unfortunate situation probably will not prevail very long. Several studies in progress have been stimulated by the prospect that ozone will be used increasingly as a water treatment chemical and by the need for more information on by-products that may be formed from ozone oxidations of water contaminants. Some of these studies have been reported in preliminary form at scientific meetings (Rice and Cotruvo, 1978). Combined with the earlier literature, they allow one to see an emerging picture of ozone by-product chemistry. Clearly, much is left to be accomplished in this area.

This part of the chapter is divided into four sections. In the first, some of the physical and chemical properties of ozone as they pertain to its use as a water disinfectant are examined. The second lists those few cases where reaction by-products from actual in-plant use of ozone have been isolated and identified. The third section examines some studies that have been conducted with model compounds. The final section discusses reactions that are thought to be possible on the basis of the known chemistry of ozone and the various substrates that occur in municipal drinking waters.

Properties of Ozone

Ozone is a gas at normal ambient temperatures. It is unstable and highly reactive (Manley and Niegowski, 1967). Ozone is one of the most powerful chemical oxidizing agents known, having a standard redox potential in water of 2.07 V at 25°C. [For comparison, the value for hypochlorous acid (HOCl) is 1.49 V]. As a result, ozone is capable of oxidizing organic and inorganic compounds—in most cases with great facility. It is also particularly adept at oxidizing carbon–carbon double bonds, other multiple bonds, aromatic compounds, and most nitrogenous and sulfurous compounds in which the element is at a low oxidation state.

Ozone is moderately soluble in water. Manley and Niegowski (1967) have reported solubility data at various temperatures; however, saturated solutions of ozone in water seldom occur due to the decomposition of ozone or its tendency to react with dissolved materials in water. In practice, ozone doses of a few milligrams per liter are most commonly used in water treatment applications.

Ozone gas is generated at the site of application because concentrated mixtures of the substance are subject to detonation. Various reports place an upper limit of 9% to 20% ozone, but in practice ozone generators usually produce 1% to 2% ozone when air is used and 3% to 5% when pure oxygen is used as the carrier (Klein et al., 1975).

Ozone is generated by electrical discharge in the air or oxygen stream (Klein et al., 1975), by photochemical processes involving ultraviolet radiation (Briner, 1959), or by other methods. It decomposes in aqueous solution by a complex mechanism yielding oxygen and a small amount of hydrogen peroxide (H_2O_2) (Kilpatrick et al., 1956; Stumm, 1954).

Decomposition is catalyzed by hydroxide (OH⁻). Therefore, it occurs more rapidly at high pH values. Most importantly, the decomposition occurs at such a fast rate in neutral to basic solutions that an active disinfectant residual cannot be maintained in a water supply distribution that uses ozone as the primary disinfectant (Falk and Moyer, 1978; Symons, 1977).

Hoigne and Bader have shown that aqueous ozone chemistry is explicable in terms of two mechanisms: one involves "direct" reactions of ozone; the other involves reactions of active hydroxyl radical intermediates (Hoigne and Bader, 1975, 1976, 1977, 1978a,b). Hoigne has pointed out that the reaction involving radical intermediates is accelerated at high pH values and may yield a variety of products, some of which may serve as radical chain carriers or as chain-terminating agents. The nature of the medium may have a profound effect on the rate of the radical reaction, particularly if it contains amines, carbonates, and organic carbon (Hoigne, 1978a).

The direct reaction of ozone with organic substrates has been the subject of numerous studies, but in most cases the solvent has not been water (Bailey, 1975). The reaction with olefin compounds has been the most studied. It is now agreed that the so-called Criegee mechanism (Criegee, 1959) explains most of the products formed. In general, aqueous ozonolysis reactions of olefins would be expected to yield ketones and carboxylic acids plus small amounts of hydroxyhydroperoxides (Bailey, 1975).

Aromatic compounds, amines, acetylenes, and many other compounds have been subjected to ozonolysis in aqueous solution. The results of these studies have been reviewed by Bailey (1975), Oehlschlaeger (1978), Maggiolo (1978), and Rice (1977). These studies are summarized below. However, few studies have been conducted over the full range of conditions that are likely to prevail in a typical water treatment plant. The strong influence of pH and interfering substances such as ammonia (NH_3) and carbonate (CO_3^-) on ozone reactions may seriously limit the effectiveness of such studies. Nonetheless, a review of the available information confirms the need for further research to determine ozone by-products.

Ozone By-Products Found in Drinking Water or Selected Nonpotable Waters

Ozone is now used in over 1,000 drinking water plants in Europe and is being incorporated into some new plants in North America, predominantly in the Province of Quebec (Miller and Rice, 1978). In view of this experience, it is remarkable that so little is known about the formation of the by-products from organic or inorganic materials in the influent water. The subcommittee surveyed leading authorities in the European water treatment industry. With the exceptions noted below, they expressed no knowledge of "before and after" ozonization studies to determine what, if any, by-products of the ozonization process may be present in treated water. Similarly, the U.S. Environmental Protection Agency (EPA) authorities in this field, as well as private and academic scientists, purport to know of no such studies with the exception of a few that are in progress.

In the waterworks in Zurich, Switzerland, investigators have studied the by-products of ozonization (Schalekamp, 1978). These studies, which were conducted with assistance from the Swiss Federal Institute for Water Resources and Water Pollution Control (EAWAG), demonstrated that a series of aldehydes [n-hexanal ($C_5H_{11}CHO$), n-heptanal ($C_6H_{13}CHO$), n-octanal ($C_7H_{15}CHO$), and n-nonanal ($C_8H_{17}CHO$)] that were present after ozonization had not been present beforehand.

The origin of these aldehydes is not fully understood; however, Sievers and co-workers (1977a), while studying ozonized secondary wastewater effluent from a treatment facility in Estes Park, Colorado, found the same compounds. They also found n-pentanal (C_4H_9CHO) and the hydrocarbons n-hexane (C_6H_{14}), n-heptane (C_7H_{16}), n-octane (C_8H_{18}), and n-nonane (C_9H_{20}). Moreover, the concentration of toluene ($C_6H_5CH_3$) apparently increased.

Removal of organics at the water treatment plant in Rouen-la-Chapelle, France, has been discussed by Rice et al. (1978). Although they did not describe the details of the analytical procedures, their data show that ozonization produces no increases in the concentrations of the several organic materials that were monitored.

Other than these three studies, little is known about the reaction products from ozonization of natural or treated waters. Chian and Kuo (1976) and Kinman et al. (1978) have reported on the ozonization of secondary treated wastewater, but they found no new compounds resulting from the ozonolysis process. Glaze and co-workers and scientists at the Research Institute of the Illinois Institute of Technology (Klein, 1978, private communication) are involved in studies that are directed to this goal, but their results are not yet available.

The apparent lack of data on this subject may be attributed to the preoccupation of trace analytical chemists with the methods of gas chromatography (GC) and combined GC-mass spectrometry (GC/MS) for the analysis of organic materials at the parts per million level and below. These methods have proven to be invaluable for the analysis of volatile compounds, particularly nonpolar compounds that may be preconcentrated by various partitioning techniques; however, they have not been perfected for the analysis of very polar compounds, which may result from oxidation processes. Nor are these methods useful for labile compounds such as peroxidic compounds, ozonization intermediates that may affect health. Thus, it appears that investigators have yet to demonstrate the important products that are produced from the ozonization of organic materials in untreated and treated waters. To do so, these investigators will presumably use techniques such as liquid chromatography, Fourier transform infrared spectroscopy, etc.

Ozonization of Model Organic and Inorganic Compounds

Rice (1977) has reviewed several studies on the reaction products from the ozonization of various organic and inorganic compounds in aqueous solution. A recent monograph by Rice and Cotruvo (1978) contains papers from a 1976 conference on the products arising from organic materials treated with ozone or chlorine dioxide (ClO_2). Together, these two references contain the vast majority of papers on this subject. No critical examinations of the reliability of the data contained in the papers have been attempted in this report.

Tables III-11 through III-18 list products of ozonization of various classes of organic compounds. In most of the studies listed, if ozone was measured at all, it was simply reported that ozone was bubbled, at a measured gas phase level, into water plus substrate. Exhausting ozone gas or decomposition by virtue of contact with the bubbler first, etc., were generally not measured. Similarly, pH was seldom measured, despite its importance in such studies.

REACTIONS WITH INORGANIC COMPOUNDS

In general, ozone oxidizes inorganic elements to a stable high oxidation state. Among the common metallic elements, iron is converted to the ferric state (Mallevialle et al., 1978) and manganese to either the IV or VII oxidation state, manganate (MnO_4^{2-}) or manganese dioxide (MnO_2), and permanganate (MnO_4^-), respectively. Ozone followed by filtration has been used to reduce iron and manganese to levels below those required by public health standards (Kjos et al., 1975). Ozone effectively removes a variety of trace metals as insoluble oxides at pH values from 7 to 9 (Netzer and Bowers, 1975). Sulfur in organic compounds often is converted to sulfate (SO_4^{2-}) (Gunther et al., 1970; Mallevialle et al., 1978), although in this and other cases the lower oxidation states of the element will result if small amounts of ozone are used.

Bromine is oxidized first to hypobromite (OBr^-) and then to bromate (BrO_3^-) (Ingols, 1978). Although hypobromite may be unstable in

TABLE III-11   Summary of Ozonization Byproducts of Organic
Compounds—Aromatic Compounds: Benzene and Its Homologs

Substrate	Products	Reference
Benzene	Glyoxal	Jurs, 1966 in Rice, 1977
	Glyoxylic acid	
	Oxalic acid	
1,3,5,-Trimethylbenzene	Methylglyoxal[a]	Cerkinsky and Trahtman, 1972
	Formic acid	
	Acetic acid	

[a]Principal product.

comparison to bromate under usual conditions, its transient existence is
indicated by the formation of bromoform ($CHBr_3$) from the ozonization
of seawater (Helz et al., 1978). Presumably one would also find iodinated
organics under the same conditions.

The ammonium ion (NH_4^+) is resistant to ozone attack, but above pH
7 ammonia is oxidized to nitrate (NO_3^-), presumably with several forms
of intermediaries, including nitrite (NO_2^-) (Hoigne and Bader, 1978b;
Huibers et al., 1969; Singer and Zilli, 1975; Wynn et al., 1973). Organic
amines have yielded both nitrate and nitrite (Rogozhkin et al., 1970).
Again, the dose of ozone could determine the relative yield of the
oxidized forms in many cases.

Ozone has been used extensively for the oxidation of free and
complexed cyanide (CN^-) to cyanate (OCN^-) (Bollyky, 1975; Garrison et
al., 1975; Mathieu, 1975; Selm, 1959).

TABLE III-12 Summary of Ozonization Byproducts of Organic Compounds—Aromatic Compounds: Polynuclear Aromatics

Substrate	Products	Reference
Phenanthrene (in aqueous methanol)	2'-Formyl-2-biphenylcarboxylic acid CHO COOH 2'-Hydroxymethyl-2-biphenylcarboxylic acid HO CH$_2$ COOH Diphenide CH$_2$—O—C=O Diphenic acid HOOC COOH	Sturrock et al., 1963

Pyrene	Acetic acid **CH₃COOH** Oxalic acid **HOOCCOOH** Plus other water soluble acids.	Kinney and Friedman, 1952
Naphthalene	Salicylic acid	Jurs, 1966
3,8-Pyrenequinone	1,2,3,4,-Benzenetetracarboxylic acid	Ahmed and Kinney, 1950

TABLE III-12 (continued)

Substrate	Products	Reference

Naphthalene-2,7-disulfonic acid
 	
	Formic acid
	HCOOH
	
	Oxalic acid
	HOOCCOOH
	
	Sulfate
	SO$_4$$^{2-}$
	
	Glyoxal
	OHCCHO
	
	Mesoxalic acid
	HOOC–C–COOH
	       =O
	
	Mesoxalic acid semialdehyde
	HOOC–C–CHO
	       =O
		Gilbert, 1976b

Inferences of Possible Ozone Reaction By-Products

As indicated above, attempts to identify new by-products from the reaction of ozone with organic materials in water have been limited to rather conventional separation and identification methods. As expected, rather conventional compounds have been identified as reaction by-products; however, some of them have important characteristics. For example, paroxon ($C_9H_{10}O_2$) from parathion ($C_{10}H_{14}NO_5PS$) is reported to be more toxic than its precursor. Nonetheless, the most important by-products from many organic substrates may have been overlooked because of shortcomings of the analytical method that was used. There is indirect evidence of the presence of these species. Carlson and Caple (1977) observed residual oxidizing species in ozonized water long after ozone would have decomposed. Moreover, analysis of ozone in water by a purge method yields only 81% of the value that was obtained by the direct iodide/thiosulfate titration procedure (Brody, 1975).

It appears that studies have not shown that many of the labile intermediates, such as hydroxyhydroperoxides, peroxides, etc., are absent in ozonized organic solutions. Investigators simply have not looked for them carefully. These by-products may be of considerable significance to human health and need evaluating in this respect.

The Criegee mechanism for the reaction of ozone with carbon–carbon double bonds (Reaction 24) predicts that a hydroxyhydroperoxide will be formed as an intermediate when water is used as the solvent (Criegee, 1959).

Moreover, Oehlschaeger (1978) reported that various polymeric peroxides form in nonaqueous solvents, but there have been no known studies to determine if this occurs in water.

$$R_2C=CR_2 \xrightarrow{\quad O_3 \quad O_3\quad} R_2C-CR_2 \longrightarrow R_2C=O + R_2C^+-O-O^- \text{ (Carbonyl oxide)}$$

$$\downarrow HOH$$

$$R_2C \begin{array}{c} \diagup OOH \\ \diagdown OH \end{array}$$

$$\text{hydroxy hydroperoxide} \qquad (24)$$

210

TABLE III-13 Summary of Ozonization Byproducts or Organic Compounds—Aromatic Compounds: Phenolics

Substrate	Products	Reference
Cresols 	Salicylic acid[a] (from o-Cresol) Maleic acid $HOOCCH=CHCOOH$ (cis) Acetic acid CH_3COOH Oxalic acid $HOOCCOOH$ Glyoxylic acid $HOOCCHO$ Mesotartaric acid $HOOC-CH(OH)-CH(OH)-COOH$ Glycolic acid $HOCH_2-COOH$	Bauch et al., 1970
Xylenols 	Same Products as from Cresols plus Biacetyl $CH_3-\overset{O}{\overset{\|}{C}}-\overset{O}{\overset{\|}{C}}-CH_3$	Bauch et al., 1970

Hydroxyphthalic acid

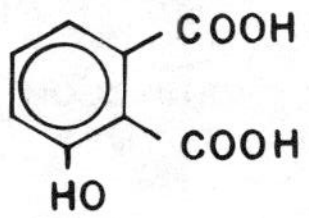

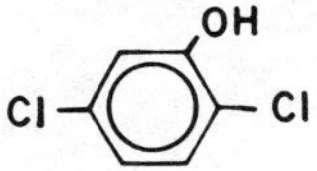

Formic acid

HCOOH

Oxalic acid

HOOCCOOH

Chloride ion

Cl⁻

Gilbert, 1976

2,4-Dichlorophenol

Chloride ion[a]

Cl⁻

Acetic acid[b]

CH₃COOH

Formic acid

HCOOH

Methylglyoxal[a]

OHC–C=O
     |
    CH₃

Gilbert, 1978

212

TABLE III-13 (continued)

Substrate	Products	Reference
4-Chloro-o-Cresol	Pyruvic acid[b] $CH_3-C=O$, $COOH$ (with $C-OH$ / carbonyl structure)	Gilbert, 1978
Phenol	Catechol[a] P-Quinone Muconic acid Fumaric acid $HOOC-CH=CH-COOH$ (trans) Oxalic acid $HOOC-COOH$	Eisenhauer, 1968
Phenol	Maleic acid $HOOC-CH=CH-COOH$ (cis) Tartaric acid $HOOC-CHOH-CHOH-COOH$ Glyoxylic acid $HOOC-CHO$	Bauch and Burchard, 1970

Oxalic acid
HOOC–COOH

| Phenol | P-Quinone, Catechol (as above) O-Quinone | Hydroquinone | Mallevialle, 1975 |

| Phenol | Catechol (as above) Resorcinol | | Spanggord and McClurg, 1978 |

| Phenol | Glyoxylic acid, Hydroquinone,[a] Catechol, Oxalic acid (as above) Glyoxal[b] **OHC–CHO** | | Gould and Weber, 1976 |

[a] Initial product.
[b] Intermediate product.

TABLE III-14 Summary of Ozonization Byproducts of Organic Compounds—Aromatic Compounds: Miscellaneous

Substrate	Products	Reference
Chlorobenzene	o-, m-, and p-Chlorophenols Chlorotartaric acid **HOOC—CH(OH)—CH(Cl)—COOH** Plus other ring ruptures products as from chlorophenols	Bauch *et al.*, 1970
Unsym-Diphenylhydrazine hydrochloride	1-Hydroxypenyl-1-phenyl hydrazine hydrochloride Diphenyl-N-hydroxyl amine	Spanggord and McClurg, 1978
	Diphenylamine Hydroxyphenyl-phenylamine	

Indole

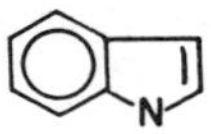

Skatole

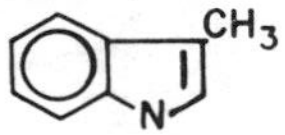

2-Amino-benzaldehyde

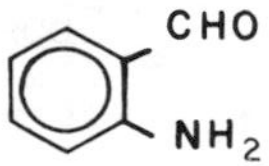

CHO
NH_2

2-Amino-benzoic acid

COOH
NH_2

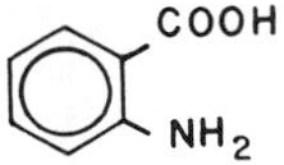

Jurs, 1966

Nitrobenzene

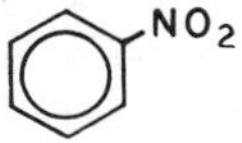

NO_2

o-, m-, and p-Nitrophenols

NO_2
OH

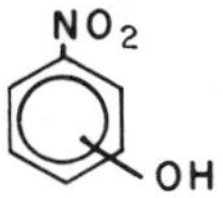

Westgate Research Corp., 1978

PCB Mixture

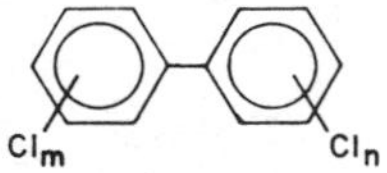

Cl_n
Cl_m

Chloro-benzoic acids

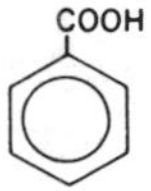

COOH
Cl

Benzoic acid

COOH

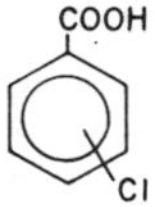

Chloride ion

Cl^-

Hydrogen peroxide

H_2O_2

Yokoyama et al., 1974

TABLE III-14 (continued)

Substrate	Products	Reference
Biphenyl 	Glyoxal **OHCCHO** Glyoxylic acid **HOOCCHO** Oxalic acid **HOOCCOOH**	Yokoyama et al., 1974
Styrene CH=CH$_2$ 	 $$H-\overset{\overset{\displaystyle O}{\|}}{C}-H$$ Formaldehyde; benzaldehyde[a] Benzoic acid	Yocum, 1978
4-Aminobenzoic acid 	Ammonia **NH$_3$** Nitrate **NO$_3^-$** Formic acid **HCOOH** Oxalic acid (as above)	Gilbert, 1976

Compound	Product	Reference
o-Toluidine	Acetic and oxalic acids (as above)	Chian and Kuo, 1976
N,N-Dimethyl-m-toluamide	Formic, acetic, and oxalic acids (as above)	Chian and Kuo, 1976
Phthalic acid	Oxalic and acetic acids (as above)	Kinney and Freidman, 1952

[a] Initial product.

TABLE III-15 Summary of Ozonization Byproducts of Organic Compounds
—Humic Acids and Similar Natural Products

Substrate	Products	Reference
Humic acid (Aldrich Chemical)	Malonic acid[a] $HOOC-CH_2-COOH$	Lawrence, 1977
	Hexanoic acid[a] $CH_3(CH_2)_4COOH$	
	Succinic acid[a,b] $HOOC-(CH_2)_2-COOH$	
	Heptanoic acid $CH_3(CH_2)_5COOH$	
	Benzoic acid[a,b] C_6H_5-COOH	
	Octanoic acid $CH_3-(CH_2)_6-COOH$	
	Glutaric acid[a,b] $HOOC-(CH_2)_3-COOH$	
	Adipic acid[a,b] $HOOC-(CH_2)_4-COOH$	

Pimelic acid[a,b]

HOOC–(CH₂)₅–COOH

Suberic acid[a,b]

HOOC–(CH₂)₆–COOH

Azelaic acid[a,b]

HOOC–(CH₂)₇–COOH

Sebacic acid[a,b]

HOOC–(CH₂)₈–COOH

1,2,3,-Propane tricarboxylic acid[a,b]

HOOCCH₂CH(COOH)CH₂COOH

Di-, tri-, tetra-, and penta-carboxylic Benzenes

1,2,3,4-Butane tetracarboxylic acid

Humic acid (Peat)	Crenic and Apocrenic acids	Shevchenko and Taran, 1966
	Oxalic acid **HOOCCOOH**	
Humic acid (Coal Derived)	Oxalic acid (as above) plus "ozone-resistant acids"	Ahmed and Kinney, 1950

[a] Also identified from ozonized lignosulfonic acids.
[b] Also identified from ozonized tannic acid.

TABLE III-16 Summary of Ozonization Byproducts of Organic Compounds—Pesticides

Substrate	Products	Reference
Parathion	Paraoxon	Gunther et al., 1970
	Paraoxon[a] (as above) 2,4-Dinitrophenol Picric acid (2,4,6-Trinitrophenol) Sulfuric acid H_2SO_4 Phosphoric acid H_3PO_4	Richard and Brener, 1976

Malathion	Malaoxon	Richard and Brener, 1978
$C_2H_5OOC\,CH_2$ $\overset{S}{\underset{}{\|}}$ $C_2H_5OOC\,CH-S-P-OCH_3$ $\underset{CH_3O}{\|}$	$C_2H_5OOC-CH_2$ O $C_2H_5OOC-CH-S-\overset{\|}{P}-OCH_3$ $\underset{OCH_3}{\|}$	
Phosalone 	Bis(chloro-6-oxo-2-benzoxazolyl-3-methyl) ether, Hydroxymethyl-3-chlorobenzoxazolone 	Richard and Brener, 1978
2,4,5-Trichlorophenoxyacetic acid 	Dichloromaleic acid[a] $HOOC-CHCl-CHCl-COOH$ Glycolic acid HCH_2COOH Oxalic acid $HOOCCOOH$ Chloride Cl^-	Weil et al., 1977

[a] Initial product.

TABLE III-17 Summary of Ozonization Byproducts of Organic Compounds—Aliphatic Compounds

Substrate	Products	Reference
2-Hydroxylpropane $CH_3CH(OH)CH_3$	Mesoxalic acid $HOOC-C-COOH$ $\parallel$ O Acetone[a] CH_3COCH_3 Oxalic acid $HOOCCOOH$ Pyruvic acid $CH_3C-COOH$ $\parallel$ O	Kuo *et al.*, 1977
Acetic acid CH_3COOH	Glyoxylic acid $CHO-COOH$ Oxalic acid (as above)	Kuo *et al.*, 1977
Propanol $CH_2CH_2CH_2OH$	Propanal CH_3CH_2CHO	Chian and Kuo, 1976
Propanoic acid CH_3CH_2COOH	Acetone (as above)	Chian and Kuo, 1976
Methylethyl ketone O $\parallel$ $CH_3CCH_2CH_2$	Acetate ion CH_3COO^-	Chian and Kuo, 1976

Compound	Products	Reference
Diethylether $CH_3CH_2OCH_2CH_3$	Ethyl acetate $CH_3CH_2OOCCH_3$; Acetate ion (as above); Acetaldehyde CH_3CHO; Methyl Formate $HCOOCH_3$; Ethanol C_2H_5OH; Acetone[b], ethyl formate[b]	Chian and Kuo, 1976
Polyethylene glycol $(-CH-CH-)_n$ OH OH	Ethylene glycol; diethylene glycol; triethylene glycol; pentaethylene glycol; organic acids; aldehydes	Yokoyama et al., 1974
Malonic acid $HOOC-CH_2-COOH$	Hydroxymalonic acid $HOOC-CH(OH)-COOH$; Ketomalonic acid $HOOC-C-COOH$ $=O$	Dobinson, 1959
Maleic acid (cis) $HOOC-CH=CH-COOH$	Glyoxylic acid[c] (as above); Formic acid[c] $HCOOH$; Glyoxal $OHCCHO$	Gilbert, 1976

TABLE III-17 (continued)

Substrate	Products	Reference
α-Terpineol 	4-(3-Oxobutanyl)-5,5-dimethyl-2-furanone 	Carlson and Caple, 1977
Oleic acid $CH_3(CH_2)_7CH=CH-(CH_2)_7$ $HOOC$	n-Nonyl aldehyde $CH_3(CH_2)_7CHO$ Octanoic acid[d] $CH_3(CH_2)_6COOH$ Suberic acid $HOOC-(CH_2)_6-COOH$ Azelaic acid[d] $HOOC-(CH_2)_7-COOH$ Azeladehydic acid[d] $OHC-(CH_2)_7-COOH$ 9,10-Dihydroxysteric acid $CH_3(CH_2)_7-CHOH-CHOH-(CH_2)_7-COOH$ 9,10-Oxyoleic acid $CH_3(CH_2)_7CH(O)CH(CH_2)_7COOH$	Carlson and Caple, 1977

		Reference
Linoleic acid CH₃(CH₂)₄CH=CH$\diagdown$CH₂ HOOC(CH₂)₇—CH=CH$\diagup$	n-Hexanal **CH$_3$(CH$_2$)$_4$CHO** n-Hexanoic acid **CH$_3$(CH$_2$)$_4$COOH** Azelaldehydic acid **OHC—(CH$_2$)$_7$—COOH** Azelaic acid **HOOC—(CH$_2$)$_7$—COOH** 3-Nonenal **CH$_3$(CH$_2$)$_4$CH=CH—CH$_2$CHO**	Carlson and Caple, 1977
Oxalacetic acid **HOOCC—CH$_2$COOH** $\Vert$ **O**	Mesoxalic acid (as above) Oxalic and Glyoxylic acids (as above)	Gilbert, 1978
Dihydroxyfumaric acid **HOOC—C(OH)=(OH)COOH**	Oxalic acid[c] (as above) Dihydroxytartaric **HOOC—C(OH)$_2$—COOH** Mesoxalic acid (as above) Mesoxalic acid Semialdehyde **HOOCCOCHO**	Gilbert, 1978
Glyoxal $\underset{H}{\overset{O}{\Vert}}C - C\underset{H}{\overset{O}{\Vert}}$	Oxalic acid (as above)	Gilbert, 1978

TABLE III-17 (continued)

Substrate	Products	Reference
Tartronic acid **HOOCCH(OH)–COOH**	Mesoxalic acid (as above)	Gilbert, 1978
Malonic acid **HOOCCH₂COOH**	Oxalic acid (as above) Mesoxalic acid (as above) Tartronic acid[e] **HOOCCH(OH)COOH**	Gilbert, 1978
Diethylamine **(C₂H₅)₂NH**	Acetaldoxime **CH₃CH=NOH**	Spangord and McClurg, 1978

[a]Initial product.
[b]Minor product.
[c]Major product.
[d]Also identified by Spangord and McClurg, 1976.
[e]Intermediate product.

EPOXIDE FORMATION

The possibility that ozone will produce potentially dangerous epoxides has been the subject of much informal speculation, but few studies on the subject have been reported. Carlson and Caple (1977) found oleic acid oxide from the aqueous phase ozonization of oleic acid, but subsequent experiments indicated that the compound results from the oxidation of the acid by peracid intermediates in the reaction mixture arising from the autooxidation of aldehydic products. No examples of epoxide formation from polynuclear aromatic compounds with aqueous ozone have been found, but the possibility that these compounds exist as minor products cannot be dismissed. Further study in this area is needed.

CONCLUSIONS

The preceding sections of this chapter summarize the results of an extensive survey of the chemistry of disinfectants that are or may be used in water treatment. Although it has been recognized since 1974 that chlorine produces potentially harmful by-products, such as the ubiquitous chloroform, little attention has been given to the other prospective disinfectants and oxidants such as ozone, chlorine dioxide, chloramines, and the other halogens, bromine and iodine. Quite apart from the question of the efficacy of these substances as alternative disinfectants, there remains the question, "Will the substitution of a disinfectant for chlorine in water treatment merely produce a different set of by-products whose effects on human health may be as significant, or more so, than those by-products known to be produced from chlorine?"

Unfortunately, a definitive answer cannot yet be given to this question. The surveys that are reported in the foregoing sections illustrate the lack of information on this subject even for the two common disinfectant chemicals, chlorine and ozone. There have been few studies in which the water of a treatment plant has been characterized before and after treatment, and, in most of these cases, chlorine was used as the disinfectant chemical. There are only two studies of water that had been treated with ozone, which is a common treatment in Western Europe, and no in-plant studies of water for which chlorine dioxide or the other halogens were used.

The authors were forced to resort to a survey of laboratory studies in which the various disinfectants were used or to works where a secondary wastewater was treated with one of the alternative disinfectants. As

TABLE III-18 Summary of Ozonization Byproducts of Organic Compounds—Miscellaneous Compounds

Substrate	Products		Reference
Caffeine	1,3-Dimethyl-2,6-dioxo-4-methylcarbamyl-S-triazine	Dimethylparabanic acid	Sievers *et al.*, 1977a

3,5-Dimethyl-2,4,6-
trioxo-S-triazine

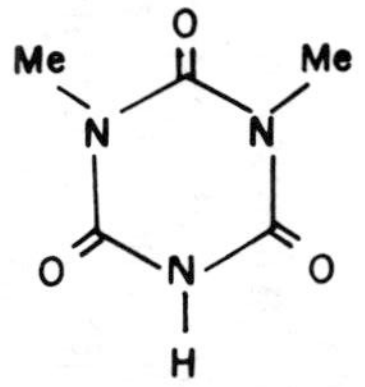

1,3-Dimethyl-
2,4-dioxo-S-
triazine

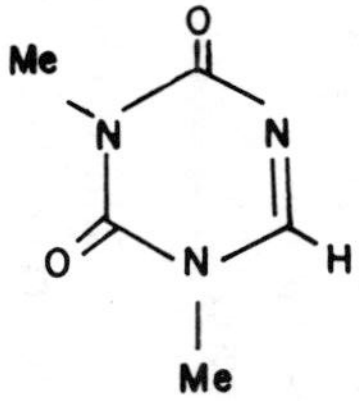

N,N′-Dimethyl-oxamide

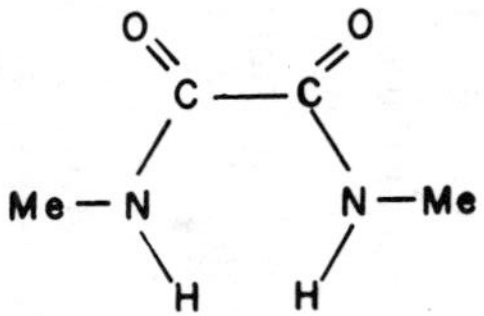

expected, these surveys showed that each disinfectant produces a set of by-product compounds that reflect the nature of the starting materials and the disinfectants that were used. Unfortunately, many of the laboratory studies were conducted under conditions that were not comparable to those in water treatment. For example, the initial concentrations of starting materials or disinfectant doses were too high, pH was too low, etc. Moreover, in most cases, the characterization of the by-products was incomplete or in other ways equivocated, so that a direct parallel could not be drawn between the laboratory results and those that could be expected in an actual water treatment plant.

Nonetheless, it is clear that each disinfectant chemical examined in this survey produces by-products that may occur in actual water treatment applications. Of particular concern are the following substances that result from the use of the various disinfectants.

• From chlorine: the trihalomethanes (THM's), trichloroacetone (CCl_3COCH_3), and other largely uncharacterized chlorinated and oxidized intermediates that are formed from the complex set of precursors in natural waters; chloramines; chlorophenols; and the largely unknown products of dechlorination.

• From ozone: epoxides that may in principle result from unsaturated substrates such as oleic acid, although none have yet been found in drinking water; peroxides and other highly oxidized intermediates such as glyoxal (OHCCHO) and methylglyoxal (CH_3COCHO) from aromatic precursors.

• From bromine and iodine: THM's and other bromine and iodine analogs of chlorinated species; bromophenols, bromoindoles, and bromoanisoles; plus the halogens themselves, which may remain in drinking water as residual.

• From chlorine dioxide: chlorinated aromatic compounds; chlorate (ClO_3^-) and chlorite (ClO_2^-), which are often present as by-product or unreacted starting material from production of chloride dioxide; and chlorine dioxide itself.

This list, incomplete as it is, is compelling in that it shows that each disinfectant produces chemical side effects that should be examined in more detail before the disinfectant is widely adopted for water treatment. It is clear that each of these disinfectants, being highly reactive chemical agents, will have inevitable side effects. Even in the case of chlorine, all of these side effects are not fully understood. This situation is due partly to the lack of systematic studies designed to evaluate by-products from each alternative disinfectant under actual water treatment conditions. But of equal importance is the need for these studies to utilize the complete spectrum of analytical instrumentation for the detection and identification of by-product compounds, not just for compounds that are amenable to extraction and GC/MS analysis. It appears that a preoccupation with these techniques has led chemists to omit from their characterizations those very polar, water-soluble components that might elude extraction and those high-molecular-weight or labile compounds that might not be detectable by GC/MS.

The subcommittee hopes that this report will stimulate future research that will avoid these deficiencies and provide more complete information on the by-products that are associated with the use of each alternative disinfectant under realistic conditions.

REFERENCES

Precursor Compounds and the Haloform Reaction

Bell, R.P., and O.M. Lidwell. 1940. The base catalyzed prototropy of substituted acetones. Proc. R. Soc. (Lond.) A176:88–113.

Black, A.P., and R.F. Christman. 1963. Chemical characteristics of fulvic acids. J. Am. Water Works Assoc. 55:897–912.

Burges, N.A., H.M. Hurst, and B. Walkden. 1964. The phenolic constituents of humic acid and their relation to the lignin of the plant cover. Geochim. Cosmochim. Acta 28:1547–1554.

Christman, R.F. 1978a. Progress Report, EPA Research Grant No. R 804430, for the period October 15, 1977, through January 15, 1978. University of North Carolina, Raleigh.

Christman, R.F. 1978b. Progress Report, EPA Research Grant No. R 804430, for the period July 15, 1978, through October 15, 1978. University of North Carolina, Raleigh.

Christman, R.F., and M. Ghassemi. 1966. Chemical nature of organic color in water. J. Am. Water Works Assoc. 58:723–741.

Christman, R.R., and R.T. Oglesby. 1971. Microbiological degradation and the formation of humus. Pp. 769–795 in K.V. Sarkanen and C.H. Ludwig, eds. Lignins: Occurrence, Formation, Structure, and Reactions. Wiley Interscience Publishers, New York.

Dubach, P., N.C. Mehta, T. Jakab, F. Martin, and N. Roulet. 1964. Chemical investigations on soil humic substances. Geochim. Cosmochim. Acta 28:1567–1578.

Fuson, R.C., and R.A. Bull. 1934. The haloform reaction. Chem. Rev. 15:275–309.

Gagosian, R.B., and D.H. Stuermer. 1977. The cycling of biogenic compounds and their diagenetically transformed products in seawater. Mar. Chem. 5:605–632.

Gjessing, E.T. 1976. Physical and Chemical Characteristics of Aquatic Humus. Ann Arbor Science Publishers, Inc., Ann Arbor, Mich. 120 pp.

Green, G., and G. Steelink. 1962. Structure of soil humic acid. II. Some copper oxide oxidation products. J. Org. Chem. 27:170–174.

Khan, S.U., and F.J. Sowden. 1972. Distribution of nitrogen in fulvic acid fraction extracted from the black solonetzic and black chernozemic soils of Alberta. Can. J. Soil Sci. 52:116–118.

Morris, J.C. 1975. Formation of Halogenated Organics by Chlorination (A Review). EPA-600/1-75-002, Office of Research and Development, U.S. Environmental Protection Agency, Washington, D.C. 154 pp.

Morris, J.C., and B. Baum. 1978. Precursors and mechanisms of haloform formation in the chlorination of water supplies. Pp. 29–48 in R.L. Jolley, H. Gorchev, and D.H. Hamilton, Jr., eds. Water Chlorination: Environmental Impact and Health Effects, Vol. 2. Ann Arbor Science Publishers, Inc., Ann Arbor, Mich. 909 pp.

Neyroud, J.A., and M. Schnitzer. 1975. Alkaline hydrolysis of humic substances. Geoderma 13:171–188.

Nissenbaum, A., and I.R. Kaplan. 1972. Chemical and isotopic evidence for the *in situ* origin of marine humic substances. Limnol. Oceanogr. 17:570–582.

Schnitzer, M., and S.U. Kahn. 1972. Humic Substances in the Environment. Marcel Dekker, New York. 327 pp.

Shapiro, J. 1957. Chemical and biological studies on the yellow organic acids of lake water. Limnol. Oceanogr. 2:161–179.

Steelink, C. 1977. Humates and other natural organic substances in the aquatic environment. J. Chem. Ed. 54:599–603.

Stevens, A.A., C.J. Solcum, D.R. Seeger, and G.G. Robeck. 1978. Chlorination of organics in drinking water. Pp. 77–104 in R.L. Jolley, ed. Water Chlorination: Environmental Impact and Health Effects, Vol. 1. Ann Arbor Science Publishers, Inc., Ann Arbor, Mich. 439 pp.

Stuermer, D.H., and G.R. Harvey. 1978. Structural studies on marine humus: a new reduction sequence for carbon skeleton determination. Mar. Chem. 6:55–70.

Whittaker, R.H., and G.E. Likens. 1973. Carbon in the biota. In G.M. Woodwell and E.V. Pecan, eds. Carbon and the Biospere. AEC Symposium Series 30:281–302. Technical Information Center, U.S. Atomic Energy Commission, Washington, D.C.

Chlorine

Andelman, J.B., and J.E. Snodgrass. 1974. Incidence and significance of polynuclear aromatic hydrocarbons in the water environment. Crit. Rev. Environ. Control 4:69–83.

Babcock, D.P., and P.C. Singer. 1977. Chlorination and coagulation of humic and fulvic acids. Proceedings of the 97th Annual American Water Works Association Conference held in Anaheim, California, May 8–13, 1977. American Water Works Association, Denver, Colo.

Barnes, D.B. 1978. Trihalomethane-forming potential of algal extracellular products and biomass. M.S. thesis. Virginia Polytechnic Institute and State University, Blacksburg.

Bell, R.P., and O.M. Lidwell. 1940. The base catalyzed prototropy of substituted acetones. 1940. Proc. R. Soc. (Lond.) A176:88–113.

Bellar, T.A., J.J. Kichtenberg, and R.C. Kroner. 1974. The occurrence of organohalides in chlorinated drinking water. J. Am. Water Works Assoc. 66(12):703–706.

Blakenship, W.M. 1978. Personal communication with R.C. Hoehn. U.S. Environmental Protection Agency, Region III, Water Supply Branch, Philadelphia, Pa.

Blumer, M., and W.W. Youngblood. 1975. Polycyclic aromatic hydrocarbons in soils and recent sediments. Science 188:53–55.

Brass, H.J., M.A. Feige, T. Halloran, J.W. Mello, D. Munch, and R.F. Thomas. 1977. The national organic monitoring survey: samplings and analyses for purgeable organic compounds. Pp. 393–416 in R.B. Pojasek, ed. Drinking Water Quality Enhancement Through Source Protection. Ann Arbor Science Publishers, Inc., Ann Arbor, Mich.

Burttschell, R.H., A.A. Rosen, F.M. Middleton, and M.B. Ettinger. 1959. Chlorine derivatives of phenol causing taste and odor. J. Am. Water Works Assoc. 51:205–214.

Carlson, R.M., and R. Caple. 1978. Organochemical implications of water chlorination. Pp. 65–75 in R.L. Jolley, ed. Water Chlorination: Environmental Impact and Health Effects, Vol. 1. Ann Arbor Science Publishers, Inc., Ann Arbor, Mich. 439 pp.

Carlson, R.M., R.E. Carlson, H.L. Kopperman, and R. Caple. 1975. Facile incorporation of chlorine into aromatic systems during aqueous chlorination processes. Environ. Sci. Technol. 9:674–675.

Christman, R.F., and M. Ghassemi. 1966. Chemical nature of organic color in water. J. Am. Water Works Assoc. 58:723–741.

Christman, R.F., J.D. Johnson, J.R. Haas, F.K. Pfaender, W.T. Liao, D.L. Norwood, and H.J. Alexander. 1978a. Natural and model aquatic humics: reactions with chlorine. Pp. 15–28 in R.L. Jolley, H. Gorchev, and D.H. Hamilton, Jr. eds. Water Chlorination: Environmental Impact and Health Effects, Vol. 2. Ann Arbor Science Publishers, Inc., Ann Arbor, Mich. 909 pp.

Christman, R.F., J.D. Johnson, and D.L. Norwood. 1978b. Progress Reports, EPA Research Grant No. R 804430 for Oct. 15, 1977, through Oct. 15, 1978.

Coleman, W.E., R.L. Lingg, R.G. Melton, and F.C. Kopfler. 1976. The occurrence of volatile organics in five drinking water supplies using gas chromatography/mass spectrometry. Pp 305–327 in L.H. Keith, ed. Identification and Analysis of Organic Pollutants in Water. Ann Arbor Science Publishers, Inc., Ann Arbor, Mich. 718 pp.

Fuchs, F., and W. Kuhn. 1976. The use of activated carbon to analyze natural waters with regard to their behaviour in waterworks filters. In H. Sontheimer, ed. Translation of Reports on Special Problems of Water Technology, Vol. 9. Adsorption. Conference held in Karlsruhe,West Germany, 1975. EPA-600/9-76-030. U.S. Environmental Protection Agency, Water Supply Research Division, Cincinnati, Ohio.

Garrison, A.W. 1978. Personal communication with R.C. Hoehn, U.S. Environmental Protection Agency, Southeastern Regional Laboratory, Athens, Ga.

Garrison, A.W., J.D. Pope, and F.R. Allen. 1976. GC/MS analysis of organic compounds in domestic wastewaters. Pp. 517–556 in L.H. Keith, ed. Identification and Analysis of Organic Pollutants in Water. Ann Arbor Science Publishers, Inc., Ann Arbor, Mich.

Gehrs, C.W., and G.R. Southworth. 1978. Investigating the effect of chlorinated organics. Pp. 329–342 in R.L. Jolley, ed. Water Chlorination: Environmental Impact and Health Effects, Vol. 1. Ann Arbor Science Publishers, Inc., Ann Arbor, Mich. 439 pp.

Giger, W., M. Reinhard, C. Schaffner, and F. Zurcher. 1976. Analyses of organic constituents in water by high-resolution gas chromatography in combination with specific detection and computer-assisted mass spectrometry. Pp. 433–452 in L.H. Keith, ed. Identification and Analysis of Organic Pollutants in Water. Ann Arbor Science Publishers, Inc., Ann Arbor, Mich.

Glaze, W.H., and J.E. Henderson, IV. 1975. Formation of organochlorine compounds from the chlorination of a municipal secondary effluent. J. Water Pollut. Control Fed. 47:2511–2515.

Glaze, W.H., J.E. Henderson, IV., and G. Smith. 1976. Analysis of new chlorinated organic compounds in municipal wastewaters after terminal chlorination. Pp. 247–254 in L.H. Keith, ed. Identification and Analysis of Organic Pollutants in Water. Ann Arbor Science Publishers, Inc., Ann Arbor, Mich.

Glaze, W.H., J.E. Henderson, IV., and G. Smith. 1978. Analysis of new chlorinated organic compounds formed by chlorination of municipal wastewater. Pp. 139–159 in R.L. Jolley, ed. Water Chlorination: Environmental Impact and Health Effects, Vol. 1. Ann Arbor Science Publishers, Inc., Ann Arbor, Mich. 439 pp.

Harrison, R.M., R. Perry, and R.A. Wellings. 1975. Review paper: polynuclear aromatic hydrocarbons in raw, potable, and waste waters. Water Res. 9:331–346.

Hase, A., and R.A. Hites. 1976. On the origin of polycyclic aromatic hydrocarbons in the aqueous environment. Pp. 205–214 in L.H. Keith, ed. Identification and Analysis of Organic Pollutants in Water. Ann Arbor Science Publishers, Inc., Ann Arbor, Mich.

Hoehn, R.C., and C.W. Randall. 1977. Drinking water disinfection and chlorinated organics formation. Proceedings AWWA Disinfection Seminar. Presented at the 97th Annual Conference of the American Water Works Association in Anaheim, California, May 8, 1977. Paper No. 11, pp. 1–18.

Hoehn, R.C., C.W. Randall, F.A. Bell, Jr., and P.T.B. Shaffer. 1977. Trialhomethanes and viruses in a water supply. J. Environ. Eng. Div., ASCE 103:803–814.

Hoehn, R.C., R.P. Goode, C.W. Randall, and P.T.B. Shaffer. 1978. Chlorination and treatment for minimizing trihalomethanes in drinking water. Pp. 519–535 in R.L. Jolley, H. Gorchev, and D.H. Hamilton, Jr., eds. Water Chlorination: Environmental Impact and Health Effects, Vol. 2. Ann Arbor Science Publishers, Inc., Ann Arbor, Mich. 909 pp.

Jolley, R.L. 1975. Chlorine-containing organic constituents in chlorinated effluents. J. Water Pollut. Control Fed. 47:601–618.

Jolley, R.L., G. Jones, W.W. Pitt, Jr., and J.E. Thompson. 1976. Determination of chlorination effects on organic constituents in natural and process waters using high-pressure liquid chromatography. Pp. 233–246 in L.H. Keith, ed. Identification and Analysis of Organic Pollutants in Water. Ann Arbor Science Publishers, Inc., Ann Arbor, Mich.

Jolley, R.L., G. Jones, W.W. Pitt, and J.E. Thompson. 1978. Chlorination of organics in cooling waters and process effluents. Pp. 105–138 in R.L. Jolley, ed. Water Chlorination: Environmental Impact and Health Effects. Ann Arbor Science Publishers, Inc., Ann Arbor, Mich.

Keith, L.H., A.W. Garrison, F.R. Allen, M.H. Carter, T.L. Floyd, J.D. Pope, and A.D. Thruston, Jr. 1976. Identification of organic compounds in drinking water from thirteen U.S. cities. Pp. 329–373 in L.H. Keith, ed. Identification and Analysis of Organic Pollutants in Water. Ann Arbor Science Publishers, Inc., Ann Arbor, Mich.

Kleopfer, R.D. 1976. Analysis of drinking water for organic compounds. Pp. 399–416 in L.H. Keith, ed. Identification and Analysis of Organic Pollutants in Water. Ann Arbor Science Publishers, Inc., Ann Arbor, Mich.

Laubusch, E.J. 1959. Standards of purity for liquid chlorine. J. Am. Water Works Assoc. 51:742–748.

Lee, G.F. 1967. Kinetics of reactions between chlorine and phenolic compounds. Pp. 54–74 in S.D. Faust and J.V. Hunter, eds. Principles and Applications of Water Chemistry. Proceedings of the Fourth Rudolfs Research Conference held at Rutgers State University, New Brunswick, N.J., 1965. John Wiley & Sons, Inc., New York.

Lee, G.F., and J.C. Morris. 1962. Kinetics and chlorination of phenol–chlorophenolic tastes and odors. Int. J. Air Water Pollut. 6:419–431.

Miller, G.W., R.G. Rice, C.M. Robson, W. Kuhn, and H. Wolf. 1978. An assessment of ozone and chlorine dioxide technologies for treatment of municipal water supplies, Part

2, Section 9. Draft Report. EPA Grant No. R 80435-01, Municipal Environmental Research Laboratory, Office of Water Supply, U.S. Environmental Protection Agency, Cincinnati, Ohio. 96 pp.

Morris, J.C. 1967. Kinetics of reactions between aqueous chlorine and nitrogen compounds. Pp. 23–53 in S.D. Faust and J.V. Hunter, ed. Principles and Applications of Water Chemistry. Proceedings of the Fourth Rudolfs Research Conference, held at Rutgers State University, New Brunswick, N.J., 1965. John Wiley & Sons, Inc., New York.

Morris, J.C. 1975. Formation of Halogenated Organics by Chlorination of Water Supplies (A Review). EPA-600/1-75-002, Office of Research and Development. U.S. Environmental Protection Agency, Washington, D.C. 154 pp.

Morris, J.C. 1978. The chemistry of aqueous chlorine in relation to water chlorination. Pp. 21–35 in R.L. Jolley, ed. Water Chlorination: Environmental Impact and Health Effects, Vol. 1. Ann Arbor Science Publishers, Inc., Ann Arbor, Mich. 439 pp.

Morris, J.C., and B. Baum. 1978. Precursors and mechanisms of haloformation in the chlorination of water supplies. Pp. 29–48 in R.L. Jolley, H. Gorchev, and D.H. Hamilton, Jr., eds. Water Chlorination: Environmental Impact and Health Effects, Vol. 2. Ann Arbor Science Publishers, Inc., Ann Arbor, Mich.

Munch, D.J., M.A. Feige, and H.J. Brass. 1977. The analyses of purgeable compounds in the national organic monitoring survey by gas chromatography/mass spectrometry. In Water Quality in the Distribution System. American Water Works Association's Fifth Annual Water Quality Technology Conference held in Kansas City, Dec. 4–7, 1977. Paper 3A–6, 5 pp. American Water Works Association, Denver, Colo.

Oyler, A.R., D.L. Bodenner, K.J. Welch, R.J. Liukkonen, R.M. Carlson, H.L. Kopperman, and R. Caple. 1978. Determination of aqueous chlorination reaction products of polynuclear aromatic hydrocarbons by reversed phase high performance liquid chromatography–gas chromatography. Anal. Chem. 50:837–842.

Pfaender, F.K., R.B. Jonas, A.A. Stevens, L. Moore, and J.R. Haas. 1978. Evaluation of direct aqueous injection method for analysis of chloroform in drinking water. Environ. Sci. Technol. 12:438–441.

Rook, J.J. 1974. Formation of haloforms during chlorination of natural waters. Water Treat. Exam. 23:234–243.

Rook, J.J. 1976. Haloforms in drinking water. J. Am. Water Works Assoc. 68:168–172.

Rook, J.J. 1977. Chlorination reactions of fulvic acids in natural waters. Environ. Sci. Technol. 11:478–482.

Rosenblatt, D.H. 1975. Chlorine and oxychlorine species reactivity with organic substances. Pp. 249–276 in J.D. Johnson, ed. Disinfection: Water and Wastewater. Ann Arbor Science Publishers, Inc., Ann Arbor, Mich. 425 pp.

Shackelford, W.M., and L.H. Keith. 1976. Frequency of Organic Compounds Identified in Water. EPA-600/4-76-062. Environmental Research Laboratory, Office of Research and Development, U.S. Environmental Protection Agency, Athens, Ga. 629 pp.

Sievers, R.E., R.M. Barkley, G.A. Eiceman, L.P. Haack, R.H. Shapiro, and H.F. Walton. 1978. Generation of volatile organic compounds from non-volatile precursors by treatment with chlorine or ozone. Pp. 615–624 in R.L Jolley, H. Gorchev, and D.H. Hamilton, Jr., eds. Water Chlorination: Environmental Impact and Health Effects, Vol. 2. Ann Arbor Science Publishers, Inc., Ann Arbor, Mich. 909 pp.

Stevens, A.A., C.J. Slocum, D.R. Seeger, and G.G. Robeck. 1976. Chlorination of organics in drinking water. J. Am. Water Works Assoc. 68:615–620.

Stevens, A.A., C.J. Slocum, D.R. Seeger, and G.G. Robeck. 1978. Chlorination of organics in drinking water. Pp. 77–104 in R.L. Jolley, ed. Water Chlorination: Environmental Impact and Health Effects, Vol. 1. Ann Arbor Science Publishers, Inc., Ann Arbor, Mich. 439 pp.

Suffet, I.H., L. Brenner, and B. Silver. 1976. Identification of 1,1,1-trichloroacetone (1,1,1-trichloropropanone) in two drinking waters: a known precursor in the haloform reaction. Environ. Sci. Technol. 10:1273–1275.

Symons, J.M., T.A. Bellar, J.K. Carswell, J. Demarco, K.L. Kropp, G.G. Robeck, D.R. Seeger, C.J. Slocum, B.L. Smith, and A.A. Stevens. 1975. National organic reconnaissance survey for halogenated organics. J. Am. Water Works Assoc. 67:634–647.

Thompson, B.C. 1978. Trihalomethane formation potential of algal extracellular products and biomass. M.S. thesis. Virginia Polytechnic Institute and State University, Blacksburg. 135 pp.

Vallentyne, J.R. 1957. The molecular nature of organic matter in lakes and oceans, with lesser reference to sewage and terrestrial soils. J. Fish. Res. Bd. Can. 14:33–82.

Chloramines

Agrawal, M.C., and S.P. Mushran. 1973. Mechanism of oxidation of aldoses by chloramine-T. J. Chem. Soc. Perkin Trans. 2:762–765.

Antelo, J.M., J.M. Cachaza, J. Casado, and M.A. Herraez. 1974. Influence of pH on the reaction of cresols with chloramine-T. An. Quim. 70:555–558; Chem. Abstr. 82:15941z (1975).

Banerji, K.K. 1977. Kinetics and mechanism of the oxidation of substituted benzyl alcohols by chloramine-T in acid solution. Bull. Chem. Soc. Jpn. 50(6):1616–1618.

Bauer, R.C., and V.L. Snoeyink. 1973. Reactions of chloramines with active carbon. J. Water Pollut. Control Fed. 45:2290–2301.

Burttschell, R.H., A.A. Rosen, F.M. Middleton, and M.B. Ettinger. 1959. Chlorine derivatives of phenol causing taste and odor. J. Am. Water Works Assoc. 51:205–214.

Chapin, R.M. 1929. Dichloroamine. J. Am. Chem. Soc. 51:2117–2122.

Colton, E., and M.M. Jones. 1955. Monochloramine. J. Chem. Educ. 32:488–489.

Corbett, R.E., W.S. Metcalf, and F.G. Soper. 1953. Studies of N-halogeno-compounds. Part IV. The reaction between ammonia and chlorine in aqueous solution, and the hydrolysis constants of chloroamines. J. Chem. Soc. 1953:1927–1929.

Crochet, R.A., and P. Kovacic. 1973. Conversion of o-hydroxyaldehydes and ketones into o-hydroxyanilides by monochloramine. J. Chem. Soc. Chem. Commun. 197(19):716–717.

Cross, C.F., E.J. Bevan, and W. Bacon. 1910. Chloramine reactions. Methylenechloroamine. J. Chem. Soc. Trans. 97:2404–2406.

Czech, F.W., R.J. Fuchs, and H.F. Antczak. 1961. Determination of mono-, di-, and trichloramine by ultraviolet absorption spectrophotometry. Anal. Chem. 33:705–707.

Dowell, C.T., and W.C. Bray. 1917. Experiments with nitrogen trichloride. J. Am. Chem. Soc. 39:896–905.

Drago, R.S. 1957. Chloramine. J. Chem. Educ. 34:541–545.

Ellis, A.J., and F.G. Soper. 1954. Studies of N-halogeno-compounds. Part VI. The kinetics of chlorination of tertiary amines. J. Chem. Soc. 1954:1750–1755.

Gmelin's Handbuch der Anorganischen Chemie. 1969. Chlor und Stickstoff. Pp. 483–500 in Gmelin's Handbuch der Anorganischen Chemie, 8. Auflage. Chlor Erganzungsband,

Teil B–Lieferung 2, System-Nr. 6. Verlag Chemie, G.m.b.H., Weinheim/Bergstr, W. Germany.

Gowda, N.M.M., A.S.A. Murthy, and D.S. Mahadevappa. 1975. Oxidation of cysteine with chlorimine-T and dichloramine–T. Curr. Sci. 44:5–6.

Gray, E.T., Jr., and D.W. Margerum. 1978. Kinetics and equilibria of chloramine species. In Abstracts of Papers of the 175th American Chemical Society National Meeting, Anaheim, Calif., March 13–17. Abstr. No. INOR 257.

Harwood, J.E., and A.L. Kuhn. 1970. A colorimetric method for ammonia in natural waters. Water Res. 4:805–811.

Hauser, C.R., and M.L. Hauser. 1930. Researches on chloramines. I. Orthochlorobenzalchlorimine and anisalchlorimine. J. Am. Chem. Soc. 52:2050–2054.

Houben, J., and T. Weyl. 1962. Halogen-Verbindungen. Pp. 760–811 in J. Houben and T. Weyl, eds. Methoden der Organischen Chemie (Houben-Weyl), 4. Auflage, Band 5, Teil 3. Geroge Thieme Verlag, Stuttgart, W. Germany.

Ingols, R.S., H.A. Wyckoff, T.W. Kethley, H.W. Hodgden, E.L. Fincher, J.C. Hildebrand, and J.E. Mandel. 1953. Bactericidal studies of chlorine. Ind. Eng. Chem. 45:996–1000.

Jander, J. 1955a. Ein Beitrag zur Kenntnis des Monochloramins. Naturwissenschaften 42:178–179.

Jander, J. 1955b. Zum Verstandnis der Chemie der Chlor-Stickstoff- und Chlor-Sauerstoff-Verbindungen. Z. Anorg. Allg. Chem. 280:276–283.

Kinman, R.N., and R.F. Layton. 1976. New method for water disinfection. J. Am. Water Works Assoc. 68(6):298–302.

Kirk-Othmer Encyclopedia of Chemical Technology. 1964. Vol. 4, 2nd ed. Wiley Interscience Publishers, New York.

Kovacic, P., M.K. Lowery, and K.W. Field. 1970. Chemistry of N-bromamines and N-chloramines. Chem. Rev. 70:639–665.

Kumar, A., A.K. Bose, and S.P. Mushran. 1975. Kinetic study of oxidation of acetophenone by chloramine-T. Ann. Soc. Sci. Bruxelles, Ser. 1, 89:567–574.

Kumar, A., R.M. Mehrostra, and S.P. Mushran. 1976a. Kinetics and mechanism of oxidation of cyclohexanol by chloramine-T. Bull. Acad. Pol. Sci., Ser. Sci. Chim. XXIV:181–185.

Kumar, A., A.K. Bose, and S.P. Mushran. 1976b. Kinetics and mechanism of oxidation of phenyalanine and serine by chloramine-T. J. Indian Chem. Soc. LIII:755–758.

Lindsay, M., and F.G. Soper. 1946. Methylenechloroamine. J. Chem. Soc. 1946:791–792.

Mahadevappa, D.S., and N.H.M. Gowda. 1975. Estimation of glutathione with chloramine-T and dichloramine-T. Talanta 22:771–773.

Mahadevappa, D.S., and N.H.M. Gowda. 1975. Estimation of glutathione with chloramine-T and dichloramine-T. Talanta 22:771–773.

Mahadevappa, D.S., and H.M.K. Naidu. 1976. Oxidation of valine, leucine, and phenyl alanine by chloramine-T. Curr. Sci. 45:652–653.

Mani, U.V., and A.N. Radhakrishnan. 1976. The oxidation of hydroxyproline by chloramine-T. Evidence discounting pryrrole-2-carboxylate as an intermediate in the reaction. Indian J. Biochem. Biophys. 13:185–186.

Margerum, W., and E.T. Gray, Jr. 1978. Chlorination and the formation of N-chloro compounds in water treatment. In Abstracts of Papers of the 175th American Chemical Society National Meeting, Anaheim, Calif., March 13–17. Abstr. No. INOR 158.

Metcalf, W.S. 1942. The absorption spectra of mono-, di-, and trichloramines and some aliphatic derivatives. J. Chem. Soc. 1942:148–150.

Morris, J.C. 1967. Kinetics of reactions between aqueous chlorine and nitrogen compounds. Pp. 23–53 in S.D. Faust and J.V. Hunter, eds. Principles and Applications of Water Chemistry. Proceedings of the Fourth Rudolfs Research Conference held at Rutgers State University, New Brunswick, N.J., 1965. John Wiley & Sons, Inc., New York.

Morris, J.C. 1978. Modern chemical methods in water and waste treatment, Vol. I. International Course in Sanitary Engineering, International Institute for Hydraulic and Environmental Engineering, Delft, The Netherlands.

Mushran, S.P., R.M. Mehrotra, and R. Sanehi. 1974a. Kinetics and mechanism of chloraminometric reactions involving some primary alcohols. J. Indian Chem. Soc. LI:594–596.

Mushran, S.P., K.C. Gupta, and R. Sanehi. 1974b. Kinetics and mechanism of oxidation of D-(-)-ribose by chloramine–T. J. Indian Chem. Soc. LI:145–148.

Naidu, H.M.K., and D.S. Mahadevappa. 1976. Oxidation of crotoyl alcohol with chloramine–T. Curr. Sci. 45:216–218.

Nair, C.G.R., and V.R. Nair. 1973. Dichloramine-T as a new oxidimetric titrant in nonaqueous and partially aqueous media. II. Potentiometric determination of hydroquinone, hydrazine, oxine, cinnamic acid, tin (II), antimony (III), thallium (I), and ferrocyanide. Talanta 20:696–699.

Natarajan, N.M., and V. Thiagarajan. 1975. Kinetics of oxidation of secondary alcohols by chloramine-T. J. Chem. Soc. Perkin Trans. 2:1590–1594.

Neale, R. 1964. The chemistry of ion radicals: The free-radical addition of N-chloramines to olefinic and acetylenic hydrocarbons. J. Am. Chem. 86:5340–5342.

Palin, A.T. 1950. A study of the chloro derivatives of ammonia and related compounds, with special reference to their formation in the chlorination of natural and polluted waters. Water Water Eng. 54:151–159.

Petrov, A.A., G.A. Galaev, and D.B. Ioffe. 1953. Halogenation and thiocyanation of aromatic amines with liquid chloramines, chloramides, alkyl hypochlorites, and organic hydroperoxide. J. Gen. Chem. USSR 23:689–692.

Ramanujam, V.M.S., and N.M. Trieff. 1977. Kinetic and mechanistic studies of reactions of aniline and substituted anilines with chloramine-T. J. Chem. Soc. Perkin Trans. 2:1275–1280.

Raschig, F. 1907. Vorlesungsversuche aus der Chemie der anorganischen Stickstoffverbindungen. Chem. Ber. 40:4580–4588.

Remick, A.E. 1942. A semiquantitative extension of the electronic theory of the English school. J. Org. Chem. 7:534–545.

Rickabaugh, J., and R.N. Kinman. 1978. Trihalomethane formation from iodine and chlorine disinfection of Ohio River water. Pp. 583–591 in R.L. Jolley, H. Gorchev, and D.H. Hamilton, Jr., eds. Water Chlorination: Environmental Impact and Health Effects, Vol. 2. Ann Arbor Science Publishers, Inc., Ann Arbor, Mich. 909 pp.

Robson, H.L. 1964. Chloramines and chloroamines. Pp. 908–929 in Kirk-Othmer Encyclopedia of Chemical Technology, Vol. 4, 2nd ed. Interscience Publishers, New York.

Saguinsin, J.L.S., and J.C. Morris. 1975. The chemistry of aqueous nitrogen trichloride. Pp. 277–299 in J.D. Johnson, ed. Disinfection Water and Wastewater. Ann Arbor Science Publishers, Inc., Ann Arbor, Mich. 425 pp.

Sanehi, R., K.C. Gupta, R.M. Mehrotra, and S.P. Mushran. 1975. Kinetics and mechanism of oxidation of D-(+)-sorbose by chloramine-T. Bull. Chem. Soc. Jpn. 48:330–332.

Shih, K.L., and J. Lederberg. 1976a. Chloramine mutagenesis in *Bacillus subtilis*. Science 192:1141–1143.

Shih, K.L., and J. Lederberg. 1976b. Effects of chloramine on *Bacillus subtilis* deoxyribonucleic acid. J. Bacteriol. 125:934–945.

Sisler, H.H., N.K. Kotia, and R.E. Highsmith. 1970. The formation of sulfur–sulfur bonds by the chloramination of thiols. J. Org. Chem. 35:1742–1745.

Srivastava, A., and S. Bose. 1975a. Determination of mercaptans and xanthates with chloramine-T and chloramine–B. J. Indian Chem. Soc. LII:214–216.

Srivastava, A., and S. Bose. 1975b. Analytical applications of *N*-haloamines *N*-haloamides for the determination of some sulfur containing functional groups. J. Indian Chem. Soc. LII:217–220.

Standard Methods for the Examination of Water and Wastewater, 14th ed. 1976. American Public Health Association, Washington, D.C. 1193 pp.

Stasiuk, W.N., Jr. 1974. Reactions of chloramines with activated carbon. Ph.D. thesis. Rensselaer Polytechnic University, Troy, N.Y. 136 pp.

Stevens, A.A., C.J. Slocum, D.R. Seeger, and G.G. Pobeck. 1978. Chlorination of organics in drinking water. Pp. 77–104 in R.L. Jolley, ed. Water Chlorination: Environmental Impact and Health Effects, Vol. I. Ann Arbor Science Publishers, Inc., Ann Arbor, Mich. 439 pp.

Symons, J.M., J.K. Carswell, R.M. Clark, P. Dorsey, E.E. Geldreich, W.P. Heffernam, J.C. Hoff, O.T. Love, L.J. McCabe, and A.A. Stevens. 1977. Ozone, Chlorine Dioxide, and Chloramines as Alternatives to Chlorine for Disinfection of Drinking Water: State of the Art. Water Supply Research Division, U.S. Environmental Protection Agency, Cincinnati, Ohio. 84 pp.

Theilacker, W., and E. Wegner. 1964. Organic syntheses using chloramine. Pp. 303–317 in W. Foerst, ed. Newer Methods of Preparative Organic Chemistry. Vol. III. (Trans. by H. Birnbaum). Academic Press, Inc., New York.

Trieff, N.M., and V.M.S. Ramanujam. 1977. Removal of odorous aromatic amine environmental pollutants by chloramine-T. Bull. Environ. Contam. Toxicol. 18(1):26–28.

U.S. Public Health Service. 1963. Inventory of Municipal Water Supplies. PHS Publication No. 1039. U.S. Public Health Service, Washington, D.C.

Wei, I.W. 1972. Chlorine–ammonia breakpoint reactions: kinetics and mechanism. Ph.D. dissertation. Harvard University, Cambridge, Mass.

Wei, I.W., and J.C. Morris. 1974. Dynamics of breakpoint chlorination. Pp. 297–332 in A.J. Rubin, ed. Chemistry of Water Supply, Treatment, and Distribution. Ann Arbor Science Publishers, Inc., Ann Arbor, Mich.

Weil, I., and J.C. Morris. 1949. Kinetic studies on the chloramines. I. The rates of formation of monochloramine, *N*-chlormethylamine and *N*-chlorodimethylamine. J. Am. Chem. Soc. 71:1664–1671.

White, G.C. 1972. Handbook of Chlorination. Van Nostrand Reinhold, New York. 744 pp.

Bromine and Iodine

Bean, R.M., R.G. Riley, and P.W. Ryan. 1978. Investigation of halogenated components formed from chlorination of marine water. Pp. 223–233 in R.L. Jolley, H. Gorchev, and D.H. Hamilton, Jr., eds., Water Chlorination: Environmental Impact and Health

Effects, Vol. 2. Ann Arbor Science Publishers, Inc., Ann Arbor, Mich. 909 pp.

Bellar, T.A., J.J. Lichtenberg, and R.C. Kroner. 1974. The occurrence of organohalides in chlorinated drinking waters. J. Am. Water Works Assoc. 66:703–706.

Berliner, E. 1966. The current state of positive halogenating agents. J. Chem. Educ. 43:124–133.

Black, A.P., W.C. Thomas, Jr., R.N. Kinman, W.P. Bonner, M.A. Keirn, J.J. Smith, Jr., and A.A. Jabero. 1968. Iodine for the disinfection of water. J. Am. Water Works Assoc. 60:69–83.

Bunn, W.W., B.B. Haas, E.R. Deane, and R.D. Kleopfer. 1975. Formation of trihalomethanes by chlorination of surface water. Environ. Lett. 10:205–213.

Chang, S.L. 1958. The use of active iodine as a water disinfectant. J. Am. Pharm. Assoc. 47:417–423.

Engel, P., A. Oplatka, and B. Perlmutter-Hayman. 1954. The decomposition of hypobromite and bromite solutions. J. Am. Chem. Soc. 76:2010–2015.

Environmental Health Directorate. 1977. National Survey for Halomethanes in Drinking Water. Department of National Health and Welfare, Health Protective Branch, Ottawa, Canada. Publ. No. 77-EHD. 119 pp.

Freund, G., W.C. Thomas, Jr., E.D. Bird, R.N. Kinman, and A.P. Black. 1966. Effect of iodinated water supplies on thyroid function. J. Clin. Endocrinol. Metab. 26:619–624.

Gilow, H.M., and J.H. Ridd. 1973. Mechanism of aromatic bromination by hypobromous acid in aqueous perchloric acid. Kinetic evidence against the prior formation of 'positive bromine.' J. Chem. Soc. Lond. Perkin Trans. 2:1321–1327.

Goodenough, R.D., J.F. Mills, and J. Place. 1969. Anion exchange resin (polybromide form) as a source of active bromine for water disinfection. Environ. Sci. Technol. 3:854–856.

Helz, G.R., and R.Y. Hsu. 1978. Volatile chloro- and bromocarbons in coastal waters. Limnol. Oceanogr. 23:858–869.

Henderson, J.R., G.R. Peyton, and W.H. Glaze. 1976. A convenient liquid–liquid extraction method for the determination of halomethanes in water at the parts-per-billion level. Pp. 105–111 in L.H. Keith, ed. Identification & Analysis of Organic Pollutants in Water. Ann Arbor Science Publishers, Inc., Ann Arbor, Mich.

Kuehl, D.W., G.D. Veith, and E.N. Leonard. 1978. Brominated compounds found in waste-treatment effluents and their capacity to bioaccumulate. Pp. 175–192 in R.L. Jolley, H. Gorchev, and D.H. Hamilton, Jr., eds. Water Chlorination: Environmental Impact and Health Effects, Vol. 2. Ann Arbor Science Publishers, Inc., Ann Arbor, Mich. 909 pp.

Johnson, J.D., and R. Overby. 1971. Bromine and bromamine disinfection chemistry. J. Sanit. Eng. Div., Am. Soc. Civ. Eng. 97:617–628.

LaPointe, T.F., G. Inman, and J.D. Johnson. 1975. Kinetics of tribromamine decomposition. Pp. 301–338 in J.D. Johnson, ed. Disinfection: Water and Wastewater. Ann Arbor Science Publishers, Inc., Ann Arbor, Mich. 425 pp.

Laubusch, E.J. 1971. Chlorination and other disinfection processes. Pp. 158–224 in American Water Works Association. Water Quality and Treatment. A Handbook of Public Water Supplies, 3rd ed. McGraw-Hill, New York.

Livingstone, D.A. 1963. Chemical Composition of Rivers and Lakes. U.S. Geological Survey Professional Paper 440-G. Washington, D.C. 64 pp.

Macalady, D.L., J.H. Carpenter, and C.A. Moore. 1977. Sunlight-induced bromate formation in chlorinated seawater. Science 195:1335–1337.

Mills, J.F. 1975. Interhalogens and halogen mixtures as disinfectants. Pp. 113–143 in J.D. Johnson, ed. Disinfection: Water and Wastewater. Ann Arbor Science Publishers, Ann Arbor, Mich. 425 pp.

Moelwyn-Hughes, E.A. 1971. The Chemical Statics and Kinetics of Solutions. Academic Press, New York. 530 pp.

Morris, J.C., S.L. Chang, G.M. Fair, and G.H. Conant, Jr. 1953. Disinfection of drinking water under field conditions. Ind. Eng. Chem. 45:1013–1015.

Pauling, L. 1960. The Nature of the Chemical Bond, and the Structure of Molecules and Crystals: An Introduction to Modern Structural Chemistry, 3rd ed. Cornell University Press, Ithaca, N.Y. 644 pp.

Rickabaugh, J.F., and R.N. Kinman, 1978. Trihalomethane formation from iodine and chlorine disinfection of Ohio River water. Pp. 583–591 in R.L. Jolley, H. Gorchev, and D.H. Hamilton, Jr., eds. Water Chlorination: Environmental Impact and Health Effects, Vol. 2. Ann Arbor Science Publishers, Inc., Ann Arbor, Mich. 905 pp.

Rickabaugh, J.F. 1977. The study of trihalomethane formation when iodine is used for disinfection of drinking water. M.S. thesis. University of Cincinnati, Cincinnati, Ohio. 110 pp.

Rook, J.J. 1974. Formation of haloforms during chlorination of natural waters. Water Treat. Exam. 23:234–243.

Rook, J.J., A.A. Gras, B.G. van der Heijden, and J. de Wee. 1978. Bromide oxidation and organic substitution in water treatment. J. Environ. Sci. Health A13:91–116.

Shackleford, W.M., and L.H. Keith. 1976. Frequency of Organic Compounds Identified in Water. EPA-600/4-76-062. U.S. Environmental Protection Agency, Environmental Research Laboratory, Athens, Ga. 629 pp.

Sugam, R.J. 1977. Chlorine degradation in estuarine waters. Ph.D. dissertation. University of Maryland, College Park, Md. 221 pp.

Swain, C.G., and D.R. Crist. 1972. Mechanisms of chlorination by hypochlorous acid. The last of chlorinium ion, Cl^+. J. Am. Chem. Soc. 94:3195–3200.

Turekian, K.K. 1971. Rivers, tributaries, and estuaries. Pp. 9–73 in D.W. Hood, ed. Impingement of Man on the Oceans. Wiley Interscience Publishers, New York.

White, G.C. 1972. Handbook of Chlorination. Van Nostrand Reinhold, New York. 744 pp.

Chlorine Dioxide

Beuermann, L. 1965. Preparation of chlorine dioxide from sodium chlorite and hydrochloric acid. Gas-Wasserfach. 106:783–788.

Bowen, E.J., and W.M. Cheung. 1932. The photodecomposition of chlorine dioxide solutions. J. Chem. Soc. Lond. 1932(Part I): 1200–1208.

Bray, W. 1906. Beitrage zur Kenntnis der Halogensauerstoffverbindungen. Abhandlung III. Zur Kenntnis des Chlordioxyds. Z. Physik. Chem. 54:569–608.

Buydens, R. 1970. Ozonization and its effects on the mode of purification of river waters. (In French) Trib. CEBEDEAU 23:319– 320, 286–291.

Dence, C.W., and K.V. Sarkanen. 1960. A proposed mechanism for the acidic chlorination of softwood lignin. Tappi 43:87–96.

Dence, C.W., M.K. Gupta, and K.V. Sarkanen. 1962. Studies on oxidative delignification mechanisms. Part II. Reactions of vanillyl alcohol with chlorine dioxide and sodium chlorite. Tappi 45:29–38.

Dowling, L.T. 1974. Chlorine dioxide in potable water treatment. Water Treat. Exam. 23(2):190–204.

Feuss, J.V. 1964. Problems in the determination of chlorine dioxide residuals. J. Am. Water Works Assoc. 56:607– 615.

Flis, I.E. et al. 1955. Trans. Leningr. Techn. Inst. Tsell, Bumazhu Prom. 16:62–67.

Fuchs, W., and H. Leopold. 1927. Humic acids. II. The action of bromine, thionyl chloride and chlorine dioxide on artificial humic acids. Brennstoff Chem. 8:101–103.

Fujii, M., and M. Ukita. 1957. Mechanism of wheat protein coloring by chlorine dioxide. Nippon Nogei Kagaku Kaishi 31:101–109.

Gall, R.J. 1978. Chlorine dioxide—an overview of its preparation, properties and uses. Pp. 356–382 in R.G. Rice and J.A. Cotruvo, eds. Ozone/Chlorine Dioxide Products of Organic Materials. Proceedings of a Conference held in Cincinnati, Ohio, November 17–19, 1976. Sponsored by the International Ozone Institute, Inc., and the U.S. Environmental Protection Agency. Ozone Press International, Cleveland, Ohio. 487 pp.

Glabisz, U. 1968. The Reaction of Chlorine Dioxide with Components of Phenolic Wastewaters—A Summary. Monograph 44. Wyd. Uczln. Politech., Szczecin, Poland. 127 pp.

Glabisz, U. 1967. Action of chlorine dioxide on monohydric phenols. Chem. Tech. (Berlin) 19:352–355.

Gordon, G., and F. Feldman. 1964. Stoichiometry of the reaction between uranium (IV) and chlorite. J. Inorg. Chem. 3:1728–1733.

Gordon, G., R.G. Kieffer, and D.H. Rosenblatt. 1972. The chemistry of chlorine dioxide. Pp. 201–286 in S.J. Kippard, ed. Progress in Inorganic Chemistry, Vol. 15. John Wiley & Sons, Inc., New York.

Granstron, M.L., and G.F. Lee. 1957. Rates and mechanisms of reactions involving oxy-chloro compounds. Public Works 88:90–92.

Granstrom, M.L., and G.F. Lee. 1958. Generation and use of chlorine dioxide in water treatment. J. Am. Water Works Assoc. 50:1453–1466.

Hodgen, H.W., and R.S. Ingols. 1954. Direct colorimetric method for the determination of chlorine dioxide in water. Anal. Chem. 26:1224–1226.

Jeanes, A., and H.S. Isbell. 1941. Chemical reactions of the chlorites with carbohydrates. J. Res. Natl. Bur. Stand. 27:125–142.

Kennaugh, J. 1957. Action of diaphanol on arthropod cuticles. Nature 180:238.

Kieffer, R.G., and G. Gordon. 1968. Inorg. Chem. 7:235–238, 239–244.

Leopold, B., and D.B. Mutton. 1959. The effect of chlorinating and oxidizing agents on derivatives of oleic acid. Tappi 42:218–225.

Lindgren, B.O., and B. Ericsson. 1969. Reaction of chlorine dioxide with phenols: formation of α,β-epoxy ketones from mesitol and 2,6–xylenol. Acta Chem. Scand. 23:3451– 3460.

Lindgren, B.O., and T. Nilsson. 1972. Lignin reactions during chlorine dioxide bleaching of pulp. Oxidation by chlorite. Sven. Papperstidn. 75:161–168.

Lindgren, B.O., and C.M. Svahn. 1966. Reactions of chlorine dioxide with unsaturated compounds. II. Methyl oleate. Acta Chem. Scand. 20:211–218.

Lindgren, B.O., C.M. Svahn, and G. Widmark. 1965. Chlorine dioxide oxidation of cyclohexene. Acta Chem. Scand. 19:7–13.

Love, O.T., Jr., J.K. Carswell, R.J. Miltner, and J.M. Symons. 1976. Treatment for the prevention of removal of trihalomethanes in drinking water. In J.M. Symons. Interim Treatment Guide for the Control of Chloroform and Other Trihalomethanes. Water

Supply Research Division, Municipal Environmental Research Laboratory, U.S. Environmental Protection Agency, Cincinnati, Ohio (App. 3).

Mallevialle, J. 1976. Ozonation des substances de type humique dans les eaux. Pp. 262–270 in R.G. Rice, P. Pichet, and M.A. Vincent, eds. Proceedings of the 2nd International Conference on Ozone Technology. International Ozone Institute, Cleveland, Ohio.

Masschelein, W. 1967. Development in the chemistry of chlorine dioxide and its applications. Chim. Ind. Genie Chim. 97:49–61.

Masschelein, W. 1969. Les oxydes de chlore et le chlorite de sodium. Monogr. Dunod 74:16–57.

Miller, G.W., R.G. Rice, C.M. Robson, W. Kuhn, and H. Wolf. 1978. An assessment of ozone and chlorine dioxide technologies for treatment of municipal water supplies. Pp. 9–57 to 9–89 in Report of EPA Grant R804385-01. Municipal Environmental Research Laboratory, Office of Water Supply, U.S. Environmental Protection Agency, Cincinnati, Ohio.

Miltner, R.J. 1977. Measurement of chlorine dioxide and related products. In Proceedings, American Water Works Association Water Quality Technology Conference, San Diego, Calif., Dec. 6–7, 1976. Paper No. 2A-5. American Water Works Association, Denver, Colo.

Otto, J., and K. Paluch. 1965. Reactions of chlorine dioxide with some organic compounds. V. Reaction of benzaldehyde with chlorine dioxide. Roczniki Chem. 39:1711–1712.

Paluch, K. 1964. The reaction of chlorine dioxide with phenols. I. Phenol and chlorophenols. II. Hydroquinone, chloro derivatives of hydroquinone, and nitrophenols. Rocznicki Chem. 38:35–42, 43–46.

Paluch, K., J. Otto, and K. Kozlowski. 1965. Reaction of chlorine dioxide with some organic compounds. VI. Reaction of benzyl alcohol with chlorine dioxide and with acidified sodium chlorite solution. Rocznicki Chem. 39:1603–1608.

Reichert, J.K. 1968a. Kanzerogene Substanzen in Wasser und Boden. XXI. Die Entfernung polyzyklischer Aromaten bei der Trinkwasser-Aufbereitung durch Chlordioxid: Quantitative Befunde. Arch. Hyg. 152:37–44.

Reichert, J.K. 1968b. Kanzerogene Substanzen in Wasser und Boden. XXIII. Die Entfernung polyzyklischer Aromaten bei der Trinkwasseraufbereitung durch Isolierung und Identifizierung der 3,4-Benzpyrenfolgeprodukte. Arch. Hyg. 152:265–276.

Robson, H.L. 1964. Pp. 35–50 in H.F. Mark, J.J. McKetta, Jr., and D.F. Othmer, eds. Kirk-Othmer Encyclopedia of Chemical Technology. Vol. 5, 2nd ed. Interscience Publishers, New York.

Rosenblatt, D.H. 1975. Chlorine and oxychlorine species reactivity with organic substances. Pp. 249–276 in J.D. Johnson, ed. Disinfection: Water and Wastewater. Ann Arbor Science Publishers, Inc., Ann Arbor, Mich. 425 pp.

Rosenblatt, D.H. 1978. Chlorine dioxide: chemical and physical properties. Pp 332–343 in R.G. Rice and J.A Cotruvo, eds. Ozone/Chlorine Dioxide Oxidation Products of Organic Materials. Proceedings of a Conference held in Cincinnati, Ohio, November 17–19, 1976. Sponsored by the International Ozone Institute and the U.S. Environmental Protection Agency. Ozone Press International, Cleveland, Ohio. 487 pp.

Sarkanen, K.V., K. Kakehi, R.A. Murphy, and H. White. 1962. Studies on oxidative delignification mechanisms. Part I. Oxidation of vanillin with chlorine dioxide. Tappi 45:24–29.

Sarkar, P.B. 1935. Chemistry of jute lignin. VII. Behaviour of organic compounds towards chlorine dioxide and its significance on the constitution of lignin. J. Indian Chem. Soc. 12:470–482.

Schmidt, E., and K. Braunsdorf. 1922. Natural proteins. I. Behavior of chlorine dioxide towards organic compounds. Ber. 55B:1529–1534.

Somsen, R.A. 1960. Oxidation of some simple organic molecules with aqueous chlorine dioxide solutions. I. Kinetics. II. Reaction products. Tappi 43:154–156, 157–160.

Spinks, J.W.T., and J.M. Porter. 1934. Photodecomposition of chlorine dioxide. J. Am. Chem. Soc. 56:264–270.

Stevens, A.A., D.R. Seeger, and C.J. Slocum. 1978. Products of chlorine dioxide treatment of organic materials in water in ozone/chlorine oxidation products of organic materials. Pp. 383–399 in R.G. Rice and J.A. Cotruvo, eds. Ozone/Chlorine Dioxide Oxidation Products of Organic Materials. Proceedings of a Conference held in Cincinnati, Ohio, November 17–19, 1976. Sponsored by the International Ozone Institute and the U.S. Environmental Protection Agency. Ozone Press International, Cleveland, Ohio. 487 pp.

Sussman, S., and J.S. Rauh. 1978. Use of chlorine dioxide in water and wastewater treatment. Pp. 344–355 in R.G. Rice and J.A. Cotruvo, eds. Ozone/Chlorine Dioxide Oxidation Products of Organic Materials. Proceedings of a Conference held in Cincinnati, Ohio, November 17–19, 1976. Sponsored by the International Ozone Institute and the U.S. Environmental Protection Agency. Ozone Press International, Cleveland, Ohio. 487 pp.

Symons, J.F., J.K. Carswell, R.M. Clark, P. Dorsey, E.E. Geldreich, W.P. Heffernam, J.C. Hoff, O.T. Love, L.J. McCabe, and A.A. Stevens. 1977. Ozone, Chlorine Dioxide, and Chloramines as Alternatives to Chlorine for Disinfection of Drinking Water: State of the Art. U.S. Environmental Protection Agency, Water Supply Research Division, Cincinnati, Ohio. 84 pp.

Taylor, M.C., J.F. White, G.P. Vincent, and G.L. Cunningham. 1940. Sodium chlorite, properties and reactions. Ind. Eng. Chem. 32:899–903.

Thielemann, H. 1972. Uber die Einwirkung von Chlordioxid auf einige polycyklische aromatische Kohlenwasserstoffe. Mikrochim. Acta 575–577.

Toussaint, M. 1972. Chlorine dioxide in drinking water treatment. Trib. CEBEDEAU 25(342):260–266.

Vilagenes, R., A. Monteil, A. Derremaux, and M. Lambert. 1977. A comparative study of halomethane formation during drinking water treatment by chlorine or its derivatives in a slow and sand filtration plant and in wastewater treatment plants. Paper presented at 96th Annual Conference, American Water Works Association, Anaheim, Calif., May 8, 1977.

White, J.F., M.C. Taylor, and G.P. Vincent. 1942. The chemistry of chlorites. Ind. Eng. Chem. 34:782–792.

Ozone Reactions and Products

Ahmed, M., and C.R. Kinney. 1950. Ozonation of humic acids prepared from oxidized bituminous coal. J. Am. Chem. Soc. 72:559–561.

Bailey, P.S. 1975. Reactivity of ozone with various organic functional groups important to water purification. Pp. 101–119 in R.G. Rice and M.E. Browning, eds. First International Symposium on Ozone for Water and Wastewater Treatment. International Ozone Institute, Waterbury, Conn.

Bauch, H., and H. Burchard. 1970. Untersuchungen uber die Einwirkung von Ozon auf Wasser mit geringen Verunreinigungen. Wasser Luft Beitr. 14:270–273.

Bauch, H., H. Burchard, and H.M. Arsovic. 1970. Ozone as an oxidant for phenol degradation in aqueous solutions. Gesund. Ing. 91(9):258–262.

Bollyky, L.J. 1975. Ozone treatment of cyanide and plating wastes. Pp. 522–532 in R.G. Rice and M.E. Browning, eds. First International Symposium on Ozone for Water and Wastewater Treatment. International Ozone Institute, Waterbury, Conn.

Briner, E. 1959. Photochemical production of ozone. Pp. 1–6 in Ozone Chemistry and Technology. Advances in Chemistry Series No. 21. American Chemical Society, Washington, D.C.

Brody, S.S. 1975. A proposed new analysis for ozone in water using a field portable chemiluminescent ozone analyzer. Pp. 84–92 in R.G. Rice and M.E. Browning, eds. First International Symposium on Ozone for Water and Wastewater Treatment. International Ozone Institute, Waterbury, Conn.

Carlson, R.M., and R. Caple. 1977. Chemical/Biological Implications of Using Chlorine and Ozone for Disinfection. U.S. Environmental Protection Agency, Environmental Research Laboratory, Duluth, Minn. Report No. EPA/600/3-77/066. 99 pp.

Cerkinsky, S.N., and N. Trahtman. 1972. The present status of research on the disinfection of drinking water in the USSR. Bull. WHO 46:277–283.

Chian, E.S.K., and P.P.K. Kuo. 1976. Fundamental study on the post-treatment of RO permeates from army wastewater. Second Annual Summary Report, Report No. UILU-ENG-76-2019. U.S. Army Medical R & D Command, Washington, D.C.

Criegee, R. 1959. Products of ozonization of some olefins. Pp. 133–135 in Ozone Chemistry and Technology. Advances in Chemistry Series No. 21. American Chemical Society, Washington, D.C.

Dobinson, F. 1959. Ozonization of malonic acid in aqueous solution. Chem. Ind. Lond. 26:853–854.

Eisenhauer, H.R. 1968. The ozonization of phenolic wastes. J. Water Pollut. Control Fed. 40:1887–1899.

Falk, H.L., and J.E. Moyer. 1978. Ozone as a disinfectant of water. Pp. 38–58 in R.G. Rice and J.A. Cotruvo, eds. Ozone/Chlorine Dioxide Oxidation Products of Organic Materials. Proceedings of a Conference held in Cincinnati, Ohio, November 17–19, 1976. Sponsored by the International Ozone Institute and the U.S. Environmental Protection Agency. Press International, Cleveland, Ohio. 487 pp.

Garrison, R.L., C.E. Mauk, and H.W. Prengle, Jr. 1975. Advanced ozone–oxidation system for complexed cyanides. Pp. 551–577 in R.G. Rice and M.E. Browning, eds. First International Symposium on Ozone for Water and Wastewater Treatment. International Ozone Institute, Waterbury, Conn.

Gilbert, E. 1976. Ozonolysis of chlorophenols and maleic acid in aqueous solution. Pp. 253–261 in R.G. Rice, P. Pichet, and M.A. Vincent, eds. Proceedings of the Second International Symposium on Ozone Technology, Montreal, Canada, May 11–14, 1975. Ozone Press International, Jamesville, N.Y. 725 pp.

Gilbert, E. 1978. Reactions of ozone with organic compounds in dilute aqueous solution: identification of their oxidation products. Pp. 227–242 in R.G. Rice and J.A. Cotruvo, eds. Ozone/Chlorine Dioxide Oxidation Products of Organic Materials. Proceedings of a Conference held in Cincinnati, Ohio, November 17–19, 1976. Sponsored by the International Ozone Institute and the U.S. Environmental Protection Agency. Ozone Press International, Cleveland, Ohio. 487 pp.

Gould, J.P., and W.J. Weber, Jr. 1976. Oxidation of phenols by ozone. J. Water Pollut. Control Fed. 48:47–60.

Gunther, F.A., D.E. Ott, and M. Ittig. 1970. The oxidation of parathion to paraoxon. II. By use of ozone. Bull. Environ. Contam. Toxicol. 5:87–94.

Helz, G.R., R.Y. Hsu, and R.M. Block. 1978. Bromoform production by oxidative biocides in marine waters. Pp. 68–76 in R.G. Rice and J.A. Cotruvo, eds. Ozone/Chlorine Dioxide Oxidation Products of Organic Materials. Proceedings of a Conference held in Cincinnati, Ohio, November 17–19, 1976. Sponsored by the International Ozone Institute and the U.S. Environmental Protection Agency. Ozone Press International, Cleveland, Ohio. 487 pp.

Hoigne, J., and H. Bader. 1975. Ozonation of water: role of hydroxyl radicals as oxidizing intermediates. Science 190:782–784.

Hoigne, J., and H. Bader. 1976. Identification and kinetic properties of the oxidizing decomposition products of ozone in water and its impact on water purification. Pp. 271–282 in R.G. Rice, P. Pichet, and M.A. Vincent, eds. Proceedings of the Second International Symposium on Ozone Technology, Montreal, Canada, May 11–16, 1975. Ozone Press International, Jamesville, N.Y. 725 pp.

Hoigne, J., and H. Bader, 1977. Rate constants for the reactions of ozone and organic pollutants and ammonia in water. Symposium on Advanced Ozone Technology. International Ozone Institute, Toronto, Ontario, Canada.

Hoigne, J., and H. Bader. 1978a. Ozone initiated oxidations of solutes in wastewater. A reaction kinetic approach. Paper presented at International Conference on Water Pollution, Stockholm, Sweden.

Hoigne, J., and H. Bader. 1978b. Ozonation of water: kinetics of oxidation of ammonia by ozone and hydroxyl radicals. Environ. Sci. Technol. 12:79–84.

Huibers, D.T.A., R. McNabney, and A. Halfon. 1969. Ozone treatment of secondary effluents from wastewater treatment plants. Federal Water Pollution Control Administration, U.S. Department of the Interior, Cincinnati, Ohio. Robert A. Taft Water Research Center Report No. TWRC-4. 62 pp.

Ingols, R.S. 1978. Ozonation of seawater. Pp. 77–81 in R.G. Rice and J.A. Cotruvo, eds. Ozone/Chlorine Dioxide Oxidation Products of Organic Materials. Proceedings of a Conference held in Cincinnati, Ohio, November 17–19, 1976. Sponsored by the International Ozone Institute and the U.S. Environmental Protection Agency. Ozone Press International, Cleveland, Ohio. 487 pp.

Jurs, R.H. 1966. Die Wirkung des Ozons auf in Wasser geloste Stoffe. Fortschr. Wasserchem. Ihrer Grenzgeb., Heft 4:40–64.

Kilpatrick, M.L., C.C. Herrick, and M. Kilpatrick. 1956. The decomposition of ozone in aqueous solution. J. Am. Chem. Soc. 78:1784–1789.

Kinman, R.N., J. Rickabaugh, V. Elia, K. McGinnis, T. Cody, S. Clark, and R. Christian. 1978. Effect of ozone on hospital wastewater cytotoxicity. Pp. 97–114 in R.G. Rice and J.A. Cotruvo, eds. Ozone/Chlorine Dioxide Oxidation Products of Organic Materials. Proceedings of a Conference held in Cincinnati, Ohio, November 17–19, 1976. Sponsored by the International Ozone Institute and the U.S. Environmental Protection Agency. Ozone Press International, Cleveland, Ohio. 487 pp.

Kinney, C.R., and L.D. Friedman. 1952. Ozonization studies of coal constitution. J. Am. Chem. Soc. 74:57–61.

Kjos, D.J., R.R. Furgason, and L.L. Edwards. 1975. Ozone treatment of potable water to remove iron and manganese: preliminary pilot plant results and economic evaluation. Pp. 194–203 in R.G. Rice and M.E. Browning, eds. First International Symposium on Ozone for Water and Wastewater Treatment. International Ozone Institute, Waterbury, Conn.

Klein, M.J., R.I. Brabets, and L.C. Kinney. 1975. Generation of ozone. Pp. 1–9 in R.G. Rice and M.E. Browning, eds. First Internatinal Symposium on Ozone for Water and Wastewater Treatment. International Ozone Institute, Waterbury, Conn.

Kuo, P.P.K., E.S.K. Chian, and B.J. Chang. 1977. Identification of end products resulting from ozonization and chlorination of organic compounds commonly found in water. Environ. Sci. Technol. 11:1177–1181.

Lawrence, J. 1977. Identification of ozonization products in natural waters. Presented at the Symposium on Advanced Ozone Technology. International Ozone Institute, Toronto, Ontario, Canada.

Lawrence, J., and F.P. Cappelli. 1977. Ozone in drinking water treatment: a review. Sci. Total Environ. 7:99–108.

Maggiolo, A. 1978. Ozone's radical and ionic mechanisms of reaction with organic compounds in water. Pp. 59–67 in R.G. Rice and J.A. Cotruvo, eds. Ozone/Chlorine Dioxide Oxidation Products of Organic Materials. Proceedings of a Conference held in Cincinnati, Ohio, November 17–19, 1976. Sponsored by the International Ozone Institute and the U.S. Environmental Protection Agency. Ozone Press International, Cleveland, Ohio. 487 pp.

Mallevialle, J. 1975. Action de l'ozone dans la degradation des composes phenoliques simples et polymerises: Application aux matieres humiques contenues dans les eaux. Tech. Sci. Munic. Revue l'Eau 70:107– 113.

Mallevialle, J., Y. Laval, M. Lefebvre, and C. Rousseau. 1978. The degradation of humic substances in water by various oxidation agents (ozone, chlorine, chlorine dioxide). Pp. 189–199 in R.G. Rice and J.A. Cotruvo, eds. Ozone/Chlorine Dioxide Oxidation Products of Organic Materials. Proceedings of a Conference held at Cincinnati, Ohio, November 17–19, 1976. Sponsored by the International Ozone Institute and the U.S. Environmental Protection Agency. Ozone Press International, Cleveland, Ohio. 487 pp.

Manley, T.C., and S.J. Niegowski. 1967. Ozone. Pp. 410–432 in Kirk-Othmer Encyclopedia of Chemical Technology, Vol. 14, 2nd ed. Interscience Publishers, New York.

Mathieu, G.I. 1975. Application of film layer purifying chamber process to cyanide destruction—a progress report. Pp. 533–550 in R.G. Rice and M.E. Browning, eds. First International Symposium on Ozone for Water and Wastewater Treatment. International Ozone Institute, Waterbury, Conn.

Miller, G.W., and R.G. Rice. 1978. Testimony before House Science and Technology Committee, Subcommittee on the Environment and the Atmosphere (transcript by private communication).

Murray, R.W. 1968. Ozone chemistry of organic compounds. Pp. 1–4 in F.R. Mayo, ed. Oxidation of Organic Compounds. III. Ozone Chemistry Photo and Singlet Oxygen and Biochemical Oxidation. Advances in Chemistry Series No. 77. American Chemical Society, Washington, D.C.

Netzer, A., and A. Bowers. 1975. Removal of trace metals from wastewater by lime and ozonation. Pp. 731–747 in R.G. Rice and M.E. Browning, eds. First International Symposium on Ozone for Water and Wastewater Treatment. International Ozone Institute, Waterbury, Conn.

Oehlschlaeger, H.F. 1978. Reactions of ozone with organic compounds. Pp. 20–37 in R.G. Rice and J.A. Cotruvo, eds. Ozone/Chlorine Dioxide Oxidation Products of Organic Materials. Proceedings of a Conference held in Cincinnati, Ohio, November 17–19, 1976. Sponsored by the International Ozone Institute and the U.S. Environmental Protection Agency. Ozone Press International, Cleveland, Ohio. 487 pp.

Rice, R.G. 1977. Reaction products of organic materials with ozone and with chlorine dioxide in water. Presented at International Ozone Institute Symposium on Advanced Ozone Technology, Toronto, Ontario, Canada.

Rice, R.G., and J.A. Cotruvo. 1978. Ozone/Chlorine Dioxide Oxidation Products of Organic Materials. Proceedings of a Conference held in Cincinnati, Ohio, November 17–19, 1976. Sponsored by the International Ozone Institute and the U.S. Environmental Protection Agency. Ozone Press International, Cleveland, Ohio. 487 pp.

Rice, R.G., C. Gomella, and G.W. Miller. 1978. Rouen, France water treatment plant: Good organics and ammonia removal with no need to regenerate carbon beds. Civil Eng. ASCE (N.Y.) 48(5):76–82.

Richard, Y., and L. Brener. 1978. Organic materials produced upon ozonization of water. Pp. 169–188 in R.G. Rice and J.A. Cotruvo, eds. Ozone/Chlorine Dioxide Oxidation Products of Organic Materials. Proceedings of a Conference held in Cincinnati, Ohio, November 17-19, 1976. Sponsored by the International Ozone Institute and the U.S. Environmental Protection Agency. Ozone Press International, Cleveland, Ohio. 487 pp.

Rogozhkin, G.I., T. Vsesayyzn, and I. Nauchno. 1970. Inta vodosnabzheniya kanalizatsii. Pp. 27–45 in Gidrotekhnicheskikh Sooruzheniy i Gidrogeologii.

Schalekamp, M. 1978. Experiences in Switzerland with ozone particularly in connection with the charge of undesirable elements present in water. Ozone Technology Symposium and Exposition. International Ozone Institute, Los Angeles, Calif.

Selm, R.P. 1959. Ozone oxidation of aqueous cyanide waste solutions in stirred batch reactors and packed towers. Pp. 66–77 in Ozone Chemistry and Technology. Advances in Chemistry Series No. 21. American Chemical Society, Washington, D.C.

Shevchenko, M.A., and P.N. Taran. 1966. Investigation of the ozonolysis products of humus materials. Sov. Prog. Chem. 32:408–410. [Trans. of Ukr. Khim Zn. 32(5):532–536.]

Sievers, R.R., R.M. Barkley, G.Z. Eiceman, R.H. Shapiro, H.F. Walton, K.J. Kolonko, and L.R. Field. 1977a. Environmental trace analysis of organics in water by glass capillary column chromatography and ancillary techniques. J. Chromatogr. 142:745–754.

Sievers, R.E., R.M. Barkley, G.A. Eiceman, L.P. Haack, R.H. Shapiro, and H.F. Walton. 1977b. Generation of volatile organic compounds from non-volatile precursors in water by treatment with chlorine or ozone. Presented at Conference on Water Chlorination, Gatlinsburg, Tenn.

Sievers, R.E., R.H. Shapiro, H.F. Walton, G.A. Eiceman, and R.M. Barkley. 1977c. High resolution gas chromatographic determination of organic compounds in ozonized wastewater. Presented at ACS National Meeting, Chicago, Ill.

Singer, P.C., and W.B. Zilli. 1975. Ozonation of ammonia: application to wastewater treatment. Pp. 269–287 in R.G. Rice and M.E. Browning, eds. First International Symposium on Ozone for Water and Wastewater Treatment. International Ozone Institute, Waterbury, Conn.

Spanggord, R.J., and V.J. McClurg. 1978. Ozone methods and ozone chemistry of selected organics in water. 1. Basic chemistry. Pp. 115–125 in R.G. Rice and J.A. Cotruvo, eds. Ozone/Chlorine Dioxide Oxidation Products of Organic Materials. Proceedings of a Conference held in Cincinnati, Ohio, November 15-17, 1976. Sponsored by the International Ozone Institute and the U.S. Environmental Protection Agency. Ozone Press International, Cleveland, Ohio. 487 pp.

Stumm, W. 1954. Der Zerfall von Ozon in wassriger Losung. Helv. Chim. Acta 37:773–778.

Sturrock, M.G., E.L. Cline, and K.R. Robinson. 1963. The ozonation of phenanthrene with water as participating solvent. J. Org. Chem. 28:2340–2343.

Symons, J., J.K. Carswell, R.M. Clark, P. Dorsey, E.E. Geldreich, W.P. Heffernam, J.C. Hoff, O.T. Love, L.J. McCabe, and A.A. Stevens. 1977. Ozone, Chlorine Dioxide and Chloramine as Alternatives to Chlorine for Disinfection of Water: State of the Art. Water Supply Research Division, U.S. Environmental Protection Agency, Cincinnati, Ohio. 84 pp.

Weil, L., B. Sttruif, and K.E. Quentin. 1977. Reaction mechanisms upon reaction of organic substances in water with ozone. Presented at the International Symposium on Ozone and Water, Berlin. International Ozone Institute, Cleveland, Ohio.

Westgate Research Corp. 1978. The continued investigation into the chemistry of the UV–ozone water purification process. Westgate Research Corporation.

Wynn, C.S., B.S. Kirk, and R. McNabney. 1973. Pilot plant for tertiary treatment of wastewater with ozone. U.S. Environmental Protection Agency, Washington, D.C. No. EPA-R2-73-146. 229 pp.

Yocum, F.H. 1978. Oxidation of styrene with ozone in aqueous solution. Pp. 243–263 in R.G. Rice and J.A. Cotruvo, eds. Ozone/Chlorine Dioxide Oxidation Products of Organic Materials. Proceedings of a Conference held in Cincinnati, Ohio, November 15–17, 1976. Sponsored by the International Ozone Institute and the U.S. Environmental Protection Agency. Ozone Press International, Cleveland, Ohio.

Yokoyama, K., S. Sato, I. Yoshiyasu, and T. Imamura. 1974. Degradation of organic substances in water, by ozone. Mitsubishi Denki Giho Tech. Rev. 48:1233–1238.

IV

An Evaluation of Activated Carbon for Drinking Water Treatment

This chapter contains the findings of the Subcommittee on Adsorption of the National Research Council's Safe Drinking Water Committee, which studied the efficacy of granular activated carbon (GAC) and related adsorbents in the treatment of drinking water. Some attention is given to an examination of the potential health effects related to the use of these adsorbents, but detailed toxicological and epidemiological implications resulting from the presence of organic compounds in drinking water are considered in separate chapters of *Drinking Water and Health*, Volume 3. The development of standards for GAC and the economic aspects of its use was not a part of this study.

The subcommittee defined "activated carbon" as a family of carbonaceous substances that are characterized primarily by their surface area, pore size distribution, and sorptive and catalytic properties. Different raw materials and manufacturing processes produce final products with different adsorption characteristics.

The use of GAC under specified conditions was proposed by the U.S. Environmental Protection Agency (EPA) as the option of choice for the control of "synthetic organic chemicals" in drinking water. During the subcommittee's study, the EPA held hearings and received written comments regarding this treatment.

The subcommittee reviewed the pertinent literature and rigorously assessed the scientific data base. Its scope of work included a review of work on:

251

- adsorption efficiency
- microbial activity on adsorbents
- physiochemical interactions
- regeneration of adsorbents
- analytical methods to monitor adsorption processes

The subcommittee considered the ability of adsorbents to remove organic compounds of concern to health and the possible products of the adsorption process. A large and diverse segment of the scientific literature, particularly that concerning recent European experience, was scrutinized. Studies that met established criteria for quality assurance and completeness of data were used as primary sources by the subcommittee. Where possible, stress was placed on studies of chemicals at nanogram to microgram per liter concentrations, which are typically found in drinking water. The subcommittee was confronted by a continual flow of new data and the need for postulation and interpretation. To ensure a thorough review of each topic, the data for each type of adsorbent were considered and reported separately.

Carbon and other adsorbents in various forms have been used for the treatment of water and as detoxifying pharmaceutical agents in medicine for many centuries. There has been an uninterrupted use of carbonaceous adsorbents since biblical times (Old Testament, Num. 19:9; Maimonides, 1185) and there have been marked changes in the nature of the adsorbent since that time (Kunin, 1974a,b).

During the twentieth century, GAC and powdered activated carbon (PAC) have been used in the United States to control taste and odors in drinking water (U.S. Environmental Protection Agency, 1978a). During the past 20 yr, research on the use of adsorbents to treat drinking water has emphasized the removal of specific organics. The removal of organic compounds from drinking water has been based primarily on the measurement of organic matter as measured by carbon chloroform extract (CCE), total organic carbon (TOC), or other group parameters. However, it has long been recognized that these group parameters provide only estimates of performance for target compounds. Studies beginning with those of Middleton and Rosen (1956) began to identify the specific organic compounds in drinking water and their removal by the carbon adsorption.

Over 700 volatile organic compounds have been identified in drinking water (U.S. Environnmental Protection Agency, 1978c). These compounds make up only a small fraction of the total organic matter (National Academy of Sciences, 1977). Approximately 90% of the volatile organic compounds that can be analyzed by gas chromatography have been analyzed, but this represents no more than 10% by weight of the total organic material. Only 5%–10% of the nonvolatile organic compounds that comprise the remaining 90% of the total organic matter have been identified.

The EPA (1978c) has categorized the organic compounds in drinking water into five different classes. Each class has distinctly different characteristics of concern to those involved in water treatment.

Class I: organic compounds that cause taste and odor and/or color problems;

Class II: synthetic organic chemicals that are present in source waters from upstream discharges or runoff;

Class III: organic compounds (precursors) that react with disinfectants to produce "disinfection by-products";

Class IV: organic chemicals that are the disinfection by-products themselves; and

Class V: natural (non-Class III) organic compounds of little direct toxicological importance.

Today there are GAC beds in U.S. water treatment plants for removal of Class I compounds. Consideration is being given to the use of GAC for removal of Class II, III, and IV compounds as data become available. Class V compounds are of interest because they may compete for adsorption sites, thereby lessening the removal of other compounds.

This report identifies the compounds that may be removed and/or added to drinking water by the adsorption process with its attendant chemical and microbial processes. It focuses on recently published lists of organic chemicals of concern to health (Interagency Regulatory Liaison Group, 1978; National Academy of Sciences, 1977, 1979; National Cancer Institute, 1978).

Each section deals with complex subjects in which there are uncertainties, inconclusive or incomplete data, and, thus, conflicting opinions. The length of each section represents only the number of studies reviewed and does not reflect the relative importance of the subjects.

ACTIVATED CARBON—A DEFINITION

"Activated carbon" comprises a family of substances, whose members are characterized primarily by their sorptive and catalytic properties. Different raw materials and manufacturing processes produce final products with different characteristics.

Activated carbon can be made from a variety of carbonaceous materials and processed to enhance its adsorptive properties. Some common materials that are used to make activated carbon are bituminous coal, bones, coconut shells, lignite, peat, pecan shells, petroleum-based residues, pulp mill black ash, sugar, wastewater treatment sludge, and wood (Weber, 1972). As is true with any production process, the quality of the final product is influenced by the starting material. In the past, activated carbons that were used for industrial applications were commonly produced from wood, peat, and other vegetable derivatives. Today, lignite, natural coal, and coke are the most frequently used sources of activated carbon due to their availability and attractive price.

The basic structural unit of activated carbon is closely approximated by the structure of pure graphite with only slight differences. The structure of activated carbon is quite disorganized compared with that of graphite because of the random oxidation of graphite layers. The regular array of carbon bonds in the surface of the crystallites is disrupted during the activation process, yielding free valences that are very reactive. The structure that develops is a function of the carbonization and activation temperatures. During the carbonization process, several aromatic nuclei with a structure similar to that of graphite are formed. From X-ray spectrographs, these structures have been interpreted as microcrystallites consisting of fused hexagonal rings of carbon atoms. The diameter of the planes making up the microcrystallite is estimated to be 150 Å, and the distance between microcrystallites ranges from 20 Å to 50 Å (Wolff, 1959).

The presence of impurities and the method of preparation influences the formation of interior vacancies in the microcrystallite. The ringed structures at the edges of the planes are often heterocyclic, resulting from the nature of either the starting material or the preparation process. Heterocyclic groups would tend to affect both the distance of adjacent planes and the sorptive properties of the carbon.

As a rule, the structure of the usual types of active carbon is tridisperse, i.e., they contain micropores (effective radii of 18–20 Å), transitional pores (40–200 Å), and macropores (500–20,000 Å). According to Dubinin (1966) only a few of the micropores lead directly to the outer surface of the carbon particle. Most of the pore structures of the particles are arranged in the following pattern: the macropores open directly to the external surface of the particle; transitional pores branch off from macropores; and micropores, in turn, branch off from the transitional pores. The specific area of the micropores usually amounts to at least 90% of the total surface area.

THE WATER TREATMENT PROCESS

GAC is typically used in a water treatment plant after the coagulation and sedimentation processes and, commonly, following preliminary disinfection steps during which chemical reactions can occur. Moreover, water is often disinfected before it passes through the GAC adsorbers in order to prevent nuisance biological growths. In many instances, the activated carbon functions as a granular filter medium for removing particulates, although in a few cases in the United States and in most instances in Europe the GAC adsorbers are preceded by filters for particulate removal.

Water is usually passed downward through packed beds of GAC. The frequency of backwashing is dependent on the amount of particulates being removed and the extent of microbial growth. Some intermixing of the GAC granules takes place during this step, although this tendency is countered by particle size stratification during backwash. While packed-bed downflow adsorbers in parallel are most commonly used, many other flow patterns, such as operation in series, upflow packed bed, and upflow expanded bed, may be used.

Regeneration of GAC is not generally practiced at water plants in the United States as it is in Europe. If the objective of GAC use is to include the removal of organic compounds in addition to those that cause taste and odor, regeneration is likely to become more common in the United States. The type of contactor selected for the GAC will be influenced by the frequency of regeneration.

After treatment of a water supply with GAC, postdisinfection is generally used to reduce the total number of bacteria, some of which may be present because of the microbial growths in adsorbers. Sufficient disinfectant is usually applied to ensure a residual in the distribution system to prevent contamination of the water. Postdisinfection is used in addition to predisinfection because aqueous oxidants that are used in preliminary disinfection steps will generally be eliminated by reaction with the GAC.

In certain instances, some synthetic resins may serve as replacements for GAC or they may be used in conjunction with GAC to provide the desired quality of water. The major difference between resins and GAC is that the resins are regenerated by application of aqueous solutions of acids, bases, and/or salts, or of nonaqueous solvents or steam, while GAC is usually thermally regenerated. In general, resins usually require a pretreatment step that is dependent upon the nature of the resins.

Powdered activated carbon (PAC) is now more commonly used in the

United States than is GAC. It generally added to control taste and odor at points in the water treatment plant, ranging from the water supply intake to just before the rapid sand filter. PAC is removed either in the sedimentation basin or by the rapid sand filter. No attempt is made to regenerate it during the water treatment. Whether PAC can be used to remove organics other than those that cause offensive taste and odor requires closer examination.

Various types of GAC and PAC are commercially available as a result of variations in the raw materials and manufacturing processes. Because the types of organic contaminants vary widely from location to location, the best carbon for one application may not be the best in another. Consequently, comparative testing for a particular water source is mandatory.

The chemical compounds entering an adsorption water treatment process consist of high-molecular-weight humic materials, lower-molecular-weight organic compounds of natural or industrial origin, and the products of previous treatment such as chlorination or ozonization. A portion of the chemicals can be removed by the clarification process and/or sorbed by the adsorbent or any microbial floc within the adsorbent bed. Some compounds may be nonadsorbable or only very weakly adsorbable.

The chemical compounds leaving the adsorption treatment process can be the same chemicals that entered the plant, or they may be products of chemical reaction or microbial action within the system. Organic compounds may appear in the effluent of an adsorption column because available adsorption sites are saturated or because they are displaced from the adsorption sites by other organics. Because adsorption is often reversible, adsorbed compounds may desorb and appear in the effluent when the influent concentrations of those compounds decrease. These phenomena may lead to the appearance of a larger concentration of a compound in the effluent than is in the influent. Thus, both the qualitative and quantitative variability of the mixture of organics entering an adsorption process affect the quality of water that can be produced by it.

GENERAL CONCLUSIONS AND RECOMMENDATIONS

Raw water sources and disinfected water supplies may contain organic compounds that have been demonstrated to be carcinogenic or otherwise toxic in experimental animals or in epidemiological studies. Also present are a large number of compounds that either have not been identified or their effects on health have not been characterized. Properly operated GAC systems can remove or effectively reduce the concentration of many of the compounds described above. Less is known about synthetic resins than about GAC, but it is known that they can be applied to remove certain types of organic contaminants.

The information available as of this date on the treatment of water with GAC provides no evidence that harmful health effects are produced by the process under proper operating conditions. However, there are incomplete studies on the possible production of such effects with virgin or regenerated carbon through

- reactions that may be catalyzed by the GAC surface;
- reactions of disinfectants with GAC or compounds adsorbed on it;
- reactions mediated by microorganisms that are part of the process; or
- by the growth of undesirable microorganisms on GAC.

Studies are also needed on the properties of regenerated activated carbons and on the adsorption of additional contaminants with potential health effects. The frequency of GAC regeneration is determined by the organic compounds in the water and their competitive interactions. The types and concentrations of organic compounds may vary widely among different locations and seasons of the year. Competitive interactions are complex and presently cannot be predicted without data from laboratory and/or pilot scale tests on the water to be treated.

While there is ample evidence for the effectiveness of GAC in removing many organics of health concern, more data are needed in the quantification of any harmful health effects related to the use of GAC. This need, however, should not prevent the present use of GAC at locations where analysis of the water supply clearly indicates the existence of a potential health hazard greater than that which would result from the use of GAC.

Clarification processes (coagulation, sedimentation, filtration) remove significant amounts of some organics, especially some types of THM precursors and relatively insoluble compounds that may be associated with particulates. In some cases, the removal of THM precursors by clarification may be sufficient to eliminate the need for an adsorption process.

ADSORPTION EFFICIENCY OF GAC

The trace organic compounds that can be removed by GAC are usually present at μg/liter quantities or less. The subcommittee considered the GAC adsorption efficiency for individual compounds and the competitive adsorption of mixtures. Since GAC is used in conjunction with other water treatment processes, the effect of pretreatments for removing trace organic compounds and their precursors were examined in depth. Hence, the following questions were addressed:

1. How efficiently does GAC adsorb individual trace organic compounds, particularly those of concern to health?
2. When processes such as coagulation, sedimentation, filtration, aeration, disinfection, oxidation, and PAC adsorption precede GAC adsorption, how is the efficiency of the GAC affected?
3. Can water that has been treated by GAC be disinfected more or less easily than water that has not been treated by GAC?
4. What is the potential for effectively using PAC to remove organics?
5. What reactions take place between oxidants that are applied as predisinfectants and the activated carbon or the compounds that are adsorbed on the activated carbon? Do these reactions result in potentially hazardous compounds that would not be present if activated carbon were not used?
6. To what extent does competitive adsorption between trace organics with potential health effects and the large concentrations of background organics, generally characterized as humic substances, influence the effectiveness of GAC?
7. To what extent does competitive adsorption among similar concentrations of trace organics with potential health effects influence the effectiveness of GAC?
8. How significant is the effect of competitive adsorption when it is compared to the effect of the reequilibration that is produced by the variable nature of the composition and concentration of trace organics in the feedwater to the GAC bed?

Removal of Selected Organic Compounds

Adsorption isotherms and small column studies that are performed in the laboratory using GAC are useful tools that have been developed to describe how specific organic chemicals can be removed in large-scale GAC applications. A considerable amount of adsorption research describing the affinities of pure compounds for the activated carbon surface has been reported in the literature during the last 15 years. Improved analytical tools have made it possible both to detect the organics at trace levels in the environment and to follow their removals in adsorption studies in the laboratory. This section of the chapter evaluates the efficiency of GAC adsorption of individual trace organic compounds, particularly those with potential health effects.

Removals of organic chemicals are discussed in the literature on the basis of laboratory and pilot-scale studies and large-scale applications. Laboratory studies are by far the most useful for describing specific organic removals since environmental factors can be more carefully controlled in them than in field evaluations. The problem of competitive adsorption is significant when environmental samples are used in experiments in which specific organic compounds are removed by adsorption. A later section of this chapter addresses this problem exclusively.

Adsorption data obtained in the laboratory are normally reported as percent removed, adsorption isotherms, kinetics of adsorption, and the results of small-scale column studies. In the following sections, these data are reviewed and the utility of each method is evaluated.

Percent Removals

Giusti *et al.* (1974) made extensive use of percent reduction as a measure of the effectiveness of activated carbon for removing organic chemicals. They added 93 petrochemicals individually at one level to one type of activated carbon and used the subsequent calculated percent reductions to test several hypotheses concerning the removal of different classes of organics by activated carbon.

There are several problems associated with using percent removal data exclusively to describe how well a particular organic compound is removed from water. The single value study results in a single point on an isotherm. Unfortunately, this single point gives no indication of how capacity varies with concentration, i.e., by the isotherm slope and shape. To be truly representative, the amounts of adsorbed compound per gram of carbon for individual organic compounds must be compared on an equal equilibrium concentration basis, which is not possible if only a single percent removal value is available.

Adsorption Isotherms

Adsorption isotherms are plots of the equilibrium relationship between the amount of organic compound that is left in solution (equilibrium concentration, C_e) and the amount of compound that is on the surface of the activated carbon (surface concentration, q).

Few studies describe the adsorption isotherms of a wide variety of organic compounds over several orders of magnitude. An EPA publication (U.S. Environmental Protection Agency, 1978c) tabulated references on the removals of some 50 organic compounds by GAC. While there are some useful data among the references cited in this work, a large fraction of the reported data is fragmentary. Generally, information is omitted, such as the number of data points used to define the isotherm or the equilibrium concentration range over which the slope and intercept of the linear isotherm are valid. Dobbs *et al.* (1978) have made significant efforts to standardize the reporting of isotherm data.

Table IV-1 lists a series of compounds for which detailed isotherms are available. No attempt has been made to list all studies that have been published. Instead, Table IV-1 presents a sample of available studies. The compounds in the table represent a wide variety of organic chemicals, including naturally occurring chemicals, industrial solvents, and compounds that have been identified in surface waters and waste streams in the United States. Dobbs *et al.* (1978) and Fochtman and Dobbs (1980) have made some of the few efforts to determine adsorption capacities for many organic chemicals of toxicological concern. In the future, the isotherm data base should be expanded much more rapidly to include the compounds that are just now being identified as toxic or potentially carcinogenic. There are significant difficulties in determining isotherms for some of these organic compounds. A major difficulty is that many compounds must be analyzed at concentrations that have previously been near the limit of detectability.

Isotherm data for the organic compounds that are listed in Table IV-1 have become available only recently, and few attempts have been made to analyze the data to determine whether general patterns exist. Figure IV-1 plots selected isotherms for compounds from Table IV-1 over seven orders of magnitude of equilibrium concentration (McGuire and Suffet, 1980).

Although the isotherms in Figure IV-1 were determined by different investigators using different techniques and different carbons, there is surprising agreement between isotherms for the same compound. Clearly, other aspects of the experimental conditions that affect the positions of the isotherms include pH, ionic strength, and temperature.

TABLE IV-1   Some Organic Compounds for Which Detailed, Wide-Range Isotherms Have Been Determined

acetone[f]
acetophenone[a]
acridine orange[a]
acridine yellow[a]
adenine[a]
adipic acid[a]
anethole[a]
o-anisidine[a]
benzene[a,h]
benzidine[h]
benzidine dihydrochloride[a]
benzoic acid[a]
benzothiazole[a]
bromochloromethane[g]
bromodichloromethane[a,g]
bromoform[a,g]
p-bromophenol[d]
5-bromouracil[a]
n-butanol[b]
(di)-n-butylphthalate[a]
carbon tetrachloride[a,g]
chlorobenzene[a]
bis (2-chloroethyl) ether[a]
chlorodibromethane[a]
chloroform[a,g]
1-chloro-2-nitrobenzene[a]
p-chlorophenol[c,f]
5-chlorouracil[a]
p-cresol[f]
cyclohexanone[a]
cytosine[a]
3,3'-dichlorobenzidine[h]
dichloromethane[g]
2,4-dichlorophenol[c,e]
dimethylphenylcarbinol[a]
2,4-dinitrophenol[a,c]
dimethyl phthalate[a]
1,1'-diphenyl hydrazine[h]
1,4-dioxane[b]
diphenylamine[a]

EDTA[a]
ethylbenzene[a]
ethylene chloride[a]
5-fluorouracil[a]
geosmin[e]
guanine[a]
hexachlorobutadiene[a]
hydroquinone[a,c]
p-methoxyphenol[c]
4,4'-methylene-bis
    (2 chloroaniline)[h]
methyl ethyl ketone[b]
2-methylisoborneol[e]
naphthalene[h]
α-naphthol[a]
β-naphthol[a]
α-naphthylamine[a]
β-naphthylamine[h]
p-nitroaniline[a]
nitrobenzene[a]
nitromethane[b]
p-nitrophenol[b,c,d,i]
N-nitrosodiphenylamine[a]
p-nonylphenol[a]
parathion[j]
pentachlorophenol[a]
phenol[a,c,i]
phenyl mercuric acetate[a]
2-propanol[f]
propionitrile[f]
sodium benzene sulfonate[d]
styrene[a]
tetrachloroethylene[g]
1,2,3,4-tetrahydronapththalene[a]
thymine[a]
trichloroethylene[g]
2,4,6-trichlorophenol[c]
uracil[a]
urea[b]
p-xylene[a]

[a] Dobbs et al., 1978.
[b] McGuire, 1977.
[c] Zogorski, 1975.
[d] Jain and Snoeyink, 1973.
[e] Snoeyink et al., 1977.

[f] Radke and Prausnitz, 1972a.
[g] Weber et al., 1977.
[h] Fochtman and Dobbs, 1979.
[i] Snoeyink et al., 1969.
[j] Weber and Gould, 1966.

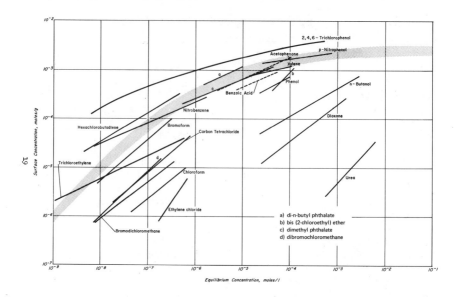

FIGURE IV-1   General and specific adsorption isotherms. From McGuire and Suffet, 1980.

McGuire and Suffet (1978) reviewed the relative importance of these and other factors on the adsorption mechanism. In general, the isotherms in Figure IV-1 were calculated for the neutral forms of the molecules.

Several investigators have shown that there can be significant differences between the adsorption characteristics of different brands of activated carbon (McGuire, 1977; Weber *et al.*, 1977; Zogorski, 1975). Pore size distribution and surface area, base material, chemisorbed oxygen and surface polarity, particle size, and hardness all affect either the capacity, kinetics, or economics of adsorption with activated carbon (McGuire and Suffet, 1978). There are significant differences between bituminous coal base carbons and coconut shell carbons. The capacity will have a significant effect on cost. Thus, the difference in isotherms for different carbons is important. However, the differences among carbons will be reflected primarily in cost, a factor not considered in this report.

The shaded area of Figure IV-1 depicts a general isotherm. At relatively high equilibrium concentrations (depending on how well a compound is adsorbed), the slope of the isotherm is relatively flat. As the equilibrium concentration decreases, the slope increases until it becomes equal to 1.0, indicating compliance with Henry's law of adsorption

(Radke and Prausnitz, 1972a). The more poorly adsorbed compounds (urea, for example) have a slope of 1.0 at high C_e values. The compounds that are more strongly adsorbed have a slope of 1.0 at much lower C_e values. For example, the isotherm for 2,4,6-trichlorophenol was determined over five orders of magnitude, and the maximum slope is only 0.592 at 10^{-8} mol/liter. Figure IV-1 also shows that for the isotherms determined on a comparative basis, substituted phenols adsorb much better than low molecular weight alkyl halides.

Our understanding of how specific organic compounds are adsorbed is generally derived from the work on well-adsorbed substituted phenols at mg/liter concentrations. Figure IV-1 indicates that the poorly adsorbed and even the moderately well-adsorbed compounds have steep slopes at the μg/liter level (1 to 10×10^{-9} mol/liter). The reduction of compound concentrations two orders of magnitude into the ng/liter range requires a much larger amount of carbon or longer column contact time than a two order of magnitude decrease at the mg/liter level. Thus, reduction to subtrace levels of these specific organics with potential health effects is more difficult than would normally be expected based on the existing level of understanding of organic compound adsorption.

Table IV-2 was compiled from studies describing the adsorption data for individual organic compounds with particular potentials for harmful health effects. The selection of compounds in the table was based on their presence on several recently published lists: Categories of Known or Suspected Organic Chemical Carcinogens Found in Drinking Water (National Academy of Sciences, 1977, p. 794), Carcinogens and Suspected Carcinogens in Drinking Water (National Cancer Institute, 1978), List of Chemicals Submitted by EPA for Evaluation by the Safe Drinking Water Committee Toxicology Subcommittee (National Academy of Sciences, 1979), and the Interagency Regulatory Liaison Group (1978). Pesticides with established maximum contaminant levels (MCL) (U.S. Environmental Protection Agency, 1975) and THM's with proposed composite MCL values (U.S. Environmental Protection Agency, 1978b) are also included in Table IV-2.

Clearly the 58 compounds and classes of compounds listed in these compilations are somewhat repetitive and overlap several types of organic chemicals. The list has been modified and edited for clarity and does not include compounds for which no data on adsorption were available. The committee attempted to provide as much specific information on the ability of a compound to be adsorbed by activated carbon as possible and convenient for a tabular format.

Several guidelines were used to select the references and the adsorp-

TABLE IV-2 Adsorption of Organic Compounds by GAC[a]

Organic Compounds	Molecular Weight	Number of Data Points	Carbon Type	Adsorption Test Method	Equilibrium Concentration Range, mol/liter	Maximum Surface Concentration, mol/g	Comments	References
Acrylonitrile	53.06	2	Unknown	Unknown	1.4×10^{-3}–9.2×10^{-3}	9.6×10^{-4}	Procedure unknown	Dahm et al., 1974
Aldrin	365	6	F300	Isotherm	2.5×10^{-9}–7.1×10^{-8}	3.0×10^{-5}		Mahon, 1979
Benzene	78.11	5	F400	Isotherm	2.6×10^{-5}–1.3×10^{-4}	3.4×10^{-3}		Fochtman and Dobbs, 1980
Benzo(a)-pyrene	252.3	2	Norit NK	% reduction	Unknown	99.8% removal	Review article	Borneff, 1979
α-BHC	290.85	Unknown	Unknown	% reduction	Unknown	80% removal	Abstract	Schmidt, 1974
γ-BHC (Lindane)	290.85	1	OU-A	% reduction	7×10^{-8}	1×10^{-4}	Translated abstract	Shevehenko et al., 1974
Bis (2-chloroethyl) ether	143.01	11	F300	Isotherm	4.2×10^{-5}–1.2×10^{-4}	1.2×10^{-3}	pH 7 and 9 data pooled	Dobbs et al., 1978
Bromodichloro-methane	163.83	7	F300	Isotherm	7.9×10^{-9}–3.5×10^{-7}	1.3×10^{-5}		Dobbs et al., 1978
Bromoform	252.75	15	F400	Isotherm	2×10^{-8}–1.3×10^{-6}	1.0×10^{-4}		Weber et al., 1977
Carbon tetra-chloride	153.82	11	F400	Isotherm	3×10^{-9}–2.6×10^{-7}	2.6×10^{-5}		Weber et al., 1977
Chlordane	764	3	F300	Isotherm	1.0×10^{-9}–2.3×10^{-8}	5.1×10^{-5}		Hansen, 1979b
Chlorobenzene	112.56	7	F300	Isotherm	1.2×10^{-5}–1.5×10^{-4}	1.5×10^{-2}		Dobbs et al., 1978
Chlorodibromo-methane	208.29	7	F400	Isotherm	7.2×10^{-9}–1.9×10^{-7}	1.5×10^{-5}		Dobbs et al., 1978
Chloroform	119.38	7	F400	Isotherm	2.8×10^{-8}–1×10^{-6}	1×10^{-5}		Weber et al., 1977
DDE	318	5	F300	Isotherm	3.5×10^{-9}–1.1×10^{-7}	1.6×10^{-5}		Mahon, 1979

Compound	Molecular weight	No.	Carbon	Method	Range	Value	Notes	Reference
DDT	354.5	2	F300	Isotherm	1.0×10^{-8}–5.9×10^{-8}	2.3×10^{-5}		Mahon, 1979
Dichlorobenzene	147.01	3	F300	Isotherm	2.7×10^{-5}–6.8×10^{-5}	1.4×10^{-3}	1,4-Dichlorobenzene	Mahon, 1979
1,2-Dichloroethane	98:96	7	F300	Isotherm	1.7×10^{-7}–6.6×10^{-7}	6.9×10^{-6}		Dobbs et al., 1978
2,4-Dichlorophenoxyacetic acid (2,4-D)	221	Unknown	Aqua Nu-char A	Isotherm	2×10^{-7}–2×10^{-6}	4×10^{-4}	Sodium salt	Aly and Faust, 1965
Dieldrin	381	6	F300	Isotherm	2.1×10^{-10}–1.7×10^{-8}	1.7×10^{-5}		Mahon, 1979
1,4-Dioxane	88.12	8	F400	Isotherm	2.5×10^{-5}–1.5×10^{-3}	2.6×10^{-4}		McGuire et al., 1978
1,1-Diphenylhydrazine	184	5	F400	Isotherm	2.2×10^{-6}–4.9×10^{-5}	8.1×10^{-4}		Fochtman and Dobbs, 1979
Endrin	381	6	F300	Isotherm	1.8×10^{-10}–3.9×10^{-8}	6.2×10^{-5}		Mahon, 1979
Halogenated phenols (e.g., pentachlorophenol)	266.4	5	F300	Isotherm	1.7×10^{-6}–2.9×10^{-5}	2.1×10^{-3}	Pentachlorophenol, pH3	Dobbs et al., 1978
Heptachlor	373.3	2	F300	Isotherm	1.6×10^{-8}–1.5×10^{-7}	3.3×10^{-5}		Mahon, 1979
Heptachlor epoxide	389	Unknown	Unknown	% reduction	Unknown	>80% removal	Abstract	Schmidt, 1974
Hexachloroethane	236.74	1	F300	Column recovery	Unknown	Amount of carbon not specified	100% removal 100 µg/liter influent	Chriswell, et al., 1977
Methoxychlor	346	Unknown	Unknown	% reduction	Unknown	>80% removal	Abstract	Schmidt, 1974
Methylene chloride (dichloromethane)	84.9	17	F400	Isotherm	1.7×10^{-5}–5.0×10^{-5}	5.8×10^{-5}		Weber et al., 1977
Nitrosamines (e.g., N-Nitrosodiphenylamine)	198.07	17	F300	Isotherm	5.0×10^{-8}–3.5×10^{-5}	2.2×10^{-3}	N-Nitrosodiphenylamine	Dobbs et al., 1978
Polychlorinated biphenyls (PCB) (e.g., Arochlor 1254)	Mixture	6	F300	Isotherm	0.5 µg/liter-37µg/liter	6.4 mg/g	Arochlor 1254	Mahon, 1979

TABLE IV-2 (continued)

Organic Compounds	Molecular Weight	Number of Data Points	Carbon Type	Adsorption Test Method	Equilibrium Concentration Range, mol/liter	Maximum Surface Concentration, mol/g	Comments	References
Polynuclear aromatic hydrocarbons	Eight compounds	—	10 types	% reduction	ppb level	Variable	99% removal; review article	Borneff, 1980
Simazine	201.69	1	OU-A	% reduction	7×10^{-7}	4×10^{-4}	Translated abstract	Shevchenko et al., 1974
Tetrachloro-ethylene	165.83	10	F400	Isotherm	6×10^{-10}–2.5×10^{-8}	6×10^{-5}		Weber et al., 1977
Toluene	92.15	4	F300	Isotherm	1.7×10^{-5}–4.8×10^{-5}	9.5×10^{-5}		Mahon, 1979
Toxaphene	412	Unknown	F300	Isotherm	5×10^{-8}–4×10^{-7}	1×10^{-4}		Hager and Rizzo, 1974
1,1,1-Trichloro-ethane	133.41	—	F300	Isotherm	2.7×10^{-6}–1.2×10^{-3}	2.7×10^{-3}		Hansen, 1979[b]
Trichloro-ethylene	131.39	7	F300	Isotherm	1.1×10^{-9}–4.8×10^{-7}	4.2×10^{-5}		Dobbs et al., 1978
2,4,5-Trichloro-phenoxypropionic acid (2,4,5-TP)	269	Unknown	Columbia LC	Isotherm	Unknown	Unknown	Follows Langmuir isotherm	Weber and Gould, 1966
Xylene	106.2	4	F300	Isotherm	1.4×10^{-5}–1.1×10^{-4}	1.2×10^{-3}	Para isomer	Dobbs et al., 1978

NOTE: All values are for neutral forms of the molecules unless stated otherwise.

[a] There are no data on adsorption by GAC of the following chemicals with possible health effects: β-BHC, bis (2-chloropropyl) ether, butyl bromide, dibromochloropropane, 1,2-dibromoethane, dichlorofluoromethane, 1,1-dichloroethene (vinylidene chloride), epichlorohydrin, ethylenethiourea (ETU), ethylene dibromide, ethylene oxide, kepone, methyl iodide, pentachloronitrobenzene (PCNB), polybrominated biphenyls (PBB), 1,1,2-trichloroethane, trichlorofluoromethane, and vinyl chloride.

[b] Personal communication with K. Hansen, Calgon Corp., March 21, 1979.

tion data that are cited in the table. Every effort was made to locate each original publication and to transcribe the data from it. In some cases, abstracts were used to obtain adsorption data. Several references contain adsorption data on the same organic compound. Well-documented adsorption isotherms were the first choice. This category was followed by selection of data based on percent reduction. The third choice was data from column tests, which indicate only that the compound is adsorbed but do not indicate sorption capacity.

Table IV-2 indicates that there are adsorption data pertaining to 40 of the 58 specific organics and classes of organic compounds. The data illustrate that a great number of the chemicals of concern are, in fact, adsorbable on activated carbon. Some of these data have been plotted in Figure IV-1; other isotherm data in Table IV-2 can be plotted in a similar fashion for comparison. One investigator claimed that some of the organic compounds being studied were not adsorbable on activated carbon (Dobbs et al., 1978). There is a conflict between the results in Dobbs et al. (1978) and Dahm et al. (1974) regarding the adsorbability of acetone cyanohydrin. Dobbs et al. (1978) listed the compound as not adsorbed by activated carbon. Dahm et al. (1974) reported percent removal values for the compound that ranged from 30% to 60%.

Equilibrium Models

Equilibrium models have the potential for predicting the adsorption capacities of wide varieties of organics on activated carbon. The information required to use such models includes thermodynamic properties of the solvents, adsorbents, and adsorbates. The following equilibrium models have been proposed to predict adsorption capacity: ideal adsorbed solution theory, Polanyi theory, solvophobic theory, and the net adsorption energy concept. These models are not equivalent in their data needs, theoretical justifications, and applications. McGuire and Suffet (1978) summarized each of these modeling approaches and listed the references that describe them. Once there is confidence in such predictive techniques, the equilibrium models can hopefully be interfaced with the mass transfer models to predict breakthrough curves of single solutes and multisolute systems.

Summary, Conclusions, and Recommendations

Existing data show that GAC will adsorb many organic compounds from water. Adsorption data for approximately 70% of the specific organics and classes of organic compounds that are suspected of being harmful to health are given in Table IV-2. Essentially, all of the compounds are adsorbable to some extent, but competitive effects are important in determining the capacity of specific water treatment applications. This is discussed in a later section.

The isotherm data base should be expanded to provide the basic data for the adsorption characteristics of chemicals that are potentially harmful to health. Experimental methods for determining isotherms and reporting of data should be standardized so that the data reported by different researchers can be compared on an equivalent basis.

More data need to be developed on the differences between adsorption kinetics for different classes of organic compounds, since the rate of adsorption is important to process efficiency. The above recommendations on standardizing experimental methods and data-reporting formats also apply to kinetic data.

EFFECTIVENESS OF PRETREATMENT FOR REMOVING SELECTED ORGANIC COMPOUNDS

Processes traditionally used to remove particulates from water also can significantly reduce organic matter. These clarification processes, which include coagulation, sedimentation, and filtration, are used at almost all surface-water treatment plants. Some organics collect on natural particles or particles that are formed during coagulation and, thus, are removed when the particles are removed. Because clarification processes remove adsorbable organic matter and consequently reduce the subsequent rate of saturation of the GAC, these processes should be used to their maximum extent. Lower loading rates will result in a lower GAC regeneration frequency, thereby lowering treatment costs, and should reduce the likelihood of displacement of organics by competitive adsorption because displacement is a function of loading. To the extent that the clarification processes remove nonadsorbable organics, they improve the quality of the water that is produced by the treatment plant and are desirable. Lowering the organic concentration by this procedure will result in a lower demand for disinfectant and lessen the likelihood of reaction of organics with the disinfectant to form undesirable end products.

Two recent reviews describe in detail many characteristics of the coagulation process in conjunction with sedimentation and filtration that are important to the removal of organics (Kavanaugh, 1978; Semmens *et al.*, 1978). The type of coagulant, coagulant dose, nature of the organic matter, and pH are especially important to the removal of organic matter as measured by dissolved organic carbon (DOC), total organic carbon (TOC), fulvic acid concentration, humic acid concentration, or color. The extent of the removals depends greatly upon the type of organic matter present. Removals as high as 95% from synthetic solutions of humic acid have been reported (Semmens *et al.*, 1978); however, typical removals are somewhat lower. TOC removals of 60% were reported for pilot scale studies of Ohio River water treatment, 25% to 40% removals from surface waters were reported in the Federal Republic of Germany, and removals up to 60% have been reported for fulvic acid, a predominant constituent of organic matter in natural waters (Kavanaugh, 1978; Semmens *et al.*, 1978).

The best removals of organic matter by coagulation are generally achieved at pH values of 5 to 6. Snoeyink *et al.* (1978) have shown that humic substances, the predominant fraction of organic matter in surface waters, are adsorbed better at these low pH values. Consequently, both coagulation and subsequent adsorption may be more effective if conducted at low pH. As reviewed by McCreary and Snoeyink (1977), adsorption isotherms before and after coagulation can be very different.

An alternative means of characterizing the organic content of water is the trihalomethane formation potential (THMFP) test, which, under a fixed set of conditions, determines the tendency to form THM's when water is chlorinated (Stevens *et al.*, 1976). Babcock and Singer (1977) found that over 70% of the THMFP was removed by alum coagulation of a humic acid solution prior to chlorination. Alum coagulation of fulvic acid also showed removal, but not as much. The EPA (U.S. Environmental Protection Agency, 1978c) reported nearly 70% removal from a particular raw water by coagulation, sedimentation, and filtration. Kavanaugh (1978) found that a maximum of about 65% removal of TOC could be achieved from a surface water in California and that the percentage THMFP removal was nearly the same, although the magnitude of the concentration of the haloforms that resulted after chlorination was highly dependent upon pH.

The importance of at least filtration as a pretreatment for GAC is illustrated by the results currently being obtained at the Jefferson Parish water treatment plant in Louisiana, where Mississippi River water is treated by prechlorination with chloramines, coagulation, and sedimentation. After sedimentation, a portion of the flow is passed through a sand filter and then through a GAC adsorber, whereas another portion is passed directly into the GAC adsorber without prior filtration. The GAC adsorber that receives the prefiltered water removes volatile halogenated organics, TOC, and THMFP much more efficiently than does the GAC adsorber that must also remove the particulates. Interpretation of the data is complicated by the failure to keep the same contact times in both beds.

Removals of specific compounds can also be achieved by the coagulation process. Sridharan and Lee (1972) demonstrated that some phenol, glycine, and citric acid could be removed by coagulation with ferric chloride. Pesticides may be adsorbed to silt (Greve and Wit, 1971) and associated with humic substances (Choi and Chen, 1976), which may also be removed by coagulation. Andelman (1973) has indicated that polynuclear aromatic hydrocarbons (PAH) usually occur in the form of particulates. The same is likely true for other organic compounds. For example, Greve and Wit (1971) observed that nearly all of the 0.2–0.6 μg/liter of endosulfan in Rhine River water was removed by clarification processes. Robeck et al. (1965) reported that nearly all of 10 ppb DDT was removed by coagulation–filtration, but nearly none of the same amount of lindane was eliminated. Thus, by achieving good particulate removal, significant amounts of selected organics may also be removed.

Reactions of chlorine, or other oxidative pretreatment chemicals such as ozone, chlorine dioxide, and permanganate, with organics may increase or decrease adsorbability. To the extent that higher-molecular-weight natural organics are converted to low-molecular-weight THM's, adsorbability is decreased (Table IV-2). Compounds such as phenol may be chlorinated during prechlorination of a water supply. When this occurs, solubility decreases and adsorbability increases when the pH of the solution is below the pK of the chlorinated phenol (Snoeyink et al., 1977). However, as chlorine atoms are substituted onto the phenol ring, the pK is lowered, i.e., the molecule becomes more acidic. It is more likely that the molecule will be ionized at the values found in natural waters; the anionic species is more soluble than the neutral species and is more poorly adsorbed. To minimize THM concentrations in product water, it is better to minimize prechlorination as much as possible and to remove THM precursors by coagulation. Adsorption may also be necessary before final chlorination. Even less is known about the effects of other oxidative pretreatments, e.g., ozone or chlorine dioxide and their influence on subsequent adsorbability.

If proper air pollution control is observed, aeration preceding adsorption may be beneficial if the water contains volatile low-molecular-weight compounds. Such compounds are adsorbed relatively weakly, and removal before adsorption should result in longer intervals between regenerations. Aeration during full-scale advanced wastewater treatment at Water Factory 21 has resulted in significant removals of volatile compounds. This process should be examined more closely at water treatment plants.

Bank filtration, which is practiced in the Federal Republic of Germany along the Rhine River, may also enhance the adsorption process (see McCreary and Snoeyink, 1977, for a review). As much as 65% to 75% reductions of DOC are attributed to the biological activity in the bank, dilution effects, and possibly some adsorption. The reduction in DOC reduces the loading on the GAC and probably allows longer intervals between regenerations, although this has not been shown by experimentation. Water quality may be degraded during filtration through the soil by uptake of iron and manganese. It would then be necessary to remove these contaminants prior to adsorption to prevent their interference with that process.

Softening and manganese removal can result in reductions of organics (McCreary and Snoeyink, 1977), as can ozonization (see below).

The subcommittee located no published case histories of the use of PAC to treat the water before GAC. Nonetheless, this possibility should not be overlooked, especially during periodic heavy loads of certain organics, which might result from spills. Carbons can be made with widely different properties. Occasionally, certain compounds in the water supply may not be well removed by the GAC that is in service, but may be removed by specific powdered carbons. The use of PAC in such cases should be investigated.

EFFECTIVENESS OF GAC AS A PRETREATMENT PROCESS FOR DISINFECTION

Disinfection efficiency is increased when GAC or other processes are used to reduce the organic content of water prior to disinfection. Moreover, during chlorination one can expect fewer side reactions resulting in the production of chlorinated organics. It should be possible to achieve a given level of inactivation of undesirable microorganisms with a lower disinfectant dose in a given period or to use a shorter contact time for the same disinfectant dose to achieve the same level of inactivation. After 25 hazen units of organic color were reduced to 5 units, Hutchinson and Ridgway (1977) observed a reduction in contact time from 65 to 28 min at pH 8.5, and from 6 to 2.5 min at pH 6.5 for 99% destruction of *E. coli* with 0.02 mg/liter of chlorine at 5°C. The reduction in time required for the same concentration of chlorine dioxide to achieve the same kill under the same conditions ranged from 13 to 10 min at pH 8.5 and from 14 to 10 min at pH 6.5. For 0.02 mg/liter of ozone concentration at pH 6.5, the contact time was reduced from 5.5 to 3.5 min, and at pH 8.5 it was reduced from 33 to 5 min.

The ozone dose that was required to produce a 3 log reduction in the standard plate count in the effluent from a GAC column in use 2 months was less than 20% of that required when no GAC was used. The chlorine dioxide dose that was required for a similar kill was reduced by a factor of 3 when GAC that was in operation for 6 months was used (U.S. Environmental Protection Agency, 1976, Appendix 3).

Nitrification may take place in GAC adsorbers when biological activity is present (see below). When this happens it is easier to use free chlorine for postdisinfection than when ammonia is present. Much more efficient destruction of bacteria and virus then becomes possible, but the likelihood of forming chlorinated organics also increases.

When the GAC adsorber removes biodegradable organic matter, not only is the disinfectant demand reduced, but also the possibilities of regrowth of microorganisms in the distribution system are decreased because the microbial food supply is reduced. Elimination of the biodegradable organic matter also increases the likelihood that residual disinfectants will persist throughout the distribution system, thereby decreasing the chances of biological growth.

Extensive biological growth in shallow beds of GAC may result in sloughing of aggregations of microorganisms into the product water. Disinfection may be more difficult if such aggregations are present, but this problem can be minimized by more frequent backwashing.

Summary, Conclusions, and Recommendations

Clarification processes (coagulation, sedimentation, filtration) remove significant concentrations of some organics, especially some types of THM precursors and relatively insoluble compounds that may be associated with particulates. In some cases, the removal of THM precursors by clarification may be sufficient to eliminate the need for an adsorption process. There is also some evidence that filtration before GAC adsorption can result in increased life of the carbon or an increase in the time between regeneration.

In some cases, chlorination before adsorption may result in improved adsorption efficiency; in others, it may decrease efficiency. The application of PAC before GAC may be advisable in specific situations.

Disinfection after GAC adsorption can be achieved with lower doses of disinfectants than if GAC were not used. By decreasing the concentration of biodegradable organic matter, the use of GAC also reduces the possibility that organism regrowth will occur in the distribution system. The subcommittee recommends that:

• Adsorption processes should be evaluated together with the clarification processes that will precede them in a water treatment plant.
• Research should be conducted on the conjunctive use of PAC and GAC.
• Research should be conducted to evaluate the aeration process for removal of volatile organic compounds during water treatment.

POWDERED ACTIVATED CARBON (PAC)

Several considerations relative to the effectiveness of PAC as the sole adsorbent for removal of organics are the same as those discussed above for GAC. In general, we can expect the same relative selectivity for the removal of organic and inorganic materials. The exceptions are those that depend upon the nature of the carbon surface because PAC usually has different properties than GAC. Lower cost materials are most often used for its manufacture, and the product usually has a much lower density. PAC is generally quite friable, but this is not important because it is usually used on a once-through basis. If friable PAC were to be regenerated, high losses undoubtedly would be observed.

The use of PAC differs from that of GAC in the point of application, the type of reactor used, the relative importance of adsorption kinetics, and the relative nature of competitive adsorption effects.

PAC is generally applied in water treatment plants at the rapid mix unit, which disperses it rapidly. The flocculation and sedimentation units, which usually follow, provide the necessary delay for many organics to adsorb. Other possible points of application include the intake and points after the rapid mix unit. The latter points are usually undesirable because of the reduced time of adsorption. If the carbon is added just ahead of the rapid filter, the contact time is only minutes or a fraction of a minute. PAC may also be applied in solids contact upflow clarifiers. In these units the PAC is suspended and the water being treated is passed through the suspension. High concentrations of PAC can be used in this type of contactor, and recycling of the PAC is possible.

When PAC is applied so that it moves through the treatment units with the water flow, it tends to equilibrate with the concentration of organics in the water treatment plant effluent. By comparison, GAC at the adsorber inlet tends to equilibrate with the concentration in the water before it comes into contact with the carbon, while GAC at the adsorber outlet tends to equilibrate with the organics in the effluent. The net result is that GAC tends to equilibrate with higher concentrations than does PAC. Because a much lower loading, i.e., mass of organic material adsorbed per mass of carbon, can be achieved at low equilibrium concentration as compared to high equilibrium concentration, more PAC than GAC is generally needed to achieve the desired removal.

To date, PAC has been used extensively in water treatment plants to remove organic compounds that cause offensive taste and odor (AWWA Committee Report, 1977). Very little has been done to evaluate its applicability to the removal of many other compounds of concern, such as THM precursors, TOC, specific chlorinated organics, etc. Some work has been performed using PAC to remove THM's, but only one carbon was used and only one type of water was treated (U.S. Environmental Protection Agency, 1976a). Competitive effects and carbon type can significantly affect results. Therefore, tests should be conducted on other types of waters and with other carbons.

Adsorption on PAC is affected by other processes. For example, when applied in the rapid mix unit the PAC is likely to become enmeshed in floc particles, thereby affecting the adsorption of certain compounds.

When PAC is applied to water containing chlorine, the carbon will act as a reducing agent and destroy the chlorine. This increases the chlorine required to achieve a given level of disinfection. There is also some evidence that the reaction with chlorine has an adverse effect on the adsorption of organics (McGuire et al., 1978; Snoeyink et al., 1974). The significance of this problem needs further evaluation. It is also not known whether the chlorine that reacts with the carbon or the organic compounds on the carbon surface produces undesirable chlorinated organics that enter the treated water.

Adsorption of molecules that diffuse rapidly should reach equilibrium with the small PAC particles in the water treatment plant. However, large molecules such as humic acid diffuse slowly, and it is very likely that adsorption equilibrium cannot be achieved in the available time.

Adsorbing molecules compete for sites on PAC just as they do on GAC. Most of the same considerations apply to both materials, but one unique difference concerns the displacement of previously adsorbed molecules. In a GAC bed, weakly adsorbed material may be displaced, sometimes resulting in an effluent concentration that is greater than the influent concentration. When PAC is used in a sludge blanket, such as in an upflow solids contact clarifier, it is expected to behave similarly, but when it is applied so that it moves through the treatment plant with the water being treated until it settles out, the effluent concentration will always be less than the influent concentration, although the percent that is removed will not be as high as when there is no competition.

Summary, Conclusions, and Recommendations

Lower loadings can be achieved on PAC than on GAC in a fixed or fluidized bed adsorber. Thus, higher doses of PAC are generally required to achieve equivalent results. PAC is also difficult to regenerate, but, because it costs less, it may be economically justified in certain applications. In general, the same types of compounds are expected to adsorb on PAC as on GAC. When PAC is applied so that it is in contact with water only a short time, it very likely does not support biological activity. Also, when PAC moves with the water being treated, effluent concentrations greater than the influent will not occur. However, when it is applied in upflow solids contact clarifiers, the time of contact between the carbon particles and the water is longer, and microbial growth may attach to the carbon particles.

More research is recommended to determine the conditions under which PAC is most effective and to ascertain whether the reaction of PAC (as well as for GAC) and its adsorbed compounds with predisinfectants will result in undesirable compounds in the treated water.

COMPETITION ON GAC

Competitive effects are created by adsorption of a wide spectrum of trace organics, which are found in water supplies and generated within the treatment process. These should be considered in order to estimate the overall efficiency of the GAC process. As shown in Figure IV-1, Table IV-2, and by the theoretical calculations of McGuire and Suffet (1980), the adsorbability of the multitude of organics that have been identified in water supplies can vary widely. Therefore, displacement of weakly adsorbed by strongly adsorbed organics is a possibility. Depending upon the relative concentrations of these organics, displacement can also lead to temporarily higher concentrations in the effluent of the GAC bed than in the influent for any given species. Thus, the degree of competition between organic compounds of potential harm to health and their competition with humic substances are considered below.

The bulk of the data illustrating the effects of competitive adsorption derives mostly from controlled laboratory experiments with two component systems. Data from a few pilot plant studies were also examined to determine if competitive effects were significant under actual operating conditions where complex mixtures of various organic contaminants are being treated. In these studies, however, it was difficult to conclude whether or not competition was responsible for earlier-than-expected breakthrough of specific organics and, in some instances, for concentrations of certain organic species in the effluent of the GAC bed being higher than in the influent. This difficulty arises because the composition and concentration of trace organics in the raw water are highly variable. Suffet et al. (1978a,b) demonstrated influent variability in studies of the effectiveness of GAC beds treating the Philadelphia water supply.

If the influent composition of organic species to the GAC bed is highly variable, then the adsorption equilibrium capacity for each organic must be continually in a state of readjustment, even when competitive adsorption is negligible. Therefore, it is reasonable to expect that desorption of an organic contaminant could occur due to reequilibration with a lower influent concentration. Such desorption thus occurs completely independent of any effect of competitive adsorption and needs to be accounted for separately. This point will be discussed further in the section entitled "Pilot Plant Studies of Competitive Adsorption."

Studies of Competitive Equilibrium Adsorption

Reported laboratory studies of competitive adsorption have been summarized in Table IV-3. In most of these studies two component systems were used. Furthermore, most of the organics tested were not suspected of having potential health effects. In many cases the range of equilibrium concentrations was much higher than the range that would be of practical concern in water treatment (mg/liter concentrations). Although these three factors limit the applicability of results, the data nevertheless provide good insight into the extent and variation of competitive adsorption. Some of the studies in Table IV-3 include mathematical modeling of fixed bed adsorbers (e.g., Crittendon and Weber, 1978a,b,c; Fritz, 1978; Hsieh, 1974; Keinath and Carnahan, 1973; Weber, 1966; Weber and Keinath, 1967; Weber et al., 1978b).

In general, the extent of competition depends upon the relative adsorption of each component in a single component system. If two components adsorb equally well, then the competition between them will also be equal and less adsorption of both will occur. On the other hand, should one component be adsorbed much more strongly, then the degree of competition will be unequal and the weaker component will be displaced to a far greater extent.

Prediction of competitive effects is not always straightforward, even in many of the oversimplified systems shown in Table IV-3. When competition involves weak organic acids, pH can be very important in determining the competing species and the resulting extent of interaction with other adsorbing organics. (See entries 1–4, 7, 10–12, 17–19, and 25–27 of Table IV-3.) Although models of competitive adsorption assume that all organics will compete for at least some, if not all, of the sites available, studies have already shown exceptions. For example, members of the alkylbenzenesulfonate family exhibit the tendency towards irreversible adsorption which in itself implies restriction of competition (see entries 3, 5, 16, 17, and 41 of Table IV-3). Also, chloroform, in competition with *p*-nitrophenol, is adsorbed far less than would be predicted from competitive adsorption models based upon the single solute adsorption isotherms, while *p*-nitrophenol is adsorbed better (see entries 37–39 of Table IV-3). This implies adsorption at different sites.

Table IV-3 shows that nitro-, chloro-, methyl- and bromo-substituted phenols have been studied in some detail in competitive systems. *p*-Nitrophenol is very strongly adsorbed compared to many organics (entries 1–14). Phenol itself is adsorbed relatively weakly and is displaced most readily in competitive systems containing substituted phenols (entries 14–19 in Table IV-3). On the other hand, the more highly substituted phenols such as trichlorophenol are strongly adsorbed in neutral form and are less easily displaced (entry 25).

While most attention has focused upon removal of the trace organics, it may also be necessary to estimate the relative sorptive behavior of humic substances, which are precursors to haloforms. This concern arises if postchlorination is a consideration. In such cases, the displacement of the humic substances by more strongly adsorbed components could control service time of the GAC bed. Entries 29–35 of Table IV-3 indicate that the concentration of humic substances has been much higher than that of the competing component in order to simulate the most likely condition to be encountered in practice. Under such conditions, some displacement of the trace organic was caused by the presence of humic substances.

Snoeyink *et al.* (1977) have shown the adsorption behavior of humic substances to vary with the molecular weight fraction. The humic substances can exhibit different degrees of competition with trace organics. Generally, humic substances are relatively weakly adsorbed. However, the much higher concentration of these organics, i.e., mg/liter, as compared with that of the trace organics of concern, i.e., μg/liter, can

TABLE IV-3 Summary of Competitive Equilibrium Studies

Entry Number	Components	Equilibrium Concentration Range	Extent of Decrease of Each Component in the Mixture[a]	Success of Competitive Adsorption Modelling	Comments	Reference
1	p-Nitrophenol (PNP)-p-Bromophenol (PBP)	$10^{-4}-10^{-2} M$	Mutual	Excellent	Both components in neutral forms. Strong competition noted.	Jain and Snoeyink, 1973
2	PNP (anion)-PBP (anion)	$10^{-5}-10^{-2} M$	PNP >> PBP	Good	Electrostatic repulsion caused by anionic charge noted to decrease adsorption. Some noncompetitive adsorption of PBP suggested.	Jain and Snoeyink, 1973
3	PNP-Benzenesulfonate (BS)	$10^{-5}-10^{-2} M$	None	Moderate	PNP in neutral form and BS in anionic form. Adsorption on different sites indicated.	Jain and Snoeyink, 1973
4	PNP (anion)-BS (anion)	$10^{-5}-10^{-2} M$	BS displaced; PNP unaffected	Poor (observed competition less than predicted)	Electrostatic repulsion caused by anionic charge noted to decrease adsorption of BS. Some adsorption without competition indicated.	Jain and Snoeyink, 1973
5	PNP-D-sulfonate (DBS)	$10^{-3}-10^{-2} M$	DBS irreversibly adsorbed	NA	Competition observed only when carbon was preloaded with PNP.	Baldauf, 1978
6	PNP-Benzoic acid (BA)	$10^{-7}-10^{-6} M$	BA >> PNP	Good	Both components in neutral form.	Baldauf, 1978; Jossens et al., 1978; Fritz, 1978
7	PNP-BA	$10^{-2}-10^{-4} M/ 10^{-2} M$	BA > PNP	Excellent	Both components in neutral form.	Rosene and Manes, 1976
8	PNP-Glucose	$10^{-2}-10^{-7} M/ 0.4-2.7M$	Glucose >> PNP	Excellent		Rosene and Manes, 1976

No.	Compound pair	Concentration range	Selectivity	Comments	Reference
9	PNP-Urea	10^{-2}-10^{-7} M	Urea >> PNB	Excellent		Rosene and Manes, 1976
10	PNP (anionic)-Aniline (neutral)	10^{-3}-10^{-2} M	PNP >> Aniline	Excellent		Baldauf, 1978
11	PNP (neutral)-Aniline (cationic)	10^{-3}-10^{-2} M	Aniline >>PNP	Excellent		Baldauf, 1978
12	PNP-p-Chlorophenol (PCP)	10^{-3}-10^{-2} M	Mutual	Excellent	Both components in neutral form. Strong competition noted.	Baldauf, 1978
13	PNP-PCP	10^{-3}-10^{-2} M	Mutual	Excellent		Jossens et al., 1978; DiGiano et al., 1978
14	PNP-Phenol	10^{-3}-10^{-2} M	Phenol >> PNP	Excellent		DiGiano et al., 1978; Fritz, 1978; Jossens et al., 1978
15	PNP-o-Phenylphenol (OPP)	10^{-3}-10^{-2} M	PNP>OPP	Excellent		Josens et al., 1978
16	Phenol-DBS	10^{-6}-10^{-4} M	Phenol >> DBS	Excellent	Some adsorption without competition suggested. Total adsorption capacity of mixture exceeded that of either maximum, single component capacity.	Weber and Morris, 1964b
17	Phenol (neutral)-DBS (anionic)	10^{-5}-10^{-4} M	Phenol >> DBS	Moderate		Crittenden and Weber, 1978c
18	Phenol-p-Toluenesulfonate (PTS)	10^{-5}-10^{-4} M	PTS >> Phenol	Moderate	Phenol in neutral form and PTS in anionic form.	Crittenden and Weber, 1978c
19	Phenol (neutral)-PBP (neutral)	10^{-4}-10^{-3} M	Phenol >> PBP	Excellent		Mathews, 1975
20	Phenol-Resorcinol	10^{-1}-1 M	Phenol > Resorcinol	Good		Radke and Prausnitz, 1972b
21	Phenol-2,4-dichloro phenoxyacetic acid (2,4 D)	1×10^{-4}M- 4×10^{-4} M	Phenol >2,4 D	Excellent		Hsieh, 1974

TABLE IV-3 (continued)

Entry Number	Components	Equilibrium Concentration Range	Extent of Decrease of Each Component in the Mixture[a]	Success of Competitive Adsorption Modelling	Comments	Reference
22	PCP-p-Cresol	10^{-5}-10^{-1} M	p-Cresol>PCP	Excellent		Radke and Prausnitz, 1972b
23	PCP-Phenyl-acetic acid	10^{-3}-10^{-2} M	PAA>>PCP	Excellent		Fritz, 1978; Jossens et al., 1978
24	OPP-Dinitro-o-sec-butylphenol (DNOSBP)	10^{-6}-10^{-5} M	OPP>>DNOSBP	Excellent		Keinath and Carnaham, 1973
25	Dichlorophenol (DCP)-Trichlorophenol (TCP)	10^{-9}-10^{-5} M	DCP>>TCP	Moderate	Both components in neutral forms. Strong competition noted, especially at higher concentrations.	Snoeyink et al., 1977
26	DCP (neutral)-TCP (anionic)	10^{-9}-10^{-5} M	TCP>>DCP	Poor (at higher concentrations competition was reverse of prediction)	Some adsorption without competition indicated; electrostatic interaction also noted.	Snoeyink et al., 1977; Murin and Snoeyink, 1979
27	DCP (anionic)-TCP (anionic)	10^{-9}-10^{-5} M	TCP>>DCP	Good	Some adsorption without competition indicated.	Snoeyink et al., 1977; Murin and Snoeyink, 1979
28	DCP-DBS	10^{-3}-10^{-2} M	Mutual	Excellent		Fritz, 1978; Jossens et al., 1978
29	Humic substances-TCP	10^{-6}-10^{-5} M 10-50 mg/liter	TCP>>Humic substances	NA	More competition noted at lower pH and higher humic substance concentration. Humics were weakly adsorbed.	Snoeyink et al., 1977; Murin and Snoeyink, 1979

281

No.	System	Concentration	Competition	Model Fit	Comments	Reference
30	Humic substances-Methylisoborneol (MIB)	10-100 mg/liter 0.1-100 μg/liter	MIB $>>$ Humic substances	NA	Even with competition MIB adsorption was very effective. More competition noted at lower MIB concentrations.	Snoeyink et al., 1977; Herzing et al., 1977
31	Humic substances-Geosmin	10-40 mg/liter 0.1-100 μg/liter	Geosmin $>>$ Humic substances	NA	Geosmin displaced to greater extent than MIB but was the more strongly adsorbed in single component system.	Snoeyink et al., 1977; Herzing et al., 1977
32	Humic substances-Benzanthracene	10-100 mg/liter 1-10 μg/liter	None	NA	Limited testing; benzanthracene did not associate with humic substances and was well removed by adsorption.	Snoeyink et al., 1977
33	Humic substances-Carbon tetrachloride	5 mg/liter/ 10^{-6} M	None	NA	No competitive interaction noted.	Weber et al., 1978b
34	Humic substances-Dieldrin	5 mg/liter/ 10^{-8}-10^{-7} M	Dieldrin $>$ Humic substances	NA	Presence of humic substances in much larger concentration than dieldrin produced a significant competitive effect.	Weber et al., 1978b
35	Humic substances-PCB (Araclor 1016)	5 mg/liter/ 10^{-8}-10^{-7} M	PCB $>$ Humic substances	NA	Same as above.	Weber et al., 1978b
36	Lignin sulfonic acids (LSA)-PNP	10 mg/liter/ 10^{-4}-10^{-7} M	Mutual	Good (simplified system description to two components)		Frick et al., in press
37	Cloroform-Bromoform	10^{-5}-10^{-3} M	Chloroform $>>$ Bromoform	Poor (Chloroform displaced more than predicted)	Little displacement of bromoform.	Baldauf, 1978
38	Chloroform-PNP	10^{-5}-10^{-3} M	Chloroform$>$PNP	Poor (chloroform displaced more than predicted)	Little displacement of PNP.	Baldauf, 1978
39	Chloroform-LSA	10-50 mg/liter	Chloroform $>>$ LSA	Poor (chloroform displaced more than predicted)	Little displacement of PNP.	Baldauf, 1978

TABLE IV-3 (continued)

Entry Number	Components	Equilibrium Concentration Range	Extent of Decrease of Each Component in the Mixture[a]	Success of Competitive Adsorption Modelling	Comments	Reference
40	Acetone-Propionitrile	10^{-4}-10^{-1} M	Mutual	Excellent		Radke and Prausnitz, 1972
41	Nitrochloro-benzene-DBS	10^{-6}-10^{-4} M	Mutual	Excellent	Some adsorption without competition.	Weber and Morris, 1964
42	BA-Glucose	10^{-3}-10^{-5} M/ 0.4-2.75 M	Glucose $>>$ BA	Excellent	Very high concentration of more weakly adsorbed component.	Rosene and Manes, 1976
43	BA-Valine	10^{-3}-10^{-5} M/ 0.6 M	Valine $>$ $>$ BA	Excellent	Very high concentration of more weakly adsorbed component.	Rosene et al., 1976
44	BA-Methionine	10^{-3}-10 M/ 0.07 M	Methionine $>$ $>$ BA	Excellent	Very high concentration of more weakly adsorbed component.	Rosene et al., 1976
45	Phthalide-Glucose	10^{-2}-10^{-5} M 0.2-0.2 M	Glucose $>$ $>$ Phthalide	Excellent	Very high concentration of more weakly adsorbed component.	Rosene and Manes, 1976
46	Phthalide-Urea	10^{-2}-10^{-5} M/ 10^{-2} M	Urea $>$ $>$ Phthalide	Excellent	Very high concentration of more weakly adsorbed component.	Rosene and Manes, 1976
47	Nitromethane (NM)-Methylethylketone (MEK)-n-Butanol (NB)-1,4 Dioxane(D)	10^{-5}-10^{-3} M	NM~MEK $>$ $>$ NB $>$ D	NA		McGuire, 1977
48	2-Chlorophenol-o-Cresol-2-Methylpyridine	10^{-4}-10^{-3} M	Mutual	NA	Total maximum adsorption capacity of mixture approximated maximum adsorption capacity of strongest adsorber in single component system.	Martin and Al-Bahrani, 1977

49	Nitrobenzene-2-Chlorophenol-o-Cresol-2-Methylpyridine-Pyridine	10^{-4}-10^{-3} M	Mutual	NA		Martin and Al-Bahrani, 1977
50	PNP-Thiourea-Acrylamide	10^{-2}-10^{-7} M/1 M/0.8 M	Mutual	Excellent	PNP displaced due to very high concentrations of other two components.	Rosene and Manes, 1977
51	Ultrawet (branched sulfonated alkyl-benzene)-Dodecyl-sulfate	~7×10^{-6} M	NA (Fixed bed dynamic testing)	NA	Sorptive capacity of each organic was reduced in fixed bed operation in comparison with that obtainable with single solute at the same concentration.	Weber, 1966
52	Sulfonated alkyl-benzene-DNOSBP-Quinine	~3×10^{-6} M	NA (Fixed bed dynamic testing)	NA	Same comments as above. Also, rates of adsorption were reduced in mixture as compared with single solute system.	Weber and Keinath, 1967
53	Sulfonated alkyl-benzene-Triethanolamine-2,4-DCP-Nonyl-phenoxypoly-ethoxyethanol	~5×10^{-4} M	NA (Fixed bed dynamic testing)	NA	Same comments as above.	Weber and Keinath, 1967
54	Phenol-Quinine-Dodecylsulfate-Sulfonated alkyl-benzene-2-sec-Butyl-4,6-dinitro-phenol-2,4-D-Nonylphenoxypoly-ethoxyethanol-Phenyl-dimethyl phosphorodiamidate	~10^{-4} M	NA (Fixed bed dynamic testing)	NA	Extent of interaction unspecified. However, significant adsorption capacity was projected in a fixed bed.	Weber, 1966

[a] In a mixture, if the adsorption of the first component is decreased more than that of the second, this is denoted by $>>$.

produce competitive displacement of trace organics. These factors suggest that competition between humic substances and trace organics will be difficult to predict unless adsorption experiments are conducted for each water source.

A relative scale of competition is produced by comparing entries in which benzoic acid (BA) adsorption has been studied. Compared to *p*-nitrophenol (PNP) (entries 6 and 7), BA is weakly adsorbed and, therefore, displaced. However, compared to glucose, valine, and methionine (entries 43–45), BA is strongly adsorbed, and only high concentrations of these competing organics can cause displacement. Thus, the competitive effect must always be viewed from knowledge of the other organics in the mixture.

More complex competition among three to eight components has been investigated by McGuire (1977), Martin and Al-Bahrani (1977), and Rosene and Manes (1977). Entries 47–54 summarize their findings (Weber, 1966; Weber and Keinath, 1967). The degree of competition observed by McGuire (1977) in a four-component system (entry 47) was not expected. Single solute isotherms showed that nitromethane and methyl ethyl ketone were much more strongly adsorbed than *n*-butanol and 1,4-dioxane at a pH of 8.0. In contrast, the degree of competition observed by Martin and Al-Bahrani (1977) agreed with the relative sorptive behavior of each of the components from single solute isotherms (entries 48 and 49).

The data in Table IV-3 were analyzed by various competitive equilibrium models, e.g., the Langmuir (Weber and Morris, 1964a) and semicompetitive Langmuir (Jain and Snoeyink, 1973) models, the ideal adsorbed solution model (Fritz, 1978; Radke and Prausnitz, 1972a), the empirical three-parameter model (Crittenden, 1976; Fritz, 1978; Mathews, 1975), the modified ideal adsorbed solution model (Baldauf, 1978; DiGiano *et al.*, 1978), and a modified Polanyi model (Rosene and Manes, 1976, 1977; Rosene *et al.*, 1976). None of these is sufficiently acceptable to predict competition among important trace organics without experimental data. However, in principle, the modified Polanyi model could be used to develop predictions based upon knowing only the refractive index, solubility, and bulk solid density of each of the competing species.

Laboratory Studies of Competition in GAC Beds

The objective of several recent studies of competitive adsorption has been to verify proposed dynamic mathematical models that can then be generally applied (Balzli *et al.*, 1978; Crittenden, 1976; Crittenden and

Weber, 1978a,b,c; Fritz, 1978; Hsieh *et al.*, 1977; Keinath and Carnahan, 1973; Merk, 1978). Model verification has been restricted mainly to two-component competition and to a range of concentrations that are considerably higher than those expected in practice for trace organics. There have been no published predictions concerning competition between high concentrations of complex humic substances and very low concentrations of chlorinated organics, which may be encountered in water treatment practice. In fixed bed experiments, Weber *et al.* (1978b) have shown evidence for displacement of carbon tetrachloride, but not dieldrin, by humic substances.

There are different assumptions regarding the mass transfer controlling step, e.g., external film versus internal pore or surface diffusion and competitive equilibria description. However, the general nature of the breakthrough behavior in studies of mathematical modeling can be predicted to be displacement of the more weakly by the more strongly adsorbed component, i.e., the chromatographic effect. The extent to which the effluent concentration of the weaker adsorbate exceeds that of the influent is determined by both the relative adsorption behavior of the two components and their influent concentrations.

There are complications in the verification of mathematical models to predict GAC bed performance, even for the simplest case of two-component mixtures. For example, Crittenden (1976) found it necessary to use the lower value of mass transfer figures for both components to account for hindrance of the flux of the faster diffusing molecule by the slower diffusion. A similar observation regarding the apparent slow rate of desorption was also made by Keinath and Carnahan (1973). Hsieh (1974) used pore diffusion coefficients that were 2 to 10 times greater than determined from independent batch experiments in order to describe the data well, although this correction was not justified by experimental evidence.

Other studies have not included mathematical modeling of competitive adsorption, but they provide interesting qualitative comparisons of competitive effects. Herzing *et al.* (1977) showed that competition occurred between a high concentration (10 mg/liter) of humic substances and a low concentration (50 μg/liter) of methylisoborneol (MIB), which is an odor-producing organic.

The complex equilibrium isotherm picture for a four-component mixture (see entry 47 of Table IV-3) was used by McGuire *et al.* (1978) to describe the breakthrough characteristics for this mixture in small GAC beds. The breakthrough curves showed that 1,4-dioxane was the most poorly adsorbed of all. In fact, halfway through the experiment there was more 1,4-dioxane in the effluent than there was in the influent, suggesting that the other three, better adsorbed compounds were competing more efficiently for the same adsorption sites. Because of the complex dynamic and equilibrium capacities of the other three compounds, it was not possible to determine clearly how they were competing on the carbon surface.

Competition in mixtures of three and five components was investigated by Martin and Al-Bahrani (1977). The extent of competition could be predicted qualitatively from the relative adsorptive behavior shown by comparing single-component, equilibrium isotherms. (See entries 49 and 50 of Table IV-3.) Continuous flow, GAC bed experiments further confirmed the same pattern of competition in which the weakest sorbate, pyridine, saturated the bed first and desorbed completely in the five-component system. The breakthrough behavior of the five organics can be ordered in terms of increasing time to reach breakthrough and decreasing magnitude of the desorption effect as follows: pyridine, 2-methylpyridine, o-cresol, 2-chlorophenol, and nitrobenzene. Obviously, the most strongly adsorbed component, nitrobenzene, did not exhibit desorption.

Pilot Plant Studies of Competitive Adsorption

Pilot plant studies have not specifically addressed evaluation of competitive adsorption. Instead, the overall effectiveness of GAC in removing specific organics with possible health effects, including the THM's, has been the focal point. Because these are pilot plant studies, the influent to the GAC bed has not been constant either in composition or in concentration of trace organics. Consequently, the net result of competitive adsorption and simple reequilibration effects is being measured in such studies.

The removal efficiencies for over 18 low-molecular-weight, volatile chlorinated and brominated organics, which are present together in a southern Florida water supply, have been measured by the EPA (U.S. Environmental Protection Agency, 1978c; Wood and DeMarco, 1980). From these measurements, estimates were made of the time for the effluent concentration to reach the influent concentration for 10 of these 18 organics in three different phases of pilot plant study (see Table IV-4). These times are necessarily approximate because the influent concentrations were highly variable and the effluent concentrations did not increase regularly with time. The EPA report did not present sufficient data to determine the importance of variations in influent concentrations.

The average concentrations of cis-1,2-dichloroethylene were at least an order of magnitude higher than those for the other components. This caused rapid initiation of breakthrough with concentrations reaching 1 μg/liter in just 3 weeks. However, this component was still relatively strongly adsorbed and effluent concentration did not equal influent concentration until the fourteenth week of operation. In contrast, vinyl chloride and 1,1-dichloroethane, while present in much lower concentrations, appeared much sooner in the effluent.

Only 1,1-dichloroethane and trichloroethylene were displaced to such an extent that effluent concentration was at some time higher than the average influent concentration. In fact, the extent of competition among these trace organics cannot be determined by the data provided in Table IV-4. Single component adsorption equilibria data are also needed. Table IV-4 also indicates apparent disparities in competitive effects for both of these two constituents. For example, comparing the average influent concentrations of the first-, second-, and third-listed test periods, it is unexplainable that the time for effluent concentration to reach the influent concentration should be shorter (and very significantly so) in the second and third test periods. Lower influent concentrations during these latter two test periods should have lessened competition if all other factors had remained constant. Such data show how difficult it can be to interpret pilot plant results.

Suffet *et al.* (1978a) reported the use of gas chromatographic profiles of 1- or 3-day composite samples and supplementary gas chromatography–mass spectrometry (GC–MS) to evaluate performance of the GAC columns. Influent and effluent samples were taken over a total of 33 weeks of pilot plant operation at the Torresdale Water Treatment Plant in Philadelphia. The two largest groups of organics that were identified were chlorinated aliphatics and aromatics, of which 19 appear on the EPA list of 129 priority pollutants (U.S. Environmental Protection Agency, 1974). Not all of these 19 compounds appeared continuously. In fact, a major conclusion of this study was that influent water quality varied considerably during the 33-week period, i.e., major GC peaks were highly transient with some periodic shifting to minor peaks while other peaks disappeared completely.

With the exception of chloroform, trichloroacetone, and toluene, GAC removed most organics to a considerable extent during 18 weeks of operation. In general, organics with lower boiling points appeared first in the effluent. However, the effluent concentration seemed to be highly variable. Some components were present in higher concentrations in the first week than in later weeks. This could be due to variations in influent concentrations. Like the EPA pilot plant study at a southern Florida waterworks, the Torresdale study also did not reveal firm evidence of displacement effects caused by competitive adsorption.

The removal of organics, whose concentrations tend to vary widely in

TABLE IV-4 Removal of Trace Organics in Pilot Plant Study of GAC[a,b]

| Component | Test Period | | | | | |
| | January 18-May 20, 1977 | | August 26-October 18, 1977 | | November 1, 1977-January 3, 1978 | |
	Average Influent Concentrations, µg/liter	Time for Effluent Concentration to Reach or Exceed Influent Concentration, weeks	Average Influent Concentrations, µg/liter	Time for Effluent Concentration to Reach or Exceed Influent Concentration, weeks	Average Influent Concentrations, µg/liter	Time for Effluent Concentration to Reach or Exceed Influent Concentration, weeks
trans-1,2-Dichloroethylene	1.3	17	1.0	7	0.63	8
1,1-Dichloroethane	0.3	13	0.3	3[c]	0.11	3[c]
cis-1,2-Dichloroethylene	29.0	14	19	7	24.5	9
Trichloroethylene	0.13	17	0.1	2	0.52	8
Tetrachloroethylene	0.06	N(17)[d]	nil	N(7)[d]	nil	N(9)[d]
Chlorobenzene	0.19	N(17)	0.8	N(7)	0.56	N(9)
p-Chlorotoluene	0.11	N(17)	0.2	N(7)	nil	N(9)
m,p,o-Dichlorobenzene	1.1	N(17)	0.3	N(7)	0.28	N(9)
Vinyl chloride	0.8	13[e]	5.4	5	7.4	2
1,2-Dichloroethane	0.11	14	5.3	7	7.9	9

[a] From U.S. Environmental Protection Agency, 1978c. Only average influent concentrations were reported for the periods indicated.
[b] See text for discussion.
[c] Apparent desorption, i.e., effluent concentration greater than average influent concentration.
[d] N( ), None found after number of days specified in parentheses.
[e] The compound was observed at first sampling after 13 weeks of operation.

the influent, can be particularly difficult to predict. For example, compounds adsorbed during periods of high concentration later are desorbed due to reequilibration with a lower influent concentration. The extent of adsorption–desorption will depend largely upon the adsorption equilibria. In the extreme case of a strongly adsorbed organic, reequilibration within a defined range of fluid phase concentration will not significantly alter the solid phase concentration. Thus, desorption is relatively unimportant. However, even in this case, almost complete disappearance of the organic in the influent will still cause desorption. Laboratory column experiments, in which a low feed concentration of carbon tetrachloride (200 μg/liter) was discontinued, have showed this desorption effect (Weber et al., 1978b). Similar results were obtained with dieldrin.

Love and Symons (1978) showed that a concentration spike of carbon tetrachloride, in which the influent concentration increased from 10 to 55 μg/liter for several weeks and then decreased to less than 1 μg/liter, caused adsorption followed by desorption. However, this produced an increase in effluent concentration that was far less than the maximum influent concentration. The effluent concentration remained at approximately 10 μg/liter for roughly 20 weeks and then dropped below the lower limit of detectability. In this example, the kinetics of adsorption-desorption probably produced a "dampening effect" during reequilibration with the lower carbon tetrachloride concentration in the influent, thereby preventing the sudden appearance of a high concentration in the effluent.

The effect of a varying influent concentration of one component on the adsorption of another component must also be considered. For example, Love and Symons (1978) showed that a "slug" of carbon tetrachloride could cause competitive displacement of chloroform, which was previously adsorbed on the GAC bed; however, the extent to which effluent chloroform concentration increased was not very significant.

In other studies, the order of appearance of various THM species in the effluent of the GAC bed has been measured. At Stuttgart, Federal Republic of Germany, the effluent concentration of chloroform exceeded the influent concentration after 55 days of operation and remained significantly higher for 14 days (Sander et al., 1977). However, this occurred for only one of the three GAC types being tested in parallel operation. This suggested that the extent of competition also depends on the type of carbon that is used. Comparisons of GAC types at Duesseldorf, Federal Republic of Germany (Poggenburg et al., 1974) and at Cincinnati, Ohio (U.S. Environmental Protection Agency, 1978c) support this argument.

Sander et al. (1977) observed that the breakthrough of dichlorobromomethane was much slower than that of chloroform. However, the concentration of dichlorobromethane entering the GAC bed was 60% less than that of chloroform. Therefore, a longer time to breakthrough is not necessarily attributable to better adsorption characteristics. Love *et al.* (1976) also compared the breakthrough behavior of haloforms with results that were similar to those obtained by Sander *et al.* (1977). Competitive adsorption may have been indicated by displacement of chloroform after 6 months of operation. A lesser displacement effect was noted for bromodichloromethane.

The removal of precursors to haloforms by GAC also was reported by Love *et al.* (1976). In the system that they studied chlorination was not used prior to the GAC. The breakthrough of the precursors that produced bromodichloromethane and dibromochloromethane occurred much sooner than that of the precursors to chloroform formation. Comparison of coal- and lignite-base carbons showed that only the coal-base carbon significantly displaced precursors to all three haloforms. This again indicates that the degree of competition can depend upon carbon type.

Observations of Competitive Effects in Full-Scale Operation

There are limited data for use in interpreting competitive adsorption in full-scale GAC systems. Sorbed phase concentration profiles have been measured for nonpolar chlorine as well as for tetrachloroethylene, hexachlorobutane, and hexachlorocyclohexane at the Duesseldorf Water Works in the Federal Republic of Germany (Poggenburg *et al.*, 1974). All of these profiles showed a decrease in concentration with depth, which did not suggest strong competitive effects. However, the adsorbed amounts of each component were considerably different and all of the sorbed phase profiles were very flat, which indicates that the adsorption of these components was relatively weak.

GAC treatment has been evaluated in full-scale testing for a total of 1 yr at the Jefferson Parish Water Treatment Plant on the lower Mississippi River (Brodtmann *et al.*, 1980). The first phase of study (February–August 1977) was distinguishable from the second phase (November–April 1978) by much higher and more variable concentrations of total THM and of precursors to the formation of the various THM species, as measured by the THMFP test.

Brodtmann *et al.* (1980) observed a strong contrast in effluent concentrations of total THM during these two phases. In the first phase, influent concentration was exceeded after 90 days of operation; after 120 days, effluent concentration was two- to fivefold higher. In the second phase, effluent concentration never exceeded influent concentration during 180 days of operation. Although the influent concentration was much lower in the second phase, the most important factor accounting for the lack of a displacement effect was most likely the more consistent nature of the influent concentration. The effluent concentration in the first phase always increased sharply whenever the influent concentration decreased sharply. This indicated that reequilibration was taking place. While Brodtmann *et al.* (1980) also pointed out that the degree of competition afforded by other organics may have been different in these two phases, they provided no evidence.

The Jefferson Parish study also showed that removal of precursors to chloroform and dichlorobromoform was not affected by displacement due to competitive adsorption and/or reequilibration with a changing influent concentration. Instead, a steady-state removal of approximately 50% was reached after 60 days of operation. Biological activity was suggested as the explanation for this.

Summary, Conclusions, and Recommendations

Dynamic situations in GAC beds can be complicated by a variety of competing species that may all have different concentrations. Table IV-2 shows the variability of adsorption of specific organics that can enter a water treatment process. In general, the relative concentrations of competing species, their degree of competition (i.e., stronger versus weaker adsorbing components), and their relative diffusive properties will influence displacement effects. Even if organics do not compete, shifts in influent concentration will cause the effluent concentration to reequilibrate with it. The extent of the reequilibration will be determined by adsorption equilibria in each case.

Competition can be anticipated between trace organics, which account for only a small fraction of the TOC, and most TOC, which is composed of humic substances originating from normal degradation processes. However, the adsorption properties of humic substances will vary, thereby making competitive interactions more difficult to predict. Table IV-4 shows examples of competitive interaction between humic substances and organics. Because the source of humic substances may be different for each water supply and may vary seasonally, pilot plant studies at specific locations over the seasons of the year will yield the most useful information on the effects of competition.

The wide spectrum of organics that have been identified in water supplies represent an equally wide spectrum of adsorption behavior. This should also lead to competition among organics of differing adsorbabilities for sites on the carbon surface. However, there is little information on the mutual reduction in adsorption capacity for competing organics in the truly multicomponent mixtures that are encountered in drinking water treatment. Data from pilot plant studies show that GAC is still effective, despite effects from competitive adsorption.

The direct information provided by the pilot plant studies seems to be an alternative to the more scientific, but as yet underdeveloped, approach that is provided by mathematical modeling of competitive adsorption. During the limited observation time in pilot plant studies, some empirical interpretation of performance can be obtained if all the major organics of concern are monitored. The results of these studies could then be used to develop a suitable monitoring program that focuses on the least adsorbable organics and/or those in highest concentration. The following conclusions can be made:

1. There are few data on the degree of competition for adsorption sites between trace organics of potential harm to health and the humic substances, which comprise the largest single fraction of organics in water supplies. It is also important to note that different sources of humic substances produced different extents of competition. There are also limited data on the degree of competition among organics of concern.

2. Organics found in water supplies exhibit a wide spectrum of adsorption behavior. Therefore, competition for adsorption sites should be expected. It is conceivable that the effluent concentrations of the more weakly adsorbed components could exceed the concentrations in the influent to the GAC bed if competitive adsorption occurred.

3. Pilot plant studies show that GAC is an effective process for removal of many organic contaminants of health concern despite whatever effects competition may have on adsorbability.

4. Pilot plant studies have shown that effluent concentrations of chloroform and, possibly, 1,1-dichloroethane and trichloroethylene exceeded influent concentrations to the GAC bed; however, from existing data, it is not possible to distinguish a displacement effect due to competitive adsorption from that due to reequilibration with a changing influent concentration.

5. Shifts in concentrations and composition of organics in the influent to the GAC bed, which then cause reequilibration, may be as important as competitive adsorption in determining effluent concentration. Because of the large number of organic components, mathematical predictions of treatment effectiveness for each component would be impractical, if not impossible.

6. Pilot plant studies over a fairly long term, e.g., conducted throughout the four seasons of the year, would seem to be necessary to evaluate the net effects of competition and reequilibration that could be

expected for organics that are potentially harmful to health under the specific conditions at each treatment facility.

More basic data are needed on the competitive interaction among trace organics of concern to health and between extremely low concentrations of these organics and the relatively high concentrations of humic substances. While it may be impossible to predict competitive effects in complex mixtures, studies of simple, two- and three-component systems can generate a relative scale of intensity of competitive interactions. Attempts to find general rules for competitive adsorption and to develop mathematical models should be continued.

Although continued research is recommended, the more immediate and pressing need is to determine whether significant displacement of any organics of health concern occurs in the operation of GAC beds that are intended for treatment of drinking water. Although trace organics of concern in the raw water supply are identified and their concentrations and the variability in their concentrations are measured, pilot plant studies will still be necessary to confirm the relative order of break-through of each contaminant and to assess the importance of any displacement effect. This displacement effect can be caused both by a variable influent composition and by competitive adsorption. Although it is difficult to distinguish between these two factors in pilot plant studies, every effort should be made to determine which is more important.

MICROBIAL ACTIVITY ON GAC

While microbial activity has long been recognized as beneficial in the operation of slow sand filters, it has only recently been given consideration as a controllable, positive feature of treatment with GAC. Electron micrographs provide clear evidence of the presence of microorganisms on the surface of GAC (Weber *et al.*, 1978a). The types and number of microorganisms will depend upon the amount and nature of the available substrates. This section evaluates this process in light of the ultimate objective of reducing the concentration of, or eliminating completely, the organic compounds that are potentially harmful to health. Hence, the following questions must be addressed:

1. To what extent does microbial activity interact with adsorption in the process of removing organic contaminants? Does it interfere with or aid removal? Does it extend bed life? How does it remove specific organics of toxicological concern?

2. What is the effect of pretreatment by ozone or chlorine on the extent of microbial activity and overall effectiveness of GAC?

3. What is the impact of microbial colonization of GAC beds on microbiological contamination of the product water? Are the number of microorganisms, including those causing disease, increased?

4. What products of microbiological activity can be expected in the finished water? Are toxicants created by microbial activity on GAC?

Interaction Between Microbial Activity and Adsorption

BIODEGRADABILITY OF ORGANIC COMPOUNDS

For the purposes of discussing the interactions between biological and physicochemical processes occurring on the GAC surface, it is convenient to divide organics into the following four categories:

1. nonadsorbable, nonbiodegradable
2. nonadsorbable, biodegradable
3. adsorbable, nonbiodegradable
4. adsorbable, biodegradable

While simple, this classification scheme is ambiguous because the term nonbiodegradable is not easily defined. Instead, Alexander (1973) has adopted the adjective recalcitrant to describe substances that persist for extended periods under all environmental conditions thus far tested. Recalcitrant organics include those that are degraded slowly or not at all in nature. Occasionally, some organics that are usually biodegradable are recalcitrant due to specific environmental causes. Alexander outlined the conditions required for biodegradation and listed 15 possible mechanisms to explain recalcitrance. While some of these may be overcome by the environment in a GAC bed, others, such as accessibility of substrate and low concentration of substrate, may not.

Attempts have been made to relate biodegradability to chemical structure (Haller, 1978; Ludzack and Ettinger, 1960; Pitter 1976; Pitter et al., 1974; Verschuren 1977). However, general rules are difficult to propose. Of all of the organic chemicals that are potentially harmful to health (National Academy of Sciences, 1977), only benzene was included in an extensive review of biodegradability studies made by Ludzack and Ettinger (1960), who concluded that benzene was resistant to biodegradation. Helfgott et al. (1977) prepared a relative index for organics that are tested. Included were some organics with potential health effects, i.e., benzene, chloroform, DDT, and vinyl chloride. They considered all four compounds to be resistant to biodegradation, but benzene has subsequently been shown to be biodegradable (Chambers *et al.*, 1963; Verschuren, 1977).

Pitter (1976) evaluated 123 organics in the aliphatic, cycloaliphatic, and aromatic classes. Of these, 21 organics were described as "biologically hard to decompose," and all were in the aromatic class. Included among these organics were dinitrobenzenes and phenols, phenyldiamines, trichlorophenol, nitroanilines, and naphthylamines. In all of the studies that were found in the literature, the experimental conditions were not those to be expected in treatment of drinking water. Most important, the concentrations of organics were in milligrams per liter rather than in micrograms per liter, and the concentrations of biomass were more consistent with biological waste treatment.

The organics that are most likely to be attacked microbially fall in the nonadsorbable, biodegradable category. In treatment with GAC, these organics could be removed by the biofilm surrounding the carbon granules without affecting the adsorption process. The adsorbable, biodegradable category of organics is of more interest because of the strong interaction expected between biological and adsorption processes. This sets GAC apart from sand or other inert media. Various researchers (Benedek, 1977; Tien, 1980; Ying and Weber, 1978) describe the removal mechanism as biodegradation in the biofilm, followed by adsorption of remaining substrate in the internal pore structure. Ying and Weber (1978) have adopted the term biosorption to describe this process. The resulting mathematical model, which has been applied to concentrations of organics as high as those found in wastewater, indicates that adsorption is responsible for removal of biodegradable organics during the initial period of GAC operation. Later, the biofilm develops enough so that biodegradation predominates. This provides for continued, steady-state removals and can explain extended bed life, particularly in wastewater treatment applications of GAC.

In water treatment, the removal of adsorbable, biodegradable organics by microbial activity, rather than by adsorption, enhances the opportunity for the GAC bed to remove the adsorbable, nonbiodegradable organics. This latter category is generally of more concern because it contains many of the synthetic organics that may be suspected carcinogens. Mathematical description of parallel removal processes for these two categories of organics has not yet appeared in the literature, although progress has been indicated. Recalcitrant organics, such as toluene sulfonate and potassium biphthalate, seem to be removed more effectively by GAC than can be explained on the basis of adsorption alone (Ying and Weber, 1978). Enhanced biodegradation is implied. Weber (1977) explained that the advantages of GAC over other media in promoting microbial activity are extension of contact time between the substrate and the microorganisms; increased concentration of substrate by adsorption; and enrichment of oxygen concentration on the surface by sorption. With regard to this third explanation, there is evidence that significant amounts of oxygen are adsorbed by GAC (Prober et al., 1975), but the availability of this oxygen to the microbial system is not clear. A further necessary condition for biodegradation is accessibility of the substrate to the microorganism. This becomes critical if the microorganisms are restricted to the outer surfaces by their size while the sorbed organics have penetrated into the macro- and micropores. This leads to the question of whether or not GAC can be regenerated biologically. The evidence thus far is incomplete and contradictory.

While the GAC bed is a suitable environment for microbial activity, questions regarding which specific organics are biodegradable and at what rate also remain unanswered by research. In addition to accessibility, the concentration of the substrate is an important factor. Clearly, many organics of concern are present in drinking water in such low concentrations that the opportunities for microbial action may be quite limited unless adsorption occurs first; however, as mentioned above, adsorption may prevent biodegradation if the substrate becomes inaccessible to the microorganism. One factor that could influence substrate availability is reequilibration when feed concentration decreases in a dynamic situation. In this case, sorbed substrate could once again become available to microorganisms. Perhaps the most reasonable picture of microbial action that emerges is that of biodegradation of easily attacked organics in the biofilm surrounding the carbon particles. Ying and Weber (1978) suggested that these are the low-molecular-weight, oxygenated organics. A certain fraction of the humic materials, which are generally known to be precursors of various chlorinated organics, may be easily degraded; however, there is evidence that other fractions are recalcitrant (Alexander, 1973; Helfgott et al., 1977). There has been no evidence to suggest that any of the suspect carcinogens are acted upon by microbial action in the GAC bed.

EVIDENCE OF MICROBIAL ACTION ON GAC BEDS IN WATER TREATMENT

Much of the recent interest on the effect of microbial activity on GAC performance stems from European research and experience. However, in all reports, removal of organics is discussed in terms of nonspecific group measurements such as potassium permanganate demand, UV absorbing substances (at 254 nm), and organic carbon. Hence, there are no specific data on biological degradation of suspect carcinogenic compounds on GAC nor on extended adsorption of such compounds on GAC as a result of biological regeneration of the surface.

A comparison of the reduction in potassium permanganate demand in slow sand filters and GAC beds was made at Bremen, Federal Republic of Germany, from March 1970 to May 1973 (Eberhardt et al., 1974). As expected, the removal of organics by adsorption on GAC was better initially than removal by slow sand filtration. However, the adsorptive capacity of GAC was exhausted over a 7-month period, and removal of potassium permanganate demand through GAC treatment gradually diminished until both the GAC and slow sand systems gave similar results. Continued microbial action was suggested by the fact that both continued to remove about the same amount of potassium permanganate demand for the next 32 months.

There were seasonal fluctuations in oxygen demand, the maximum occurring in summer (up to 7 mg/liter) and the minimum in winter (down to 1 mg/liter). The investigators concluded that biological activity predominated in summer and adsorption in winter. Part of the oxygen demand in summer was attributed to bioregeneration of the GAC surface. In a closed loop experiment, in which the same batch of water was continuously cycled through a GAC bed, both oxygen consumption and carbon dioxide production continued at a steady level of approximately 5 mg/liter for 2 months. Eberhardt et al. assumed that the production of carbon dioxide resulted from bioregeneration of the GAC surface. Accordingly, this carbon dioxide production is equivalent to 1.4 mg/liter of organic carbon being removed at steady state in a contact time of 30 min. During actual operation of the GAC beds during the last 9 months of the 3-yr pilot plant study at Bremen, the carbon dioxide production was equivalent to removal of approximately 1.4 mg/liter organic carbon.

Hutchinson and Ridgway (1977) reported that GAC beds have been installed in many waterworks in England in order to reduce residual organics. The fact that the GAC beds were still in service after several years of continuous operation was offered as evidence for the importance of removal of organics by microbial action. However, other than successful reduction of taste and odors, measurements of specific organics and their removal have not been reported. Similar conclusions may be drawn from a summary of the performance of plant installations in the Plains Region of the American Water Works System (Blanck, 1978).

A pilot study at Miami, Florida (Symons, 1980; Wood and DeMarco, 1980) indicated that removal of specific low-molecular-weight, chlorinated organics may have been enhanced by biological activity. This could be due to biodegradation of other adsorbable, biodegradable organics, which decreased the rate at which the sorptive saturation capacity was reached. The contact time before such an effect could be measured was similar to that observed by Eberhardt *et al.* (1974), i.e., approximately 20 min.

Cairo *et al.* (1980) studied contact times of up to 60 min in pilot plant studies at the Torresdale plant in Philadelphia. After 22.5 min of contact time, service time increased greatly beyond that explainable by adsorption. However, service time was measured in terms of satisfying a criterion for removal of TOC. When measured by a criterion for removal of trihalomethanes (THM's), there was no disproportionate increase of service time with contact time. These results do not support the contention that removal of adsorbable, but easily degradable, organics increases adsorption of haloforms.

In studies of long-term operation (180 days) of full-scale GAC beds at the Jefferson Parish Water Treatment Plant, which is located on the lower Mississippi River, Brodtmann *et al.* (1980) observed that a relatively steady-state removal of organic precursors to chloroform production was reached after approximately 60 days of operation. Regardless of the influent concentration of these precursors, which varied by a factor of two, the removal of them approached a steady-state level of approximately 50%, suggesting that biological activity was responsible.

At Jefferson Parish, the approach to a steady-state removal of organics, which could be interpreted as being produced by microbial activity, was also measured by other group parameters. The approximate steady-state removals of TOC, fluorescent substances, and UV-absorbing substances were 30%–50%, 65%, and 60%, respectively. These percentages were reached after periods ranging from 50 to 80 days.

Two other studies of microbial activity on GAC without preozonation provided only limited data on organics removal. Schalekamp (1976) reported on pilot and full-scale operation of GAC beds treating the water of the Lake of Zurich in Switzerland. At the Lenng plant, GAC beds removed approximately 1 mg/liter chemical oxygen demand (COD) throughout 7 months of operation. However, the continual increase in carbon loading, as measured by dimethylformamide (DMF) extract, suggests that adsorption was continuing during the entire period of operation. A similar situation existed at the Moos water works in Zurich, where carbon loading was still very low after 3 yr of bed operation. Neither the Lenng nor Moos plants can provide meaningful information on the removal of organics before the microorganic contaminants are analyzed further.

Pilot plant evaluation of microbial activity on GAC at Wiesbaden, Federal Republic of Germany, showed a decrease in total carbon of 1.2 mg/liter and a decrease in oxygen of 1.5 mg/liter (Klotz *et al.*, 1976). An attempt was made to determine the contribution of biological activity in removal of organics by operating two GAC beds in parallel, with one bed receiving water that was sterilized by passage through a membrane filtration system. However, firm conclusions cannot be drawn from this experiment because of uncertainties regarding the reliability of the sterilization system.

There has been no evidence to suggest that microbial action removes specific organics that would otherwise escape GAC treatment. On the other hand, it appears that service life of a GAC bed can be extended by microbial action if performance is measured by removal of total organics, e.g., total organic carbon, UV absorbance, or potassium permanganate demand.

Effect of Pretreatment by Ozone and Chlorine on Microbial Action

PREOZONIZATION IN WATER TREATMENT

Whether or not preozonization converts nonbiodegradable to degradable organic compounds, which are then removed by microbial activity on GAC, is open to debate. Rice *et al.* (1978) and Sontheimer *et al.* (1978) have implied that preozonization enhances microbial action on GAC in water treatment, and Guirguis *et al.* (1978) reached a similar conclusion in studies of GAC in wastewater treatment. However, the conclusions of Guirguis *et al.* (1978) have been challenged by Randtke (1978) and by Weber (1978), and results at other wastewater treatment facilities (Water Factor 21 and Lake Tahoe) indicated little enhancement of microbial activity by preozonization (Culp and Hansen, 1978).

The evidence for enhanced microbial activity with preozonization is largely indirect because there are few, if any, measurements of ozonization products and their biodegradability in studies of GAC treatment in waterworks. However, the overall positive effects of preozonization on organics removal have been reported at three full-scale waterworks located at Duesseldorf and Muelheim in the Federal Republic of Germany and at Rouen-la-Chapelle in France, as well as at pilot plant plants in Bremen, Federal Republic of Germany, Amsterdam, the Netherlands, and Morsang-sur-Seine in France (Benedek, 1977; Miller *et al.*, 1978). In all these evaluations, the removal of organics has been measured using group characteristics.

Only a few investigators have examined the effectiveness of oxidation and/or coagulation steps preceding GAC. For example, in the study by Eberhardt *et al.* (1974) at the Bremen pilot plant the overall removal of organics by ozonization and GAC was slightly better than by slow sand filtration. (Both systems receiving the same pretreated water.) However, much of the improvement could be traced to the chemical oxidation step rather than the GAC beds. Ozone oxidation accounted for most of the decrease in UV-absorbing substances, as should be expected from the nature of oxidation reactions with ozone.

In pilot plant studies at the Amsterdam waterworks, GAC performance, as measured by removal of UV-absorbing substances, was definitely improved as a result of preozonization (Miller et al., 1978; van Lier et al., 1976). However, the UV absorbance had been reduced 50% by chemical oxidation prior to adsorption. Data reported by Miller et al. (1978) for the Muelheim plant indicate that UV extinction was reduced from 6.1 to 1.8 m^{-1} by preozonization, as compared to a reduction from 6.8 to 4.4 m^{-1} without preozonization. (Extinction is expressed in terms of a light path length of 1 m.) These reductions occurred through flocculation and rapid sand filtration.

In agreement with pilot plant results, full-scale testing of preozonization at the Muelheim plant produced significant reductions in dissolved organic carbon (DOC) through ozonization, flocculation, and rapid sand filtration (Sontheimer et al., 1978). The decrease in DOC was 1.2 mg/liter as compared with 0.7 mg/liter when breakpoint chlorination was practiced.

The role of ozone in enhancing microbial activity on GAC is uncertain from the available data. In several studies, depletion of oxygen through the GAC bed was taken as evidence for biodegradation of organics. However, simultaneous nitrification, which consumes oxygen, was a significant factor. In addition, it is conceivable that ozonization, which produces supersaturation with respect to oxygen, could also have caused subsequent deoxygenation due to stripping. These two factors possibly influenced the conclusion reached by Eberhardt et al. (1974) that microbial activity on GAC was enhanced by ozone. Admittedly, microbial activity, rather than adsorption, must be considered as the mechanism involved in continued removal of organics by these GAC beds over an extended period of operation. However, from the data of Eberhardt et al. (1974), who reported GAC treatment with and without preozonization, it is difficult to say that significant improvement in removal of organics occurred within the GAC bed when it was preceded by ozonization.

One of the most significant findings regarding the effect of ozonization on GAC bed performance was reported by Sontheimer et al. (1978) from studies at the Muelheim waterworks. A nearly steady-state removal of approximately 80% of the UV-absorbing substances was obtained in pilot plant GAC beds after preozonization. However, in parallel operation of the full-scale plant, in which breakpoint chlorination was followed by preozonization and GAC beds, the removal of the absorbing substances decreased very rapidly. This indicated that the chlorinated organics that were formed in the plant, or their subsequent oxidation products, were less biodegradable and/or less adsorbable than in the unchlorinated one. The extension in life of the GAC bed after preozonization can be explained partly by the reduced concentration of UV-absorbing substances reaching the GAC bed, which was caused by more effective coagulation and oxidation processes. Nevertheless, the more or less steady-state removal by the GAC bed after several months of operation still forces the conclusion that biological activity was important. Approximately 1.5 mg/liter DOC was removed during the last 7 months of the pilot plant study after a contact time of 30 min (Jekel, 1977). The extent to which microbial action reduced organics agrees with the findings of Eberhardt et al. (1974).

The effect of microbial activity can also be measured indirectly by comparing DOC removal across the GAC bed with the DOC loading on the GAC bed (Sontheimer, 1974). At the Duesseldorf waterworks, a much higher value of DOC loading was anticipated based on the DOC removal than could be measured by extraction of polar and nonpolar organics from the GAC. This suggested that the microbial activity had removed sorbed organics; however, Sontheimer also indicated that loss of volatile DOC and failure to measure nonextractable organics could have been important factors accounting for DOC, which was removed.

Benedek (1977) compared the rates at which organics were removed in pre- and postozonized GAC systems in pilot plant studies at the Morsang-sur-Seine waterworks in France. The GAC beds had a contact time of 16 min and were in service without regeneration for approximately 1 yr. Both treatment schemes removed a similar amount of organics as measured by group characteristics. Hence, there was no significant beneficial effect of preozonization. However, the ozone concentration was only 0.3–0.4 mg/liter after 10 min of ozone contact, and the water had been chlorinated prior to treatment. Data from the pilot plant showed a decline in the rate of uptake of organics by GAC over 1 yr in both the pre- and postozonized systems. The attainment of a more or less steady rate of uptake in each system was attributed to biological activity. While this rate was somewhat higher in the preozonized system, Benedek (1977) concluded that the difference in rates was not significant. These rates compared quite closely to the range that was measured by Eberhardt et al. (1974) at the Bremen pilot plant study. A factor affecting conclusions concerning enhanced biodegradability by ozonization is the possible presence of less degradable chlorinated organics, which were formed as a result of prechlorination.

The effect of preozonization on the removal of precursors to the formation of THM's can be deduced from studies at the EPA pilot plant study in Cincinnati, Ohio (U.S. Environmental Protection Agency, 1978c). Ozonized and unozonized Ohio river waters were fed to GAC beds operating in parallel. The THM formation potential (THMFP) test showed that the ozone–GAC system removed more precursors of THM's (U.S. Environmental Protection Agency, 1978c). This indicates that ozone was able to oxidize the precursors, which were then either adsorbed or biodegraded on GAC. Without ozone, much of the humic material could be recalcitrant. This has also been suggested by microbial studies that were conducted at the Water Research Center in Medmenham, England (Hutchinson and Ridgeway, 1977) and by the studies of Helfgott *et al.* (1977). Addition of ozone could have converted these humic materials to more readily biodegradable forms. With an ozone dose of only 1 mg/liter and a GAC contact time of 9 min, removal of TOC by GAC treatment was consistently and significantly better in the preozonized system over 10 months of operation without regeneration. While effluent concentrations increased rather steadily in both systems, complete saturation was not reached in either. However, the data did not indicate a leveling off of TOC in the preozonized system, which is expected when microbial activity becomes the primary organic removal mechanism.

EFFECT OF OZONE ON ORGANICS

Chapter III, which was prepared by a subcommittee of the Safe Drinking Water Committee, includes published data on the identification of specific end products of ozonization in waterworks treatment. It suffices here to state that more polar organics such as carboxylic acids, catechols, and aldehydes can be expected. Further conclusions regarding the biodegradability of these end products can only be reached indirectly from examination of pilot plant and full-scale operations.

Dosages of ozone of up to 25 mg/liter were not able to reduce THM concentrations (Love *et al.*, 1976). Similar findings were obtained in pilot plant studies of GAC beds in which ozonization of the effluent failed to reduce the THMFP. However, as noted earlier, measurements after GAC contact indicated that the addition of ozone prior to GAC reduced the THMFP (U.S. Environmental Protection Agency, 1978c). This suggests that ozone can oxidize the THM precursors to more adsorbable species but cannot alter the original precursors to eliminate chlorination reactions.

Ozonization has been shown to produce less adsorbable organics (Benedek, 1977). This can be caused by production of more polar organics such as carboxylic acids, catechols, and aldehydes. Reductions in adsorptive capacity on GAC (as measured by DOC) were also reported by Kuhn *et al.* (1978a,b) in studies of ozonized water from the Lake of Constance in the Federal Republic of Germany, where the applied ozone dosage ranged from 0.45 to 3.5 mg/liter. On the positive side, the combination of ozonization and coagulation seemed to produce very good removals of UV-active organic substances. This process has been successfully implemented at the Muelheim waterworks for DOC reduction (Sontheimer *et al.*, 1978).

EFFECTS OF PRECHLORINATION ON MICROBIAL ACTIVITY IN GAC BEDS

For chlorination to have a detrimental effect on microbial growth within a GAC bed, residual chlorine must be present. The catalytic dechlorination reaction on GAC counteracts this problem (Suidan *et al.*, 1977). A mathematical description of the dechlorination reaction on GAC shows that with a very short contact time (0.6 min), at an application rate of 4 gpm/ft^2 and a chlorine dose of 5 mg/liter, residual chlorine would reach 0.5 mg/liter in approximately 10 days and 1 mg/liter in 40 days. Extrapolating this result to the more usual contact time of 15 min, which is needed for adsorption and biological activity, the rate of advancement of the chlorine residual front would be such that 25 days are required for a value of 0.5 mg/liter to be reached in the first 10% of the bed length. This "breakthrough time" for chlorine residual is proportionally increased with lower feed concentration of free chlorine and longer bed lengths.

The effect of the dechlorination reaction on GAC in a water treatment plant has been reported by Schalekamp (1976). He noted a 50% breakthrough of chlorine, i.e., 0.25 mg/liter, in water from the Lake of Zurich after 25 days of operation at a contact time of just 0.3 min. These data suggest that prechlorination may ónly impede bacterial activity if very long GAC service times are used. Referring to the brewing industry's experience with dechlorination, Eberhardt (1976) reported that while removal of chlorine was effective, the GAC process was much maligned because of its inability to prevent bacterial growths, which were unacceptable in the product water.

More direct evidence of microbial activity on GAC with prechlorination in waterworks has been given by Schalekamp (1976), Klotz *et al.* (1976), and Mueller and Bernhardt (1976). With simultaneous measurements of chlorine residual, bacterial counts, oxygen, carbon dioxide, and TOC, Klotz *et al.* (1976) showed that there was no influence of chlorine on microbial activity below a free residual of 0.1 mg/liter. Values lower than this occurred near the top of the GAC bed. In pilot plant studies at Breman, Eberhardt *et al.* (1974) also noted that oxygen consumption was similar with and without prechlorination. A somewhat opposite view was given in another report by Eberhardt (1976). He stated that chlorination would disturb microbial activity by creating less biodegradable, chlorinated organics. Similar reasoning was given by Miller *et al.* (1978) when explaining the lack of microbial activity on GAC at the Duesseldorf waterworks. They reasoned that the Rhine River contains chlorinated organics that are not degraded by bank filtration and eventually reach the GAC beds where adsorption, but not microbial activity, occurs. Such a conclusion was supported by measurements of chlorinated organics by Steiglitz *et al.* (1976).

Sontheimer *et al.* (1978) showed that polar chlorinated organics were produced by breakpoint chlorination at the Muelheim waterworks. In parallel operation of preozonized GAC beds, with and without breakpoint chlorination, they demonstrated clearly that GAC in the latter system was much more effective in removal of UV-absorbing organics over many months. They concluded that microbial activity on GAC was far more effective if prechlorination was not practiced. Moreover, its enhancement by preozonization depends upon the organics that were present in the treatment process prior to this step.

Therefore, the effects of prechlorination on microbial activity appear to be twofold. The impairment of bacterial growth was relatively minor because the dechlorination reaction in GAC beds greatly reduces free chlorine. However, the more important effect may be the formation of less biodegradable, chlorinated organics prior to treatment with GAC. The extent of formation of chlorinated organics should depend upon the chlorine dosage and the organic species that are present. An additional consideration would be the relative adsorbability of chlorinated organics as compared with their precursors. There are general rules to predict this effect.

Microbial Activity on GAC in Wastewater Treatment

From pilot plant studies at Pomona, California, Parkhurst *et al.* (1967) determined that adsorption capacity could not be completely exhausted even after very long service times. More detailed investigations of microbial degradation on GAC were provided by Weber *et al.* (1970, 1972) in other pilot plant studies that addressed the benefits of microbial activity more directly. Comparison studies of GAC and nonsorptive, bituminous coal clearly showed that more TOC removal and microbial growth occurred on GAC. This suggested that microbial activity was in some way interrelated with the adsorption process. Besik (1973) proposed that the rate of microbial activity in a GAC bed should be even higher than that in a conventional biological treatment process because the substrate adsorbed on the activated carbon is much higher than in the liquid. The interplay between microbial degradation and adsorption was recently confirmed by Maqsood and Benedek (1977).

The denitrification research of Jeris *et al.* (1974) also demonstrated the advantage of GAC over sand in promoting microbial activity. In this study, they were unable to achieve significant growth on sand particles. However, using fresh activated carbon, they observed excellent growth and subsequent nitrate removal 2 weeks after start-up.

Because the concentration of biodegradable organics is far greater in wastewater than in water supplies, the extent of microbial activity on GAC beds used in wastewater after either conventional primary or secondary treatment should also be greater. Ying and Weber (1978), Peel and Benedek (1975), and Andrews and Tien (1975) have all reviewed the evidence for microbial degradation and have reported that from 25% to 78% of the TOC that was removed in various GAC facilities could be attributed to this mechanism. The estimated rate of biodegradation based upon TOC in wastewater applications of GAC is approximately one order of magnitude greater than in water treatment applications (Benedek, 1977).

The effect of preozonization is unclear. Enrichment of sorbed oxygen, enhancement of biological activity, and increased or decreased adsorbability of organics have not been addressed carefully. Guirguis *et al.* (1978) discussed the results from pilot plant operation of a preozonization–GAC system at the Cleveland Westerly physical–chemical wastewater treatment plant. Excellent COD and biochemical oxygen demand (BOD) removals were obtained through 1 yr without regeneration. In addition to oxygen enrichment by ozonization, they proposed that some organics were converted to more adsorbable and more biodegradable forms. However, the basis for reaching these conclusions has been challenged by Randtke (1978) and by Weber (1978). An earlier report by Guirguis *et al.* (1976) showed no decrease in BOD after ozonization. Results obtained at the Water Factory 21 Pilot Plant in Orange County, California (Culp and Hansen, 1978) conflicted with those from the Cleveland Westerly plant. Ozonization of unchlorinated trickling filter effluent followed by GAC contact produced no enhancement of COD removal, while ozonization of unchlorinated activated sludge effluent only increased COD removals by 30%. The investigators noted microbial activity on GAC in both ozonized and unozonized systems. In another study (Culp and Hansen, 1978), ozonization (10 mg/liter) of activated sludge effluent at the Lake Tahoe Advanced Waste Treatment Plant almost doubled the bed life of the GAC for COD removal, yet chlorine residuals (1–2 mg/liter) were present in the carbon column effluent. Instead of biological action, the positive effects of ozone were attributed to oxidation reactions.

Microbial Contamination of Product Water

Microorganisms, mainly bacteria, adsorb to GAC and will colonize filter beds. They assimilate nutrients that are adsorbed to the GAC and dissolved nutrients, thereby growing to relatively high densities. Currently, the prevention of this microbial colonization is impractical.

This section will discuss what is known about the adherence and growth of microbes on GAC beds and the effect of bed contamination on the microbial content of effluent water.

ADHERENCE OF MICROBES TO GAC

Marshall (1976) and Daniels (1972) both presented excellent discussions of the factors influencing the attachment of microbes to surfaces. The mechanism of attachment remains unclear; adsorption due to electro-chemical double-layer effects, as well as mechanical adhesion, have been proposed. The nature of the microorganisms and the adsorbant are also very important. Adsorption isotherms of mixed bacteria (genus and species unspecified) to GAC were reported by Klotz et al. (1976). At bacterial concentrations of 10^7 to 10^8/200 ml of buffer, up to 90% of the bacteria were adsorbed. At bacterial concentrations greater than 10^{10}, the system tended toward saturation. Dead bacteria were adsorbed somewhat more efficiently than live bacteria. No data are available on the adsorption or selective adsorption of individual bacterial species. However, Marshall (1976) has shown that adhesion of bacteria can be dependent upon their ability to produce suitable bridging polymers.

BACTERIAL GROWTH ON GAC BEDS

Standard plate count methods for bacteria from crushed and homogenized GAC have been used for quantitation. The total number of living and dead bacteria has also been determined by microscopy. The temperatures used for growth of the bacteria vary from 22°C (Eberhardt et al., 1974) to 27°C (Klotz et al., 1976). There are few data on the optimal time of incubation. Eberhardt et al. (1974) found colony counts from 2,700–5,200/ml after 72 hr of incubation, depending on the amount of preozonization. Incubation periods of 7 and 10 days have been reported (Klotz *et al.*, 1976; Miller *et al.*, 1978), but, generally, 20-day incubations at 22°C yield the highest numbers of bacteria.

Van der Kooij (1978) showed that the bacterial counts in GAC beds reached maximal numbers in 20 to 30 days, i.e., approximately 10^8 colony-forming units per gram of GAC at 25°C. While fewer colonies formed on sand than on unactivated carbon, the differences were not as great as reported earlier (Van der Kooij, 1976). He concluded that these bacteria were not able to utilize sorbed organics on GAC. Only the larger surface area of GAC was used to explain higher colony counts. Both GAC and sand beds showed a decline in bacteria over the 10-month period. He postulated that this was caused by a shift in population to uncountable bacteria (Van der Kooij, 1976).

In another study of the microbial growth in GAC beds, Benedek (1977) showed that the total microbial burden varied as a function of filter depth. Microbe levels of $10^7/cm^3$ of GAC were found on the surface. This fell to 10^6 bacteria per cm^3 at 40 cm (Benedek, 1977).

Although the water velocity through the GAC bed and the content of organic nutrients in the water would be expected to influence the microbial growth, there are few data available on these potential effects. In studies of velocities ranging from 4 to 20 m/hr, Klotz *et al.* (1976) observed that the initial growth rate in the bed was slower at higher velocities and that the final counts were lower with lower velocities. By comparing operation of a slow sand filter at 0.3 m/hr and a GAC bed at 3.5 m/hr, Van der Kooij (1978) showed that colony counts were two orders of magnitude lower at the lower filtration rate. Love and Symons (1978) stated that the concentration of bacteria depends on the length of time the GAC sits idle, the concentration of bacteria in the applied water, the amount of TOC, bed depth, temperature, and hydraulic application rate. Unfortunately, they provide none of the data from which these conclusions were made.

Studies on denitrification in fluidized beds may offer insight into factors affecting microbial growth on support media. Jeris *et al.* (1974) showed that even a threefold increase in upflow velocity was insufficient to promote sloughing-off of bacteria in such a way that a steady-state biofilm thickness could be achieved. In later studies, Jeris and Owens (1975) also found that prolonged shutdowns were not detrimental to microbial activity. Oxygen transfer limitations may inhibit activity but only when TOC is very high as in the case described by Jeris *et al.* (1977).

There are no compelling data showing that preozonization of water has a significant impact on the microbial growth in GAC beds. Benedek (1977) reported that ozonization increased the growth of aerobic bacteria by 1/2 log. This may or may not be significant. Miller *et al.* (1978) stated that ozonization discourages the growth of anaerobic organisms and destroys slime-forming organisms, but they provided no data.

THE EFFECT OF GAC COLONIZATION ON MICROBIAL CONTENT OF THE EFFLUENT

Studies of the microbial numbers in effluents of operational and pilot GAC filters are not comparable because different culture techniques were used by the investigators. In general, the data indicate that detachment of bacteria from the bed, which results in contamination of the effluent, is a negligible problem. However, there are also notable exceptions. For example, Ford (cited in Love and Symons, 1978) studied a pilot plant in the United Kingdom and found that over a 5-yr period the effluent of GAC contained more bacteria than the effluent of a sand filter. Twenty-five percent of the GAC effluent samples contained more than 500 bacteria/ml.

The experience with GAC in Germany and Switzerland has been interpreted as favorable. During the 3-yr pilot plant study at Bremen (Eberhardt *et al.*, 1974), plate counts remained below 50/ml (assumed as a 2-day, 22°C test) with the exception of two brief periods in spring and summer of 1971 when very high plate counts were measured. A 7-day, 27°C plate count test was used in pilot plant studies at Wiesbaden (Klotz *et al.*, 1976). Much higher counts, ranging from 10^5 to 10^6/ml, were reported in these studies. This may have been caused by the much longer incubation time used. However, in full-scale operation, counts over a 3-yr period were much lower, i.e., on the order of 100/ml.

High initial plate counts were measured during treatment of reservoir water by ozonization and GAC contact (Mueller and Bernhardt, 1976). Counts remained at 5,000/ml for 12 months, 800–1,000/ml for 6 months, and finally decreased to less than 10/ml for 5 months. Initial counts in the treatment of reservoir water were higher than in groundwater. This was attributed to the higher organic carbon content of the reservoir compared to that of the groundwater (0.8 versus 0.3 mg/liter). The fecal indicators, *Escherichia coli* and *Pseudomonas* sp., were absent as were strains of streptomycetes. The Dohne plant at Muelheim reported effluents containing as many as 3,700 bacteria/ml (Sontheimer *et al.*, 1978); however, these were reduced to less than 10/ml by ground passage. At the Lenng, Switzerland, waterworks, Schalekamp (1976) reported plate counts of less than 50/ml (3-day, 20°C test) in the effluent of GAC beds; however, in pilot plant tests, he found higher counts (from 1,000 to 10,000/ml) throughout 3 months of operation. Backwashing of the full-scale GAC beds twice per week was thought to be responsible for the lower counts. Similar findings were reported by Hansen (cited in Love and Symons, 1978), but conflicting results were obtained by Sylvia *et al.* (cited in Love and Symons, 1978) at the Lawrence, Massachusetts, waterworks, where a transient increase in numbers of bacteria in the effluent was observed following backwash.

In other studies, 15 months of pilot testing at the Amsterdam waterworks showed that GAC beds without preozonization produced bacterial counts of less than 1,000/ml. A 3-day incubation test at 22°C was used (Van Lier *et al.*, 1976). Also in the Netherlands, Den Blanken (1978) found that the effluents of experimental GAC columns contained 10^2 to 10^4 bacteria/ml. In the United States, GAC effluents from a pilot plant processing Ohio River water contained less than 10^2 bacteria/ml (Love and Symons, 1978). Similar results were repoted by McElhaney and McKeon (1978) in pilot studies at Philadelphia; however, they observed an initial 5-week period of much higher counts. Finally, at the Rouen waterworks, which consists primarily of preozonization, GAC contact, and postozonization, colony counts in the finished water varied markedly. However, all counts over a 6-month period were less than 600 bacteria/ml, and most were less than 100 (Miller *et al.*, 1978).

SPECIATION OF BACTERIA ON FILTER BEDS AND IN EFFLUENTS

Few data are available on the species of bacteria colonizing GAC beds and even less are available on relative numbers. Some statements, unaccompanied by data, have been written indicating that "five or six different types of colonies could be recognized" and that "two genera, *Flavobacterium* and *Xanthomonas*, were identified" (U.S. Environmental Protection Agency, 1978c). Maqsood and Benedek (1977) stated that *Pseudomonas* and *Flavobacterium* were the most prevalent genera of bacteria on GAC that was used in wastewater treatment. Den Blanken (1978) found representatives of *Acinetobacter, Pseudomonas, Caulobacter, Corynebacterium, Flavobacterium, Alcaligenes, Actinomyces, Bacillus, Planctomyces,* and *Moraxella.*

Some isolated strains of *Pseudomonas* and coryneforms could produce color- and odor-producing substances and antibiotics; however, these were considered adsorbable by GAC. For all practical purposes, only *Bacillus, Caulobacter,* and nonpigmented *Pseudomonas* were found in the effluents. Love and Symons (1978) reported the work of Parsons, who classified the bacteria in the effluent of a pilot plant in Miami, Florida. The organisms identified were strains of *Pseudomonas, Enterobacter agglomerans, Acinetobacter, Alcaligenes faecalis, Moraxella,* and *Flavobac-*

terium. In pilot plant studies at the Philadelphia waterworks, McElhaney and McKeon (1978) identified 10 species of *Pseudomonas.* They pointed out that while none of these were pathogenic, some could become "opportunistic pathogens." This theory demands further research.

Products of Microbiological Activity

In the operation of GAC, microorganisms proliferate actively on the carbon surface for up to several months. The resulting biochemical capabilities of the established microbial community lead to the mineralization of organic matter with the formation of carbon dioxide and microbial cells. The published research does not indicate which compounds are or are not acted upon by such microbial activity and what compounds may be generated as a consequence of bacterial growth. Attention has been focused on bulk organic materials in water and not on discrete classes of molecules.

Of potential importance also is the recent finding that some normally biodegradable compounds may be destroyed very slowly or not at all at very low concentrations (Boethling and Alexander, 1979). Hence, chemicals at low concentrations may not be destroyed on GAC or, if small amounts are released, may not be destroyed by subsequent biodegradation.

MICROBIOLOGICALLY PRODUCED LOW-MOLECULAR-WEIGHT TOXICANTS

During the last few years, it has become evident that bacteria and other microorganisms form a large number of compounds that are or may be environmental pollutants. The formation of these compounds can be shown readily in microbial cultures that are tested in the laboratory or in model ecosystems, but some have also been found in nature. The production of these toxic chemicals is not restricted to microbial populations developing at low oxygen tensions or under completely anaerobic conditions, and many are produced in maximal quantities when the oxygen supply is high. A few of the products have gained considerable attention because of their potency and the frequency of their production. A few are only now emerging as significant environmental problems.

Microbially produced toxicants have not been identified in the treatment of drinking water by GAC. They are listed here only to illustrate the potential of microbial systems to create such problems. Methylation of mercury is widely recognized as a serious environmental problem that occurs in many environments in which bacteria develop.

Little organic matter is required for the process, and bacteria are involved. Hydroxylamine, a potent mutagen, can also be formed in culture media by microorganisms. Not only has it been observed in several natural bodies of water, but its formation can be catalyzed in waters by microorganisms (Verstraete and Alexander, 1973). Pesticides or molecules related to pesticides are also acted upon microbiologically to give new toxicants. A vast body of literature attests to the ability of bacteria and other heterotrophic microorganisms to convert these chemicals to new inhibitors or to products of great toxicity to humans, animals, and plants than the precursor molecules (Alexander, 1974). In laboratory models of natural water systems, polynuclear aromatic hydrocarbons have been generated both by bacteria (Knorr and Schenk, 1968) and algae (Andelman and Suess, 1970).

No definitive studies have been made to confirm that nitrosamines can be produced on GAC. However, the precursors to their formation are widespread and have been found in a number of waters. They can also be produced microbiologically in nature. The organic precursors are secondary or tertiary amines, which are natural products that are also found in industrial effluents and in agricultural pesticides. Bacteria also form such amines. The inorganic precursor of nitrosamines is nitrite, only low levels of which are required for the process to occur. Nitrite is formed during nitrification, which occurs on GAC, as well as during denitrification and nitrate reduction. Consequently, the precursors are ubiquitous and are likely to enter or be formed on GAC. Moreover, the process of combining the two precursors into the final toxin is easily accomplished in water, sewage, or soil (Ayanaba and Alexander, 1974; Mills and Alexander, 1976), and the reaction may be affected by microorganisms through their own activities or by organic materials formed microbiologically (Ayanaba and Alexander, 1973; Mills and Alexander, 1976).

Many refractory compounds are subject to cometabolism, although they are not totally biodegraded to yield carbon dioxide. Cometabolism refers to the capacity of microorganisms to degrade compounds that they cannot use as a nutrient source and, thus, cannot totally mineralize. As a result, organic products are generated—products that are usually related structurally to the original chemical; e.g., metabolites formed from DDT, aldrin, heptachlor, PCB's, and triazine herbicides. Although there are no studies of cometabolism on the GAC surface, it seems plausible that refractory organic molecules entering water from agricultural, industrial, or domestic operations or generated as a result of chlorination could be acted upon. This would give rise to products that are themselves not suitable substrates and are not attacked readily by microorganisms on

GAC. If these products of cometabolism are not adsorbed and removed from the flowing water, they will appear in the effluent.

HIGH-MOLECULAR-WEIGHT TOXINS—ENDOTOXINS

Since GAC columns are colonized by Gram-negative bacteria, there is concern that lipopolysaccharide endotoxins may be synthesized by these bacteria and may be eluted into the finished water. Complex lipopolysaccharides are found in the outer membrane of all Gram-negative bacteria (Freer and Salton, 1971), and many, but not all, of these lipopolysaccharides possess potent endotoxic activity (Hofstad and Kristoffersen, 1970).

Absorption and Toxicity   The dramatic toxicities of endotoxin, such as the production of fever, shock, or Shwartzman's phenomenon (a hemorrhagic reaction), are observed after parenteral administration. Far less is known about the absorption of endotoxin from the intestinal tract or the pathological consequences of absorption. The few data on the intestinal absorption of endotoxin suggest that the amount absorbed is minute. Gans and Matsumoto (1974) assayed endotoxin absorption in lead-sensitized rats. They found that when 5 mg of endotoxin was placed in the Thiry-Vella fistula in rats, only nanogram amounts were absorbed. Even when the rats were subjected to osmotic shock, the amount absorbed from the fistula, although increased, was so small that "it was unlikely to be of any significance" in normal animals. On the other hand, some investigators consider endotoxin absorption to be very injurious in certain circumstances. Fine and his colleagues (Schweinberg and Fine, 1960) have proposed that the endotoxin that is produced by the resident flora of the gut is absorbed continuously and is detoxified in the liver and in the spleen to render it harmless. However, during shock states detoxification is ineffective, and the absorbed endotoxin is thought to be directly responsible for a state of irreversible shock. This theory has not been accepted universally (Shands, 1975).

Endotoxin has also been proposed as a causal factor in the production of liver injury and cirrhosis. Suppression of the microbial flora of the gut prevents the development of cirrhosis in rats on a choline-deficient diet (Broitman *et al.*, 1964). The addition of endotoxin to the drinking water reverses this protective effect. In addition, animals on a choline-deficient diet become very susceptible to the lethal and hepatotoxic effects of endotoxin (Nolan and Ali, 1968). More recently, Nolan (1975) proposed that endotoxin absorption may contribute to liver diseases in the alcoholic and perhaps to the liver diseases found in obesity bypass patients.

Measurement of Endotoxin Although lipopolysaccharides can be measured chemically, endotoxins can be measured only by biological assay. Most of the tests for activity are time-consuming and expensive, e.g., pyrogenicity and lethality tests. The limulus lysate test developed by Levin and Bang (1964) is without doubt the most sensitive test for endotoxin. It is sensitive in the nanogram to picogram range (Yin *et al.*, 1972). It is a rapid test, and, unlike other biological tests for endotoxin, it is suitable for testing many samples simultaneously. For reasons of economy, efficiency, and sensititvity, it is currently the test of choice.

Measurements of Endotoxin in Drinking Water The amount of endotoxin in drinking water has been measured with the limulus lysate test. DiLuzio and Friedmann (1973) tested tap water that was obtained from a variety of sources. They found endotoxin concentrations ranging from 1 μg to 10 μg/ml in water from Denver, Colorado; Mobile, Alabama; and San Francisco, California. Jorgensen *et al.* (1976) measured endotoxin levels varying from <0.625 ng/ml to 500 ng/ml in drinking water from 10 cities. These authors opined that the high levels found by DiLuzio and Friedman were erroneous. Jorgensen *et al.* (1976) also suggested that endotoxin levels may be higher in water that had been treated by GAC. On the other hand, Love and Symons (1978), who conducted a 7-month pilot plant study for the EPA, found that the concentration of endotoxin in the effluent of a GAC bed was less than the concentration in the input. The maximal level in the finished water was 11 ng/ml. These data indicate that GAC filtration does not result in excess endotoxin in finished water. Furthermore, the data may be interpreted to suggest that GAC may adsorb lipopolysaccharide endotoxins, but more work is needed to verify this.

Summary, Conclusions, and Recommendations

1. No direct evidence has been given for removal of specific organics of potential harm to health by microbial activity. Only one study (at the Jefferson Parish Water Works, which was reported by Brodtmann *et al.*, 1980), implied that precursors to THM formation were removed by microbial action. An indirect benefit of microbial activity may be the lengthening of GAC service time by removing organics that would otherwise occupy adsorption sites; but this in itself does not imply more effective removal of organics of health concern.

2. While operation of GAC beds for 6 months to 2 yr without regeneration has shown that microbial activity removes organics, as measured by group parameters such as TOC, potassium permanganate demand, COD, and UV-absorbance, the efficiency of biodegradation is less than that of adsorption, i.e., biodegradation to remove approximately 1.5 mg/liter TOC requires about 30 min of GAC contact (Benedek, 1977; Eberhardt et al., 1974; Jekel, 1977), while adsorption only requires approximately 10 to 15 min.

3. Pilot and full-scale tests of preozonization have shown that organics are efficiently removed through the total system, including the flocculation and adsorption steps; however, the ability of microbial action to aid in removal of specific organics of potential harm to health has not been reported. Thus far, one study, at the EPA Cincinnati pilot plant (U.S. Environmental Protection Agency, 1978c), implied that precursors to THM formation were somehow altered by ozonization in such a manner that their removal was made more effective.

4. The role of ozone in promoting microbial activity remains unclear. Conversion of organics to more biodegradable forms and addition of oxygen to the biofilm are two possibilities. On the negative side, evidence shows that ozone may decrease the adsorbability of some organics.

5. While prechlorination does not stop microbial growth on GAC, there is some evidence to suggest that it results in formation of organics that are much more resistant to biodegradation on the GAC surface.

6. The bacteria that have been reported to grow on GAC beds are considered nonpathogenic. Increases in bacteria in the effluent may be controlled by backwashing.

7. Microorganisms can generate a variety of highly potent, low-molecular-weight toxicants in culture. Studies of models of several environments and some natural systems indicate that toxicants may be, or are indeed, formed. Such products may also be produced on GAC. However, there is a lack of information regarding the identification of organics in the effluent of GAC beds. Thus, while no evidence exists, the possibility that microbial end products of concern enter the finished water cannot be ruled out.

8. The endotoxin content of water that has been filtered through GAC is either not increased or not significantly increased. The measured levels are very low and should pose no risk.

Thus far, evidence of microbial activity in GAC beds has largely been indirect. Of special importance is the identification of organics that are biodegraded. If these are not potentially harmful to health, then more investigation is needed to determine whether microbial action has actually extended or improved the adsorption of other organics that are potentially harmful to health. This may result if fewer of the internal adsorption sites are occupied because of biodegradation at the surface. Related to this concern about extended removal of organics is the unresolved question of bioregeneration. More careful investigation is needed to determine if adsorbed organics, which are more resistant to biodegradation, can be acted upon by microbes.

The role of ozonization in promoting microbial action needs much further elucidation. This would involve studies to determine the changes in biodegradability and adsorbability that are brought about by ozonization of specific organics that could affect public health. There are similar concerns regarding the practice of prechlorination.

If the use of GAC is to become widespread, research is necessary to identify the factors that are responsible for the initiation of microbial growth on the GAC surface and the microbiological generation of organic compounds on the carbon. Attention should be given not only to the compounds that are present and retained in the bed, but also to those that are released and could appear in the effluent. Research should be directed toward compounds generated from innocuous, natural precursors, as well as toward those that may be formed as a result of microbial action on synthetic industrial waste, agricultural pesticides, household effluents, and compounds that are formed as a result of chlorination of water. The investigations should identify the specific organic molecules thus formed and not simply the quantity of organic carbon that is emitted from GAC. The toxicological significance of such compounds and the possibility of their occurrence in concentrations sufficiently high to be of concern should be assessed.

Although it is unlikely, the possibility that some pathogens may be able to colonize GAC beds should be tested. Of primary importance are enteric pathogens such as *Salmonella, Shigella, Vibrio, Yersinia enterocolitica,* and the enterotoxigenic *Escherichia coli.*

PRODUCTION OF NONBIOLOGICAL SUBSTANCES BY OR WITHIN THE GAC BED

One potential source of chemical breakthrough from a GAC column can be the chemical changes on GAC surfaces. This section evaluates the significance of this potential source of toxic organic chemicals in drinking water. To do this, the subcommittee addressed the following questions:

1. To what extent does the carbon interact with chemical species on the GAC column and produce chemicals of potential health concern. Does the carbon catalyze reactions or enter into reactions producing new chemicals?

2. What is the impact on reactions at the GAC surfaces that is caused by metals incorporated into GAC?

3. What is the potential for release of chemicals of concern that are formed on GAC?

4. What is the potential health effect of the release of carbon fines during operation of a GAC system?

Carbon as a Catalytic Surface

Few studies have addressed the ability of carbon to catalyze reactions producing new chemical components and their subsequent release to water that is being purified for human consumption. Emphasis has been placed on adsorption and removal. Ishizaki and Cookson (1974) suggested that carbon could mediate chemical changes during water purification, resulting in the release of compounds not originally found in the water. The chemical changes that are mediated by carbon are not only the result of oxidation and reduction reactions, but can stem from catalysis on the carbon surface. The use of carbon as a surface catalyst and catalyst support in industrial processes is well documented.

Catalysis on nonuniform surfaces such as activated carbon is not well understood. Most probably, there are only a few types of catalytically effective adsorption sites on activated carbon. Exceptions would be carbons that have been specially prepared to enhance their catalytic properties. As a result, sites contributing strongly to catalysis may contribute virtually nothing to adsorptive capacity.

While heterogeneous catalytic reactions may be complex, three individual steps can be identified. These are adsorption, surface reaction, and desorption. Heterogeneous reactions are usually sensitive to methods of preparation. The active sites on the catalytic surface are not necessarily distributed randomly. It appears that the bulk of the reactions that can be catalyzed by activated carbon are caused by the surface oxides and other impurities in the carbon structure. In most carbons, these surface functional groups would represent a small fraction of the available adsorptive sites.

Cookson (1978) has discussed the surface groups on activated carbon and their influence on adsorption and catalysis. Although many investigators have reported the above-mentioned acidic oxides to be likely inhabitants of the carbon surface, there is still no completely documented description. Thus, none of the proposed catalytic mechanisms for carbon have been proven.

A variety of interrelationships can occur between adsorption and catalysis. It appears that a number of catalytic systems have their own peculiarities, making generalization not feasible at this time. Because of the limited amount of data on adsorption to activated carbon from water and catalysis, one is handicapped when attempting to draw specific conclusions. Although data are limited, no toxic chemicals have been reported to be formed by catalysis on GAC. The oxidation reactions catalyzed by GAC yield products that are found in water supplies and would be expected in drinking water processed without the application of GAC.

ORGANIC REACTIONS MEDIATED BY CARBON

Carbon catalyzes the oxidation of sulfide in solution, glucose in the presence of phosphoric acid, oxalic acid, malonic acid, amino acids, phenylthiocarbamide, ascorbic acid, uric acid and its derivatives, and mercaptans (Garten and Weiss, 1959; Ishizaki and Cookson, 1974; Larsen and Walton, 1940; Rideal and Wright, 1925, 1926; Weiss, 1962).

Weiss (1962) reported that one of the first studies illustrating the ability of carbon in aqueous solutions to catalyze reactions with organic materials was conducted by Warburg in 1921. Utilizing aqueous suspensions of charcoal, Warburg outlined the aerial oxidation of amino acids to organic acids and ammonia. Further work illustrated that the adsorption of the amino acid on the carbon surface was an important step in the catalyzed sequence. In 1926 Rideal and Wright showed that an aqueous suspension of sugar charcoal catalyzed the oxidation of oxalic acid. These early investigators also reported that the reaction could be inhibited by a number of compounds, including amyl alcohol, cyanide, thiocyanate, chloroform, aniline, and acetone. These compounds all appeared to act as poisons and probably inhibited the reaction by combining with iron that was contained in the charcoal. Garten and Weiss (1959) proposed a mechanism for the oxidation of these organics by chromenelike structures on the carbon surface. These interpretations need confirmation with modern techniques.

The proposed oxidation of oxalic acid by activated carbon involves the adsorption of oxalate at the site of the carbonium ion on the carbon. An electron can pass from the oxalate into the carbon, resulting in the removal of oxygen as a monovalent peroxide anion. This anion captures the proton that is released simultaneously from the oxalate anion to form hydrogen peroxide. This reaction is possible, since the single electron remaining on carbon has resonance stability. The hydrogen peroxide liberated during the reaction can further oxidize organic components.

Garten and Weiss (1959) illustrated the oxidation of malonic acid by activated carbon under acid conditions. The oxidation mechanism of malonic acid appears to differ from that of oxalic acid, but no mechanism has been proposed. The investigators provided the following oxidation equation, which is based on oxygen uptake and carbon dioxide production during the reaction.

$$2CH_2 (COOH)_2 + O_2 \rightarrow 2CH(OH) (COOH)_2 \qquad (1)$$

$$2CH(OH) (COOH)_2 + O_2 \rightarrow 2CHOCO_2H + 2CO_2 + 2H_2O \qquad (2)$$

The aerial oxidation of ascorbic acid is also catalyzed by activated carbon. Garten and Weiss (1959) observed that some carbons were unable to catalyze the reactions, and others had considerable effect. Carbons that were prepared at 900°C supported the greatest catalytic activity. This suggests that the basic oxide of the carbon may be involved.

Rideal and Wright (1926) reported that in aqueous solutions substances containing but one polar group, such as alcohol, formic acid, and the higher fatty acids, do not undergo oxidation at the surface of charcoal. Substances containing two adjacent polar groups, such as α-amino acids, phenylthiocarbamide, and oxalic and malonic acids, are readily oxidized by carbon.

The catalytic activity of carbon under more alkaline conditions probably involves the quinone–hydroquinone surface groups. These groups can function as electron acceptor sites that facilitate the chemisorption of electron donors on the surface of the carbon. Under alkaline conditions, the formation of the semiquinones would mediate the transfer of electrons to chemisorbed oxygen. This enables the quinone to play essentially the same role as the carbonium ions of basic carbons and acid solutions.

The catalytic activity of carbons in alkaline solutions has been demonstrated for the oxidation of uric acid, its 1-methyl and 7-methyl derivatives, and mercaptan (Ishizaki and Cookson, 1974; Weiss, 1962).

The oxidation of mercaptans to disulfides by activated carbon in aqueous suspensions has been documented by Ishizaki and Cookson (1974). The adsorption of mercaptan on carbon is a complex phenomenon, because the adsorption of mercaptan and disulfide on the carbon parallel the conversion of the former, as indicated by the following equation:

$$2BuSH + \frac{1}{2}\,O_2 \rightarrow (BuS)_2 + H_2O \qquad (3)$$

where BuSH = n-butyl mercaptan and $(BuS)_2$ = butyl disulfide.

The oxidation of mercaptan to disulfide is catalyzed by activated carbon. This catalytic effect is significantly reduced by outgassing at elevated temperatures. Two proposed mechanisms might explain the catalytic nature of activated carbon. One mechanism involves the participation of quinone groups. In this mechanism, the disulfide formation would arise via a redox reaction involving the formation of thiol radicals and semiquinone anions.

The second mechanism is due to metal ions on the surface of the carbon. By outgassing the carbon at elevated temperatures (900°C) and analyzing the metals released, it was determined that the commercial activated carbon contained 0.041 mg of copper per gram of carbon (Ishizaki and Cookson, 1974). The amount of iron was considerably lower, indicating that this commercial carbon was probably impregnated with copper during regeneration. The catalytic activity of carbon in the oxidation of mercaptans can involve both quinone groups and metals on the carbon's surface. One mechanism does not exclude the other, but it is likely that both occur at the same time. Ishizaki and Cookson (1974) proposed a combined mechanism.

Commercial activated charcoal catalyzes the oxidation of potassium urate (Larsen and Walton, 1940). It increased the rate of autoxidation of potassium urate in water solutions of activated carbon. The degree of oxidation that normally occurred in 15 hr was achieved in 10 min in the presence of activated carbon.

Impurities incorporated in activated carbon during regeneration greatly influence its catalytic behavior. Rideal and Wright (1926) studied the influence of nitrogen and iron on carbon's catalytic activity in the oxidation of oxalic acid. When both iron and nitrogen were incorporated into the carbon, the iron–carbon–nitrogen complex produced a carbon with a specific activity that was 800 times that of the original activated carbon. When iron alone was used, the iron–carbon complex produced a carbon with a specific activity that was 50 times that of the original carbon. These studies, along with those of temperature influences, clearly illustrate the effect that activation and regeneration procedures have on carbon's catalytic behavior. Thus, the history of activated carbon prior to regeneration is important. The adsorption to carbon of various metals and other ions could result in the incorporation of these materials as impurities on the carbon surface, resulting in a carbon with greater catalytic activity than that of the virgin material.

Reactions with Disinfectants

Activated carbon serves as a very effective reducing agent for residual chlorine in aqueous solution. These reactions have been the object of a number of studies. Magee (1956), in particular, indicated that free chlorine would react as follows:

$$HOCl + C^* \rightarrow C^*O + HCl \tag{4}$$

If the reaction takes place at high pH, the following reaction is expected:

$$OCl^- + C^* \rightarrow C^*O + Cl^- \tag{5}$$

In these reactions, the asterisk (*) indicates the carbon surface. The specific types of surface oxides that form have not been well characterized, but they probably include such groups as phenolic-OH, carbonyl, and carboxyl. These reactions were found to be generally descriptive in that a short time after startup, within the limits of sensitivity of the chloride analysis test, the total chlorine entering the bed was equal to that leaving. As the extent of the carbon oxidation increased, the level of acidic oxides on the surface also increased and the adsorbability for simple phenols decreased (Snoeyink et al., 1974).

Bauer and Snoeyink (1973) proposed the following monochloramine and dichloramine reactions:

$$NH_2Cl + H_2O + C^* \rightarrow C^*O + NH_3 + HCl \tag{6}$$

$$2NH_2Cl + 2C^*O \rightarrow 2C^* + N_2(gas) + 2H_2O + 2Cl^- \tag{7}$$

$$2NHCl_2 + H_2O + C^* \rightarrow C^*O + N_2(gas) + 4HCl \tag{8}$$

Studies with nitrogen trichloride have not been conducted to date, but Atkins et al. (1973) presented evidence indicating that it also reacts very rapidly with activated carbon.

However, Reactions 1–5 do not completely describe the oxidation phenomena, because carbon dioxide is observed in the effluent of the reactor after a certain amount of oxidation (Magee, 1956). As the reaction increases further (up to 1–4 g of free chlorine as Cl_2 per gram of carbon), the oxidation of the carbon has become so extensive that a resulting end product produces a visible dark color in the aqueous solution. This extent of reaction is not expected to occur within 2 to 3 yr under typical operating conditions at a water treatment plant (i.e., chlorine enters the carbon adsorber at a concentration of 1 to 2 mg/liter or less). The GAC will probably be replaced or regenerated prior to this time, although additional investigation is needed on this subject. Some preliminary identification work on the solution with the dark color has indicated that several purgeable organics, including volatile halogenated organics, are present. Much of the dark color remained after purging the sample. Further work is needed to identify the composition of that material (Snoeyink and McCreary, 1978). Regeneration of the carbon prior to the production of the dark color should result in the volatilization of many of the oxidation products and surface oxides, thereby preventing the formation of undesirable end products.

When activated carbon is used at a water plant, organics collect on its surface. Chlorine residual can now react either with the activated carbon surface or with the adsorbed organics. Whether a significant amount of chlorinated organics is formed by the reaction of chlorine with adsorbed organics and whether such organics, if formed, can be eluted from the bed are questions that must be answered.

There have been few studies on the reaction of ozone with activated carbon. The nature of this reaction is of less importance, because, when ozone is used as a predisinfectant, its half-life is such that a relatively small amount, or none, will enter the GAC adsorber. Dietz and Bitner (1972) reported that, when some ozone entered the adsorber, it reacted very readily with the carbon. The reaction consisted of the following three steps taking place, depending upon the amount of ozone that had reacted:

$$C^*_xO + O_3 \rightarrow C^*_xC_{y+1} + O_2 \tag{9}$$

$$C^*_xO + O_3 \rightarrow C^*_{x-1}O_{y+1} + CO_2 \tag{10}$$

$$C^*_xO + O_3 \rightarrow C^*_{x-2}O + CO_2 + CO \tag{11}$$

These reactions show that oxides of unspecified types, O_2, CO, and CO_2, may form as reaction products. They account for the observed initial weight increase and, after a certain amount of reaction, the weight loss of the carbon. Dietz and Bitner (1972) also found evidence that the ozone converted some of the smaller pores to larger pores, with little change in total surface area, and that surface oxides formed at the entrance to the micropores, which resulted in partial blockage of those pores.

Chlorine dioxide, one of the alternative disinfectants to chlorine, is also a strong oxidizing agent that is probably reduced very readily by GAC. However, there is little information on the reaction of chlorine dioxide with carbon and/or adsorbed organics and whether any undesirable end products might be formed by such reactions. This subject requires research if chlorine dioxide is to be used as a predisinfectant at a water plant.

Dissolved oxygen also reacts with activated carbon. Prober *et al.* (1975) found uptakes of 10 to 40 mg of oxygen per gram of carbon for commercially available carbons. They noted that equilibrium had not been achieved at these loadings. The uptake resulted in an increase in acidic surface oxides. Only approximately 5% of the amount taken up could be eluted as oxygen. The reaction between oxygen and carbon is important, because it indicates that not all oxygen that is removed during adsorption can be attributed to biological activity and that the nature of the carbon surface may be altered during the adsorption process.

INORGANIC REACTIONS MEDIATED BY CARBON

The catalytic properties of activated carbon can result in the oxidation of inorganic compounds in air contact systems. The acidic oxides on the carbon surface are known to be responsible for many of these catalytic oxidations. Such systems may not be applicable to aqueous solutions because of the possible influence of adsorbed water. For this reason, reactions in the gas are not discussed here.

Studies that consider aqueous systems are few. As is true with organics, the catalytic activity of carbon has not been studied specifically. Most of the available information can be classified as conjecture that is based on extrapolations from observations gathered from adsorption studies with inorganics.

Several investigators have studied the removal of iron from aqueous solutions by treatment with activated carbon (Ford and Boyer, 1973; George and Chaudhuri, 1977; Huang, 1978; Stumm and Lee, 1961). They reported that the oxidation of ferrous ions accelerates in the presence of activated carbon. Their results suggest that carbon can act as a catalyst and that the presence of surface groups can greatly influence the rate of catalytic activity. Puri (1970) reported that the catalytic activity of a carbon that contained oxygen surface groups was more than two orders of magnitude greater than the activity of a carbon that was devoid of these groups.

Huang (1978) reported that the adsorption of Hg^{2+} on activated carbon also involves adsorption accompanied by a reduction of mercury on the surface of the carbon. The activation procedure for activated carbon plays a major role in determining the mechanisms of mercury adsorption and reduction.

This catalytic effect of carbon is greatly influenced by the techniques of its preparation of activation. The effect of activation temperature on a carbon's catalytic potential with inorganics is clearly illustrated by the work of Larsen and Walton (1940). These investigators studied the catalytic activity of activated carbon for oxidizing stannous chloride in solution. The carbons were activated at temperatures ranging from 350°C to 850°C. The speed of reaction was greatly influenced by activation temperature, indicating maximum catalytic activity at 575°C. The reaction rates decreased rapidly for carbons that were activated at temperatures above 650°C and below 450°C.

Unfortunately, the undefined nature of the trace metals in water supplies makes it extremely difficult to predict the efficiency of carbon to adsorb metals (Huang and Wu, 1975; Kunin, 1976). For example, many of these metals are bound or complexed with the various organic substances in water, thereby forming complexes that are completely unrelated to the simple ionic states that have been reported for these metals in classical texts on inorganic chemistry.

The problem becomes even more complicated if we consider the thermal regeneration phase of the cyclical process that is associated with the use of carbon. In most systems, carbon is regenerated thermally under controlled conditions by "burning off" the adsorbed organic substances. Under these conditions, the metals, except perhaps mercury, remain in the carbon. These metals accumulate in the carbon. How they affect the adsorptive properties of carbon is not clear.

Chemical Changes Mediated by Adsorbed Compounds

ORGANIC REACTIONS

The subcommittee could find no information concerning a situation in which one adsorbed organic component mediated a reaction with a second. This does not mean that such reactions do not exist or occur on carbon. Investigators simply have not directed research toward this area. Reactions mediated by adsorbed organics are expected to be insignificant.

Various organic chelates will adsorb on carbon and improve the carbon's ability to adsorb various metals such as copper and mercury (Huang, 1978). The presence of these surface metal ions may increase carbon's catalytic activities as discussed in the following section concerning inorganics.

INORGANIC REACTIONS

In the chemical industry, a number of chemical reactions are mediated by adsorbed inorganic compounds on carbon. An example of such a catalyst is palladium on activated carbon. When activated carbon is soaked in a dilute solution of palladium chloride and hydrochloric acid for several hours and then washed, the palladium ions adsorb on the activated carbon and the chloride ions are completely washed from the carbon surface. Catalysts prepared with activated carbon in this manner have demonstrated excellent catalytic activity for liquid-phase hydrogenation of benzene at room temperature (Morikawa *et al.*, 1969). Despite these uses of activated carbon for catalytic reactions, there is a poor understanding of its behavior as a catalyst.

Methods used to prepare activated carbon catalyst include impregnation, precipitation, and adsorption. Impregnation normally involves the heating of the ion to be impregnated on the carbon surface. This may be performed after the ion is first adsorbed on carbon from solutions. The precipitation method involves the precipitation of the specific ion on the carrier. In the adsorption method, ions are deposited on the carbon surface by physical or chemical adsorptive forces. Many of the methods for preparing activated carbon catalysts are similar to processes occurring in water treatment and carbon regeneration. Thus, the importance of the above carbon–metal catalyses in water purification is unknown. Since metals are placed on carbon surfaces during regeneration procedures, this area needs more investigation.

Potential for Release of Catalytic Products

The formation of new organic or inorganic components as a result of carbon catalytic activity can result in enhanced adsorption or their release to solution. The use of activated carbon as a catalyst for industrial purposes is successful only when high yields of the product are obtained. It follows that a significant release of catalyzed products does occur. While examining adsorption of mercaptan on activated carbon, Ishizaki and Cookson (1974) illustrated that activated carbon catalyzed the oxidation of mercaptan to disulfide. They confirmed that the disulfide competes with mercaptan for sorption sites on activated carbon. Adsorption equilibrium constants were established for both the mercaptan and disulfide. In light of this information, it appears that any product that is produced by carbon's catalytic activities would be released to solution in accordance with their adsorption equilibrium and the competitive nature of other solutes in the water phase.

There has been no documentation of organics produced by activated carbon that are potential health hazards. Nitrosamine formation on activated carbon may be similar to that for ion-exchange resins (Fiddler and Kimoto, 1979). This area has not been investigated.

For inorganic components, the potential for release appears to be less than that of organic compounds. Most studies have indicated that carbon has a great affinity for inorganic species. The use of activated carbon for treating raw surface waters would not be expected to release significant amounts of inorganic components.

Carbon Fines

Because GAC is friable, fines can be released. The amount of release will depend upon the properties of the activated carbon. Consequently, traces of finely divided particles form constantly and could enter the treated water. McCarty et al. (1979) have reported continual bleed-off of carbon fines, primarily of those ranging from 2.5 to 25 μm diameter, from a GAC column utilized in an up-flow, countercurrent, packed bed contractor at Water Factory 21 Advanced Wastewater Treatment facility in Orange County, California. Operation of the column in a gravity downflow mode tended to arrest the process. Total particle counts were 4 times as high in the upflow mode even at 0.2 m/min.

The carbon itself should pose no health problems because of its inertness; however, the carbon particle may have adsorbed and concentrated compounds on its surface which may be released upon ingestion. There are essentially no reliable data on the association and release of adsorbed substances or on fate or the toxicity of the substances after release from carbon fines.

Summary, Conclusions, and Recommendations

Catalysis on the surface of activated carbon most likely involves localized defects that are caused by impurities in the carbon structure or through the adsorption of metals, oxides, and other substances. When adsorption is accompanied by catalytic reactions, kinetic and equilibrium interpretations of the system become extremely complex. A variety of interrelationships can occur between adsorption and catalysis. A number of catalytic systems have their own peculiarities making generalization difficult. Because of the limited amount of data on adsorption on activated carbon from water and catalysis, one is handicapped when attempting to draw specific conclusions. In addition, generalizations are extremely risky, making it difficult to project the possible significance of catalysis in adsorption on activated carbon from water. This subject needs further research.

Activated carbon serves as a catalyst for some reactions in water systems, e.g., oxidization, reduction, and polymerization. These reactions can produce organic and inorganic species that were not originally present. These can be released to the water solution and behave as typical solutes in that they adsorb, desorb, and compete for adsorpton sites.

The studies dealing with adsorption of organics and inorganics have frequently utilized detection procedures that would not provide observation of catalyzed reactions if such were occurring. At this time, we can only conclude that such reactions are possible. However, little can be said concerning the degree of their occurrence during water purification and their possible impacts on public health. There is no doubt that future studies must attempt to clarify the uncertainties that exist.

Carbon may undergo significant changes via its patterns of use and regeneration. The studies that have been reviewed in this chapter point to the effects of adsorbed ions on carbon's catalytic activity for a number of reactions. It would follow that carbons used in the treatment of wastewater may adsorb significant quantities of various metals that become incorporated in the carbon structure during regeneration procedures. Thus, the recycling and regeneration of activated carbon could result in a material that is radically different from the virgin material. This may indicate the need for a control program that is related to carbon monitoring and the use of carbon in the water purification industry.

Industrial secrecy surrounding the manufacture of activated carbon and the varied industrial applications make it difficult to regulate carbon quality for water purification without the implementation of specific quality requirements and the monitoring and control of carbon for water use. Without doubt, this matter demands additional attention. A research evaluation program and controls for carbon use should be adopted until results of future studies indicate that they are unnecessary.

The subcommittee concludes that:

1. The limited amount of data on catalysis by activated carbon makes it impossible to provide specific conclusions on the potential significance of toxic organic production. Nontoxic products have been produced by catalysis on activated carbon during adsorption from water.

2. Chlorine, chlorine dioxide, and ozone react readily with carbon and may react with compounds adsorbed on carbon. There is no evidence to indicate that such reactions, under the conditions that exist in water treatment plants, will or will not produce potentially hazardous compounds.

3. Metals on GAC increase the catalytic potential.

4. Reaction products can be released to the water solution. They behave as typical solutes in that they adsorb, desorb, and compete for GAC sites.

5. Catalytic properties of activated carbon depend upon its method of preparation, surface characteristics as determined by previous uses with particular emphasis on adsorbed metals, and regeneration.

6. Past studies on GAC adsorption have not used techniques that would provide observation of catalyzed reactions if such were occurring.

The subcommittee recommends that:

1. Additional studies should be conducted to assess the potential of GAC-catalyzed reactions for both virgin and regenerated carbons.

2. Studies should be directed toward the need for regulating the quality of carbon that is used in water purification.

3. Techniques should be developed for measuring carbon's catalytic potential and applied as a quality control method.

4. The catalytic potential of producing toxic products by metals that become incorporated onto the carbon surface as a result of use and regeneration must be evaluated.

5. Studies should be conducted to determine levels of carbon fines that pass into drinking water and their biological significance.

6. Research is needed to identify the end products of reactions between activated carbon and disinfectants, especially chlorine and chlorine dioxide. Moreover, the interaction of oxygen with the carbon surface must be evaluated.

REGENERATION OF GAC

In the United States, activated carbon has been used in the treatment of potable water primarily to control taste and odor. The first major GAC installation in this country was built in Hopewell, Virginia, in 1961. Since then, GAC has been installed in approximately 60 potable water supply systems to control taste and odor. However, use for this purpose has generally not required GAC regeneration.

The widespread use of GAC will require effective regeneration of spent carbon for economic utilization. This section contains a detailed presentation of the factors that are involved with carbon regeneration technology. Specifically, the character of the original source material, how the GAC source material was utilized, the methods of producing the GAC, and the regeneration of GAC are reviewed. The following questions are addressed:

1. Does the nature of the regeneration process change the adsorption properties of carbon? Are such changes significant to health?
2. Does the spent carbon's past use affect its properties after regeneration? Is this history significant to health?
3. How does GAC change during storage?
4. Does virgin or regenerated carbon contain substances that can be leached into water? Are these substances of significance to health?
5. Does the volatilization of pollutants resulting from the regeneration of spent GAC present risks to health?

The Dependence of Surface Chemistry on Preparation

The adsorptive properties of activated carbon are influenced by the regeneration procedure and contaminating ions. The activated carbon source material has been described in the introduction. Disturbances in the elementary microcrystalline structure, which are caused by such factors as the presence of imperfect (partially burnt-off) graphite layers, changes the arrangement of the electron clouds in the carbon skeleton. As a result, unpaired electrons appear. This condition influences the adsorptive properties of activated carbon, especially for polar or polarizable substances. Another type of disturbance is the presence of hetero atoms in the carbon structure.

Activated carbon contains chemically bonded elements such as oxygen and hydrogen. These elements can be contained in the starting material and remain as a result of imperfect carbonization, or they can become chemically bonded to the surface during activation. In addition, the activated carbon contains ash, which is not an organic part of the product. The ash content and its composition vary widely with the kind of activated carbon (Anderson and Emmett, 1947; Kipling, 1965). The adsorption by activated carbon of electrolytes and nonelectrolytes from solution is significantly influenced even by small amounts of ash (Blackburn and Kipling, 1955). The presence of oxygen and hydrogen has a great effect on the properties of activated carbon. These elements combine with atoms of carbon by chemical bonds. They differ from the ash by forming an organic part of the chemical structure of the activated carbon.

Because of the importance of oxygen on carbon's adsorption and catalytic properties, the influence of regeneration on their reaction is discussed below. However, most other chemical groups on carbon have not been well documented. The few studies that were performed did not have the benefit of modern techniques.

When oxygen is adsorbed on a carbon surface, it undergoes a chemical change, even at room temperature. Nitrogen and other gases that are adsorbed on charcoal are easily removed as such. However, oxygen is removed as carbon dioxide only by heating the charcoal at high temperatures. Rhead and Wheeler (1912, 1913) pointed out that oxygen combines with the carbon to form a physicochemical complex, C_xO_y, of variable composition. This complex decomposes upon heating giving a mixture of carbon monoxide and carbon dioxide.

There are several methods by which oxygen surface complexes can be formed during regeneration. They may be classified into two major groups: methods utilizing oxidizing gases and those involving oxidizing solutions. The most common oxidizing gases are oxygen (Hart et al., 1967), water vapor (Smith, 1959), carbon dioxide (Puri, 1970), and oxides of nitrogen. Some of the oxidizing solutions are acidified potassium permanganate, nitric acid, a mixture of nitric and sulfuric acids (Puri, 1970), chlorine water, and sodium hypochlorite (Behrman and Gustafson, 1935; Donnet et al., 1961, 1963).

Commercial Regeneration Procedures

During the purification of waters and wastes, impurities in the solutions collect in the pores of the carbon. After a while, contaminants begin to break through the GAC bed, and the spent carbon must be reactivated. Various regeneration techniques that have been developed over the years include thermal, chemical, solvent, vacuum, biological, and wet (steam) oxidation methods. Of these methods, thermal regeneration is the most common. These methods of regeneration are reviewed by Lombana and Halaby, 1978; Von Dreusche, 1978; and Inhoffer, 1978.

The compounds adsorbed during water treatment should be removed by thermal regeneration, thereby making GAC a most attractive alternative. While carbons can be regenerated, documentation is needed for changes due to regeneration in hardness, pore size distribution, ash and metal ion buildup, and adsorbability for compounds present in water supplies.

The thermal regeneration of spent carbon is one of the most important factors involved in the economic consideration of activated carbon treatment of water. The adsorbed organic materials are volatilized or oxidized at a high temperature during this process. Ideally, this would be done in such a manner that a maximum amount of adsorbed organics are driven off with a minimum change in the adsorptive properties of the carbon. The success of reactivation depends on a number of factors, including carbon temperature, duration of activation, and the activating gas mixture. Presently available GAC can withstand repeated regeneration and reuse as shown in the field of wastewater treatment.

Two other methods of regeneration that have been successfully used with activated carbon involve chemical solvents and steam. In the first method chemical solvents are added to the carbon bed to desorb the adsorbed material. The solvent is then passed through the carbon bed in the direction opposite to that of the service cycle until the adsorbate is removed. The bed is then drained of the solvent, and the regenerated carbon is ready to be returned to stream.

If the carbon has been used to remove adsorbates with low boiling temperatures, it can sometimes be regenerated with steam. The steam is passed through the carbon bed opposite to normal flow. It is then either vented to the atmosphere or condensed and recovered. To avoid air pollution, condensation and recovery are preferable. Approximately 3 to 5 lb of steam are needed to remove each kilogram of adsorbate that is collected by the carbon.

These latter two methods have not enjoyed widespread acceptance. They are not as effective as thermal removal from carbon of the many different compounds that adsorb during water treatment.

Influence of Regeneration on Adsorption

Various regeneration procedures and their influence on the surface structure of carbon have been discussed above. Since regeneration procedures have a major influence on carbon surface chemistry, it follows that adsorption and catalytic potential can be changed greatly by the regeneration procedure. A number of studies illustrate that nonpolar paraffinic compounds, which are hydrophobic, will adsorb preferentially on carbon that is free from acidic surface oxides (Cookson, 1978). Acidic sites adsorb water, thereby hindering the adsorption of these organics. Acidic functional groups are found on carbon under specific temperature ranges and in the presence of certain reactivation gases. Several studies have suggested that aromatic adsorbates interact with carbonyl type groups on the carbon surface (Cookson, 1978). This interaction is believed to involve the formation of an electron donor-accepter complex of the solute ring structure containing carbonyl groups. The surface density of these chemical groups is also influenced by regeneration procedures.

The presence of metals on the surface of carbon has a significant effect on the adsorption of molecules with localized excess electrons. It appears that the attractive forces that are exerted by the surface metal can increase the rates of adsorption by several orders of magnitude (Cookson, 1978). Regeneration procedures not only affect adsorption properties but also can influence the catalytic behavior of carbon as discussed above. Carbon's potential to catalyze reactions would appear to increase when used carbon is regenerated for reuse. Carbon may adsorb significant quantities of various metals that can become incorporated in the carbon's structure during regeneration procedures. Thus, the recycling and regeneration of carbon can result in a material significantly different from the virgin activated carbon. This catalytic potential should be studied to determine if it is significant.

Sufficient data are not available to determine the difference in adsorption between regenerated and virgin GAC. These data are urgently needed to evaluate the total GAC process since regeneration is an integral part of the process.

CHEMICAL CHANGES DURING STORAGE

During storage, activated carbon undergoes chemical changes as a result of reactions with atmospheric oxygen. The reactions that occur at room temperature bring about an aging process in which the atmospheric oxygen reacts chemically with the carbon surface. This oxygen resides in the chemical structure of carboxyl or lactone type groups (Hart *et al.*, 1967; Smith, 1959). This aging process is expected to reduce the adsorption capacity of carbon for a large number of organic compounds that are found in water (Cookson, 1978). No other chemical changes that are expected to occur during storage would significantly influence any characteristics of the adsorbent.

LEACHING OF CHEMICALS FROM GAC

The extraction and leaching of chemicals from virgin activated carbon have been studied by a few investigators. Again, information is very limited, and few analytical studies have been performed with modern separation and identification techniques such as gas chromatography/mass spectrometry (GC/MS).

A few analytical studies have addressed the leaching of polycyclic aromatic hydrocarbons (PAH) from GAC. The release of PAH from virgin activated carbon has been demonstrated by Borneff (1980). Table IV-5 lists the compounds and concentrations that have been detected. The highest total amount of PAH that has been found on a virgin activated carbon is 250 μg/kg. The largest amount of carcinogenic polycyclics is 37 μg/kg. Fitch and Smith (1979) analyzed two activated carbons and several carbon blacks. They also found insignificant amounts of PAH on the activated carbons, but significant amounts were extracted from some carbon blacks. The procedures used to make carbon blacks differ greatly from those used to make activated carbons. Consequently, the difference in PAH content is not surprising. It is not anticipated that PAH would be released to drinking water in concentrations that are potentially harmful to health, because the total amount is so small and they are strongly adsorbed to activated carbon. Clearly, additional research is needed on virgin activated carbons, as well as regenerated carbons, so that the leaching potential of toxic chemicals can be evaluated completely.

Reference can be made to nitrosamine formation or leaching from resins (Fiddler and Kimoko, 1979). The possibility of nitrosamines leaching from carbon should be investigated.

Activated carbon used for treating raw surface waters would not be expected to release significant inorganic components. Love and Symons (1978) observed insignificant releases of metal ions when they exposed activated carbon to tap water. They also illustrated that the leaching of inorganic ions from activated carbon is unlikely and would probably occur only under stressed conditions.

Pollution Control During Carbon Regeneration

The removal of the adsorbates during regeneration presents another problem—the treatment and disposal of these moieties.

The thermal regeneration of carbon presents the most obvious of problems—the volatization of the adsorbates and the need to restrict their entry into the atmosphere. The disposal of the hot gases leaving a furnace requires an afterburner, wet scrubber, and dust collector.

The afterburner is used to burn gases that are driven off the carbon or formed during oxidation of the impurities. This is a refractory-lined chamber fitted with a burner and excess air injection system. The normal temperature range of operation of the afterburner is 900°C to 1,800°C. An ample supply of excess air (50%) must be available to accomplish this burning (Lombana and Halaby, 1978).

A wet scrubber usually follows the afterburner in the treatment scheme for two reasons: to collect the dust, which cannot be combusted in the afterburner, and to cool the gases so that they can be passed through the induced-draft fan. The scrubber is generally made of stainless steel in order to avoid corrosion. Baghouses are also used to remove particulates when air pollution regulations are less stringent and wet scrubbers are not used.

There are some examples of air pollution control systems in operation. As reported by Directo *et al.* (1977), a multihearth furnace used to regenerate carbon that is spent during sewage treatment operations at Pomona, California, discharged flue gases containing both particulate and odorous substances. The air pollution control system at this facility, which consists of a baghouse, was designed to remove 99% of the incoming particulate load. Data indicate that it only removed about 25%; particulate emissions were quite high, averaging 0.3 kg/hr. Odors were detected during the reactivation operations at the facility. This was confirmed by analytical testing, which detected three odor units per liter.

Studies in a similar vein performed in Kyoto, Japan, examined a number of compounds (Anonymous, 1977). The system was composed of an afterburner and scrubber following the regeneration furnace. Careful analysis of the data shows that, while dust and odor are reduced by the afterburner, the concentrations of sulfurous acid gas and nitrous oxides are increased. The scrubber was ineffective in the removal of nitrous oxides, but did remove sulfurous acid, gas, and dust. In addition, the scrubber increased the odor. However, this was due to the use of secondary effluent for scrubbing. These tests were repeated on carbons that had undergone a second and third reactivation cycle. Following the afterburner, these concentrations were reduced considerably. These studies were also performed with carbons used in wastewater treatment.

In brief, two general categories of exhaust emissions must concern the operators of regeneration facilities. These are particulates and gaseous

TABLE IV-5 Leaching of Polycyclic Aromatic Hydrocarbons from Virgin Activated Carbon

Activated Carbon	Type	Polycyclic Aromatic Hydrocarbons Detected, $\mu g/kg^a$											
		I	II	III	IV	V	VI	VII	VIII	IX	X	S	S++
Carboraffin C[b]	Powdered	80.0	—	—	1.2	—	0.8	—	0.8	—	—	83	1
Brillonit norm,[b]	Powdered	100	—	—	—	—	—	—	—	—	—	100	—
EPN-A-Kohle[c]	Powdered	28	—	—	—	—	—	—	—	—	—	28	8
Gerdit[d]	Powdered	53.6	12.4	—	5.2	1.2	2.8	—	4.0	1.2	—	68	—
Gerdit[d]	0-0.5 mm	110	—	—	12.4	9.6	—	—	10.0	2.4	—	157	37
Gerdit[d]	1-2.0 mm	216	—	—	21.2	3.6	8.4	—	5.2	2.4	—	257	27
Gerdit[d]	2-4 mm	81.6	—	—	3.2	2.0	—	—	2.0	0.8	—	90	6
Hydraffin 118 ff[b]	Powdered	1.2	—	—	—	—	—	—	—	—	—	1	—
Hydraffin BD[b]	0.5-2.5 mm	60	3.6	3.6	8.0	1.2	0.8	—	2.4	0.8	20.0	100	16
Hydraffin BD[b] (extra)	0.5-1.5 mm	3.6	—	—	—	—	—	—	—	—	—	4	—
Hydraffin LW[b]	0.5-3.0 mm	40	—	8.0	3.2	0.8	0.8	—	1.2	0.8	20.0	75	13
Hydraffin LW[b] (extra)	0.5-3.0 mm	80	—	—	2.4	—	1.6	—	0.8	0.4	—	85	3
Hydraffin TC[b] Spez I/II	0.5-2.5 mm	28	—	—	1.2	0.8	0.8	—	0.8	—	—	32	2

Material		I[a]	II	III	IV	V	VI	VII	VIII	IX	X	S	S++
KD-A-Kohle[c]	Powdered	80	—	—	—	—	—	—	—	—	—	80	—
Norit FND[e]	<5 μm 25%, 5-10 μm 6%	28	—	—	—	—	—	—	—	—	—	28	—
Norit P[e]	10-20 μm 12%, 20-50 μm 26%	1.6	—	—	—	—	—	—	—	—	—	2	—
Norit NK[e]	50-75 μm 13%, 75-90 μm 3%	—	—	—	—	—	—	—	—	—	—	—	—
Norit FNA[e]	>90 μm 15%	—	4.0	1.6	0.4	0.8	—	—	0.8	0.4	—	48	6
Norit RBWII[e]	Rods Φ = 1.6 mm	40	—	2.0	—	0.8	—	—	0.8	—	—	64	2
Olit normal[b]	<0.2 mm	60	12.0	4.0	1.6	3.2	—	—	2.8	1.6	—	93	27
R₄-A-Kohle[c]	Granul.	60	8.0	—	—	—	—	—	—	—	—	—	—
A-Kohle Nr. 2186[f]	<0.2 mm	2.8	—	—	—	—	—	—	—	—	—	3	—

[a] I fluoranthene
II benzo (a) anthracene
III benzo (j) fluoranthene
IV benzo (b) fluoranthene
V benzo (a) pyrene
VI benzo (ghi) perylene
VII perylene
VIII benzo (k) fluoranthene
IX indeno (1,2,3,-dc) pyrene
X pyrene
S sum of polycyclics I-X
S++ sum of carcinogenic polycyclics

[b] Produced by Lurgi GmbH, Frankfurt/Main.
[c] Produced by VEB-Chemiefasewerk, F. Engels.
[d] Produced by A. Jägersberg, Hamburg.
[e] Produced by Norit Corp., Amsterdam.
[f] Produced by E. Merck AG, Darmstadt.

NOTE: From Borneff, 1979.

emissions. Particulate emissions are probably most easily controlled via mechanical alterations to the regeneration system. For example, the stirring of carbon within a furnace is a major cause of particulate emission. No stirring of the carbon minimizes entrainment of fines, which results in low particulate emissions.

Gaseous emissions can include sulfur oxides, nitrogen oxides, hydrochloric acid, hydrocarbons, and other organic species. Unfortunately, there have been no studies measuring the gaseous emissions resulting from the regeneration of carbon by modern separation and identification techniques. There is a pressing need for research in this area to confirm the type of chemicals that are discharged, their amounts, and health significance.

Summary, Conclusions, and Recommendations

1. Regeneration procedures influence GAC chemical properties. This in turn will also influence adsorption, catalytic properties, and leachable chemicals. No significant health problems have been documented, but definite conclusions cannot be made because of insufficient data.

2. The previous use of a GAC and the amount of adsorbed contaminants will influence the chemical surface properties that develop during regeneration. There is inadequate information with which to evaluate the effect of these contaminants on adsorption, catalysis, and leaching.

3. The leaching of metals from carbon to water appears to be slight. The amounts leached are not known to produce adverse health effects.

4. The leaching of toxic organics from carbon to water has not been studied sufficiently to draw general conclusions. Although small amounts of PAH's have been detected, they do not appear to leach readily. The analytical studies are few and various regenerated carbon types must be evaluated.

5. Pollutants are discharged during GAC regeneration. Many studies have measured the oxides, hydrocarbons, and particulate matter present, but few have characterized the discharge sufficiently to evaluate health effects from volatilizing organics.

The subcommittee recommends that:

1. Regeneration procedures must be evaluated to determine their influence on adsorption capacity, catalytic potential, leaching of metals

and toxic organics, and volatilization of toxic discharges during regeneration.

2. The effect of various adsorbed contaminants on the properties of regenerated GAC (both metals and organics) must be evaluated in terms of carbon's adsorption and catalytic properties after regeneration.

3. Studies are needed to evaluate the potential for leaching toxic organics from operating carbon columns. Different carbons should be evaluated from this point of view for PAH's, nitrosamines, and other organic compounds of potential harm to health.

4. Gases that are discharged during regeneration should be characterized completely with particular attention given to pollutants of potential harm to health.

5. Consideration should be given to testing and regulations for controlling the regeneration process and history of the carbon to be used in drinking water purification if research shows that it is necessary.

ADSORPTION EFFICIENCY OF OTHER ADSORBENTS

This section contains an evaluation of the ability of other adsorbents to adsorb trace organic compounds during the treatment of drinking water. Two distinctly different processes are considered. One is the use of polymeric adsorbents, which include pyrolyzed polymers such as Ambersorb XE-340 (Rohm and Haas Co.) to remove low-molecular-weight organic compounds of potential harm to health. The other is the use of anion exchange resins to remove humic material.

The following questions are addressed:

1. What is the physical and chemical stability of the resins? What reactions take place between oxidants applied as predisinfectants and resins or compounds adsorbed on resins? Do these reactions result in potentially hazardous compounds that would not be present if resins were not used?

2. How well do polymeric adsorbents adsorb individual trace organic compounds, particularly those that are potentially harmful to health? What is the selectivity of the resin for single organic compounds?

3. What is the degree of competition on polymeric adsorbents between organic compounds with potential health effects, and how does the interaction with humic substances affect the competition?

4. What is the potential benefit of using ion exchange resins as a treatment method to remove organic matter before chlorination?

TABLE IV-6   Typical Properties of Amberlite Polymeric Adsorbents

Resin Type	Chemical Nature	Helium Porosity Volume		Surface Area, m²/g	Average Pore Diam., Å	Skeletal Density, g/cm³	Nominal Mesh Sizes
		%	cm³/g				
Nonpolar[a]							
XAD-1	Polystyrene	37	0.69	100	200	1.06	20-50
XAD-2	Polystyrene	42	0.69	330	90	1.08	20-50
XAD-4	Polystyrene	51	0.99	750	50	1.09	20-50
Intermediate Polarity[a]							
XAD-7	Acrylic ester	55	1.08	450	80	1.25	20-50
XAD-8	Acrylic ester	52	0.82	140	250	1.26	20-50
Synthetic Carbonaceous Adsorbent[b]							
XE-340	Polystyrene (partially pyrolyzed)			400	6-40 Å 18 Vol % 40-100 Å 13 Vol % 100-300 Å 69 Vol %	1.34	20-50

[a] From Kunin, 1976.
[b] From Rohm and Haas Co., 1977.

5. What effects on reactions within the bed are caused by the ion exchange resin or anions or cations that are on the surface of the ion exchange resin?

6. How effective are the regeneration processes? Does regeneration cause any health-related problems?

The concerted effort to develop resin adsorbents has been aided by recent advances in polymer chemistry. Efforts have been directed toward the removal of the humic materials from surface and shallow well-water supplies. The humic materials are a problem, particularly in the production of the high-purity water for power utilities and the electronics industries (Applebaum, 1968). Until recently, much of the experience with synthetic resins for potable water concerned the use of cation exchange resins to soften potable water. These water-softening resins remove few of the organics.

Resinous Adsorbents

The available synthetic resins may be classified into the following three major groups:

1. *Ion Exchange Resins.* These are cross-linked polyelectrolytes that are capable of removing ionic species via an ion exchange process; however, they may also function as adsorbents in removing organics or metal chelates. These structures may be formed from cross-linked polymers derived from styrene, acrylates, phenols, and pyridines (Kunin, 1972).

2. *Nonionic Polymeric Adsorbents.* These adsorbents are nonionic, high-surface-area, cross-linked copolymers of styrene, phenol, or acrylate (Table IV-6). Some are hydrophobic; others are hydrophilic. In essence, the macroreticular particle is composed of microspheres that are linked together, creating a continuous network of fine or large pores.

3. *Synthetic Carbonaceous Adsorbents.* Recently, synthetic carbonaceous adsorbents have been offered commercially. These are the products of the partial pyrolysis of nonionic polymeric adsorbents. They are still in the developmental stage (Slejko and Meigs, 1980).

STABILITY

The stability of the ion exchange resins and polymeric adsorbents is of major importance because their useful life affects the economic evaluation of processes involving their use. Their useful life may be limited by either physical or chemical degradation (Kunin, 1972).

PHYSICAL DEGRADATION

The adsorbents may degrade physically (attrition) into smaller particles either by abrasion or osmotic forces. Although the adsorptive properties of a resin are not affected by attrition (indeed, some of these properties may be improved), attrition is undesirable since it leads to losses of material, excessive pressure drops, and passage of finely divided adsorbent particles into the treated water. The design of the process and equipment are of paramount importance because they can affect the attrition of a resinous adsorbent (Kunin, 1972).

CHEMICAL DEGRADATION

An adsorbent resin can deteriorate chemically in several ways. First, the basic chemistry of the structure may be irreversibly altered due to oxidative reactions resulting from contact with oxygen, chlorine, peroxides, ozone, etc. (Kunin, 1976). Oxidation may destroy the activity of ion exchange resins and alter the nature of the active surfaces of adsorbents.

Second, adsorbent and ion exchange resins may be poisoned due to the irreversible adsorption of some organic and even some inorganic compounds. For example, some anion exchange resins, particularly the strongly basic resins with small pores, can be poisoned after exposure to high levels of humic materials (Abrams, 1975; Kunin, 1976). Apparently, the large molecules enter the pores of the anion exchange resin and are retained because they have a high affinity for the ion exchange sites and low rate of diffusion within the resin.

Third, pores of some adsorbents may become clogged by various colloids that are present in water supplies. These colloids may be siliceous or may contain highly dispersed particles of humic acids. Hydrous oxides of iron, aluminum, and manganese may be precipitated on the surface and in the pores of adsorbents because of only minor changes in pH and oxygen levels.

The effects of chemical deterioration of synthetic resins may be minimized by selection of proper adsorbent, removal of oxygen and chlorine from water to be treated by addition of sulfites, use of optimized or tailored regeneration conditions, use of restorative procedures such as treatment of the adsorbent with chemicals (salt, acid, alkali, etc.), and use of proper pretreatment of the influent. With proper care, the useful life of a resinous adsorbent may be prolonged.

Removal of Humic Substances by Ion Exchange Resins

For approximately 75 yr, ion exchange resins have been used extensively to treat water for a wide range of applications including water softening, water dealkalization, deionization, and removal of color (removal of humic substances), metals, nitrates, ammonia, and cyanides. The use of ion exchange resins for treating potable water has been limited primarily to the softening (removal of calcium and magnesium) of water with cation exchangers both on a municipal scale (Kunin, 1972) and in several million homes (Gulbrandson *et al.*, 1972). The cation exchanger does little to remove organic matter. The major disadvantage of the process involves the disposal of the waste salt regenerant. There is sufficient evidence indicating that the spent regenerant may be recycled a number of times without treatment and almost indefinitely by treating the waste brine with ozonization or hydrogen peroxide (Kunin, 1973). However, the reactions of these regenerants and their products have not been examined.

The use of ion exchange resins other than cation exchange resins for treating potable water has been quite limited. In some isolated cases, deionization or demineralization systems (combinations of cation and anion exchange resins) have been used to prepare potable water from brackish water (Clifford and Weber, 1978; Kunin, 1972; Kunin and Downing, 1971). Although the major objective has been the removal of salinity, some TOC was also removed.

There are data on the use of anion exchange resins for the removal of humic matter from water supplies. These data concern long-term studies using systems as large as 1–5 million gallons per day (MGD). Throughout the world, the technique has been used widely in various power utilities (Kunin 1973, 1976). In general, ion exchangers can remove from 50% to 95% of the humic matter. Some communities have used this technique to remove excess quantities of nitrates contaminating well water supplies (Clifford and Weber, 1978).

In view of the success that has been achieved with ion exchange resins to remove humic substances from water for various industrial purposes (Davis, 1977; Hinrichs and Snoeyink, 1976), it is logical that the technology be given consideration for the processing of drinking water prior to the chlorination process. This step could materially reduce the haloform concentrations in finished water. In essence, the water would be processed by deep beds of strongly basic anion exchange resins that would be regenerated with brine in a manner similar to the way municipal waters are softened with cation exchange resins.

TABLE IV-7   Adsorption of Humic Acids by Anion
Exchange Resins

Resin	Humic Acid Removed, %	
	pH 2.2	pH 7
IRA-410[a]	97	70
IRA-910[a]	92	52
A-57[b]	79	22
A-30B[b]	71	44
ES-340[b]	82	59

[a] Produced by Rohm and Haas Co.
[b] Produced by Diamond Shamrock Co.

ADSORPTION ISOTHERMS AND COLUMN STUDIES

Davis (1977) studied the adsorption of commercially available humic
acids at pH 2.2 and pH 7 by a series of anion exchange resins in batch
equilibrium studies. Results are summarized in Table IV-7. Strong base
anion exchange resins IRA-410 and IRA-910 removed more than
intermediate strength base anion exchange resins A-57, A-30B, and ES-
340 and weak anion exchange resins Statabed 93 (Rohm and Haas Co.).
Cation exchange resins had little or no affinity for humics.

In column tests, IRA-68 (intermediate anion exchange resin) removed
36%–46% of one fraction of the humic acids in a column study at pH 2.2
(Davis, 1977). Only 30% of the exchange capacity could be regenerated
with sodium hydroxide. Utilizing a second fraction of the humics,
complete removal was accomplished but only 64% was recovered by
sodium hydroxide. These data confirm earlier work of Bonsack (1962).

Boening et al. (1980) compared the adsorption of commerical humic
substances on Diamond Shamrock A-7 and ES-561 weak base anion
exchangers with that on Rohm and Haas IR-904 and IR-458 strong base
anion exchange resins. They also compared XAD-2, XAD-8, XE-340,
and five brands of GAC with the ion exchangers by isotherm and small
column studies. The anion exchange resins A-7, IR-904, and IR-458
adsorbed the humic substance better than GAC, whereas the weak base
resin ES-561 was comparable to GAC. Column tests on soil fulvic acids
and leaf fulvic acids confirmed these data. The investigators observed
that the adsorption capacity was a function of the source of organics.

The XAD-2, XAD-8, and XE-340 resins adsorbed only small amounts of humic material. Adsorption on ES-561 was best at pH 8.3 as compared to pH 7.0 and pH 9.5. Clearly, IR-904 was superior to the other resins at all pH's and maintained its capacity between 5.5 and 9.5. Whether the resins can be regenerated with an acceptable loss of capacity remains to be determined. The authors expressed concern about the fouling of strong base resins. Although weak base exchangers have a lower capacity, their use should not be ruled out, since they may regenerate more easily and regeneration is critical for the use of anion exchangers.

PILOT PLANT STUDIES

Kolle (1976) described how the strong base anion exchanger Lewatit, MP-500 A (Bayer, Leverkusen) removed natural color from groundwater at a water treatment plant in Fuhrberg, Federal Republic of Germany. The groundwater contained iron, manganese, sulfate, and humic substances. Traditional water treatment with aeration and permanganate oxidation reduced the dissolved organic carbon from 9 to 6 ppm while removing the metals. During pilot column tests at Fuhrberg, high bacterial growth during lime treatment was an added problem. New or regenerated anion exchange filters removed 58% of the 6-9 ppm dissolved organic carbon that was present initially. This was reduced to 40% after 5,000 bed volumes at an EBDT of 1.1 min. When the organic carbon was lowered, the bacterial growth decreased. Full-scale testing to develop additional data was recommended to confirm these findings.

Gauntlett (1975) tested MP 500 A resin on treated water from the Thames River in England. His results showed that the resin had a much lower capacity for organic carbon than did a GAC tested in parallel. He also observed that fresh GAC was better than regenerated base anion exchange resins for the removal of total organics as well as dodecyl benzene sulfonate, 2,4-dichlorophenol, and γBHC (benzene hexachloride) from coagulated and filtered water from the Th. mes. Lewatit MP 500 A, Amberlite XE-258, Permutit TR strong base anion exchange resins, and MP 62 weak anion exchange resins, were used at a quarter of the EBDT of 6.25 min for GAC. The strong base resins were better than the weak base resins, confirming the laboratory data presented above.

Jayes and Abrams (1968) applied a weak base anion exchange resin, Durolite A-7 (Diamond Shamrock Co.), for removal of natural color at Lawrence, Massachusetts. The resin was quite effective except when highly colored water was being treated. Under these conditions rapid breakthrough occurred. Regeneration was accomplished with 2% sodium hydroxide. These investigators estimated a resin life in excess of 200 cycles of adsorption–regeneration. Tilsworth (1974) compared strong base anion exchange resins Rohm and Haas IRA-400, Durolite S-37, Dowex SA 1273.1, and Dowex 11 with GAC for the removal of TOC, COD, and color from lake water and shallow pond water in Alaska. The flow rate through the 3-ft column was 1 gal/min/ft^3. Variability of the influent confused the evaluation of breakthrough data. In general, GAC was shown to be superior to the resins for removal of color, TOC, and COD.

Wood and DeMarco (1980) studied the removal on XE-340, GAC, and IRA-904 anion exchange resins of purgeable organics and THM precursors from raw groundwater, after lime-softening and in finished water. Since TOC analysis did not correlate consistently with THMFP, it was not a good basis for comparison.

The THMFP in the influent to the columns varied in raw water from 600 to 868 μg/liter, in lime-softened water from 394 to 580 μg/liter, and in finished water from 274 to 451 μg/liter. The lime-softening process removed an average of approximately 30% of the THM precursors. Subsequent chlorination and sand filtration removed approximately 24% more. However, this last 24% removal was probably due to conversion of THM precursors to THM's.

Table IV-8 summarizes the pilot plant data. With a 75-cm-deep bed of an adsorbent, IR-904 resin removes more THM precursors (50%) than GAC or XE-340 from raw and lime-softened water, but GAC removes slightly more from finished water. Lime-softening removes approximately as much of the THM precursors as 75 cm of GAC or XE-340 and 60% as much as IR-904 resin. An important fact to consider is that, during raw water application, a 150-cm-deep bed of IR-904 allows 100 μg/liter THM precursors to pass through at startup compared to only 12 μg/liter leakage for 75 cm of GAC. GAC was more effective than other adsorbents in removing precursors from finished water. Dechlorination did not occur on the IR-904 resin used as a postcontactor. The effluent from this process indicates an apparent catalytic effect between chlorine and organcs absorbed on the resin.

In this study IR-904 resin did not remove any of 22 purgeable chlorinated organic compounds (19 GC peaks) after lime-softening and chlorination. In fact, the level of halogenated organic compounds increased after finished drinking water entered the resin column. These compounds included chloroform (1.75 X); bromodichloromethane (1.13 X); trichloroethylene (10 X); 1,1,1-trichloroethane, 1,2-dichloroethane, and carbon tetrachloride (1.5 X); chlorobenzene (1.4 X); and o- and p-dichlorobenzene (2.7 X). The GAC and XE-340 removed volatile organics while removing the THM precursors. GAC is the most

TABLE IV-8   Removal of THM Precursors by Pilot Columns of XE-340, IR-904, and GAC after Different Stages of Water Treatment at Hialeah, Florida[a,b]

Pilot Columns	Average THMFP Removal			
	Total THMFP Entering Column, g	Percent at End of Run	Vol. Basis, g/column at 49 days	Weight Basis, g/100 g at 49 days
Raw water				
GAC	7.1	29(119)[c]	0.99	0.56
XE-340	7.1	24(119)	0.71	0.33
IR-904	2.6	46(49)	1.21	0.44
IR-904[d]	2.6	55(49)	1.43	0.26
Lime-softened water				
XE-340	5.0	4(119)	0.09	0.04
IR-904	1.7	32(49)	0.55	0.21
Finished water				
XE-340	3.8	0(119)	0.00	0.00
IR-904	1.2	13(49)	0.19	0.07
GAC	1.2	18(49)	0.23	0.13

[a] Wood and DeMarco, 1980.

[b] Based on breakthrough data for a bed depth of 75 cm.

[c] Number of days in parentheses.

[d] Bed depth of 150 cm.

successful adsorbent that has been tested for removal of THM precursors from this water. Wood and DeMarco (1980) determined that it appears best to use GAC as an adsorber before final chlorination for combined removal of THM and THM precursors.

Regeneration of Anion Exchange Resins

Regeneration and disposal of spent regenerant solution are major concerns involving resin use. A strong brine and/or alkali regenerant is used for strong base anion exchange resins.

Kolle (1976) accomplished regeneration with two bed volumes of 20 g/liter sodium hydroxide and 100 g/liter sodium chloride. The solution was reused. For every 25,000 volumes of processed water, he estimated that one volume of spent regenerant would be produced. This is a very small volume.

Gauntlett (1975) found the weak base resins to be more readily regenerated, although ammonium hydroxide solution with recovery of ammonia for reuse was not as successful as regeneration with sodium hydroxide.

Kunin (1972) presented evidence indicating that spent regenerant can be recycled a number of times without treatment and almost indefinitely by treating the waste brine with ozone or hydrogen peroxide.

Growth of Microorganisms on Ion Exchange Resins

Daniels (1972) reviewed the adsorption of microorganism onto ion exchange surfaces. He described the attachment of microbes as an ion exchange process between the resin surface and the particular microbial species. The process is a function of the isolectric point of the bacteria, the pH of the media, and the form of the ion exchanger. The specific situation for drinking water application has yet to be studied.

Nitrosamines and Ion Exchange Resins

The following levels of nitrosamines have been found in deionized water: N-nitrosodimethylamine (NDMA): 0.03–0.34 μg/liter (Fiddler et al., 1977); $\leq$0.25 μg/liter (Cohen and Bachman, 1978); 0.01 μg/liter (Gough et al., 1977); N-nitrosodiethylamine, 0.33–0.88 μg/liter (Fiddler et al., 1977).

Gough et al. (1977) found 125 μg/kg NDMA in a prewashed batch of anion exchange resin after extraction with solvent. The authors suggested that the nitrosamine was present as a resin impurity. Angeles et al. (1978) detected NDMA in the effluent from a column containing mixed strong anion and cation resins (previously washed to neutrality with distilled water) after a 1-N sodium nitrite solution was passed through it. The cationic resin was in its H^+ form and the anionic resin was in its OH^- form. They postulated that NDMA was formed by cation-acid-catalyzed nitrosation of the amine/ammonium functional group on the strong anion resin during the deionization process. Fiddler and Kimoto (1979) studied the source of nitrosamines and ruled out the acid-catalyzed nitrosation mechanism previously suggested by Angeles et al. (1978) since the presence of NDMA occurred only when anion resins were used. They also observed that anion and cation resins did not accumulate NDMA. In addition, trace levels of metal ions did not significantly enhance the formation of NDMA.

Fiddler and Kimoto (1979) concluded that the source of nitrosamine in municipal drinking water that had been exposed to deionizing resins appeared to be associated with low levels of nitrate and an unknown soluble substance(s) that promoted nitrosamine formation during the deionization process. The unknown substance(s) could be removed by degassing techniques or by activated carbon treatment. The formation of nitrosamines on activated carbon may also be possible, but this area has not yet been investigated. Nitrosamines can accumulate on GAC by treatment of water containing nitrosamines (Borneff, 1980).

Adsorption Efficiency of Polymeric Adsorbents

Adsorption isotherm data, percent removal data, kinetic data, and small column data are determined to evaluate the adsorbent characteristics. This section reviews available polymeric resin data for low-molecular-weight organic compounds of potential concern to health (Table IV-2).

PERCENT REMOVAL DATA

Chriswell et al. (1977) compared the ability of XAD-2 resin and a GAC (Filtrasorb 300) to adsorb 100 representative compounds from water at 100 μg/liter concentrations. They passed 1 liter of the spiked tap water through small-scale columns at a flow rate of 10 ml/min. Their general conclusion was that, under these conditions and under the criterion of percent removal, the XAD-2 was superior for analytical purposes. Only C_{14} to C_{20} hydrocarbons and C_5 and C_7 fatty acids, as well as benzenesulfonic acid, were poorly adsorbed to the extent of showing less than a 50% removal. Also, the resin more readily released its adsorbed organics into an organic solvent so that they could be analyzed.

Van Rossum and Webb (1978) compared the ability of XAD resins 2,4,7,8 and mixtures of two and three resins to adsorb microgram amounts of 13 nonpolar trace organics from distilled and tap water at a flow rate of 1.2 liter/hr. Recovery ranged from 65% to 76%. A mixture of XAD-4/XAD-8 was the most effective. In a second study of five polar organics (acids, phthlates, alcohols, and phenols), the effectiveness of the adsorption was XAD-4 > XAD-2 > XAD-7 > XAD-8. Percent breakthrough studies of 50 μg/liter of 24 organics (spiked into tap water) on XAD-2 and XAD-4/8 shows phthlates, bis(2-chloroethyl)ether and n-hexadecane breakthrough in both columns. XAD-4/8 was, on the average, 5% better than XAD-2.

TABLE IV-9 Available Data on Adsorption of Selected Organic Compounds on Resin Adsorbents

Organic Compounds	Molecular Weight	Number of Data Points	Resin Type	Adsorption Test Method	Equilibrium Concentration Range, mg/liter	Maximum Surface Concentration, mg/g	Comments	Reference
Chloroform	119.4	—	XE-340	Isotherm	<1-3	75	No data points	Neely, in press
Choloform	119.4	—	XAD-4	Isotherm	<1-23	27	No data points	Neely, in press
Bromodichloro-methane	147.8	—	XE-340	Isotherm	<1-5	95	No data points	Rohm and Haas Co., 1977
Dieldrin	381	—	XE-340	Isotherm	≈0.6-19	≈20	No data points	Rohm and Haas Co., 1977
Dieldrin	381	—	XAD-4	Isotherm	≈1.2-10	≈8	No data points	Rohm and Haas Co., 1977
2-Chloroethyl ether	143	1	XE-349	% reduction	5	33.3	Reported as volumetric capacity	Rohm and Haas Co., 1977
2-Chloroethyl ether	143	1	XE-347	% reduction	5	14.3	Reported as volumetric capacity	Rohm and Haas Co., 1977
2-Chloroethyl ether	143	1	XE-348	% reduction	5	26.7	Reported as volumetric capacity	Rohm and Haas Co., 1977
Chloroform	119.4	9	XE-340	Isotherm	4-200	≈6	Unchanged by 10 mg/liter of humic substances	Chudyk et al., in press

ADSORPTION ISOTHERMS

Isotherm data on XAD-1 and XAD-2 has been published by Gustafson and Lirio (1968) for many compounds of environmental concern, but are not included on the list of compounds of potential health concern in Table IV-2. The compounds studied included fatty acids, amino acids, sulfonates, tannic acid, and phenols.

Table IV-9 contains the available adsorption isotherm data for a number of organic compounds. It provides specific information on the ability of a compound to be adsorbed by resins. Chudyk et al. (1979) tested a neutral styrene–divinylbenzene (SDVB) resin, XAD-4, and the carbonaceous resin XE-340 against several different GAC materials for the adsorption of 2-methylisoborneol (MIB) from water. In terms of adsorption isotherms, the capacity of both resins for MIB was found to be less than that of the carbon with the lowest activity, but the presence of 10 mg/liter of humic acid did not affect the resin capacity in the equilibrium concentration range of 0.1 to 10 μg/liter, whereas it did affect the GAC. They also determined that the isotherms of chloroform on the carbonaceous resin and the lowest capacity carbon were approximately the same and were unchanged by the presence of 10 mg/liter of a commercially available humic acid. On the basis of these isotherms, the authors also reported that they could predict the relative efficiency of removal of MIB by bench scale columns.

Neely (1980) describes a model for the removal of chloroform from water by XE-340 where the resin macropores allow low-molecular-weight organics to diffuse to the micropores, while large molecules or humic substances cannot enter the micropores. Neely presents evidence to suggest that the high adsorptive capacity of XE-340 for chloroform is due at least partially to *absorption*. This capacity is shown to be from 3 to 5 times greater than that shown by five activated carbons that were tested simultaneously. Using the general shape of the isotherms of chloroform on XE-340 and XAD-4 and one or two measurements of capacity, he interpolated the capacity of a series of adsorbents at 2 ppm equilibrium concentration. The chloroform capacities for the polymeric resins followed the trend XAD-1 > XE-225A = XAD-4 > XAD-2 and XE-340 > XE-348 > XE-347 for carbonaceous resins.

COLUMN STUDIES—SMALL SCALE

Gustafson and Lirio (1968) studied the breakthrough of phenol and alkyl benzene sulfonate (ABS) in small columns. Phenol breakthrough followed the order XAD-1 < XAD-2 < GAC at a flow rate of 2 gal/ft^3/min; ABS followed the order XAD-4 $\approx$ GAC $<$ XAD-2. Isotherms showed ABS adsorption was less on XAD-1 $<$ XAD-2 $<$ GAC. This indicates a size effect expressed as column kinetics.

Thurman *et al.* (1978a) determined the chromatographic capacity factor (solute adsorbed/solute void volume) of over 20 compounds of different functionality for analytical method development at a flow rate of 0.12 liter/hr until saturation. XAD-8 favors aromatic over aliphatic compounds and CH$_3$ $>$ COOH $>$ CHO $>$ OH $\geq$ NH$_2$. The log of the capacity factors was inversely correlated with the log of the solubilities in water. Thurman *et al.* (1978b) reported capacities of 55 μmol/g XAD-2 and 80 μmol/g for XAD-8 when soil fulvic acid was adsorbed. Capacities of XAD-2 $>$ XAD-8 for acids, but phenols showed XAD-8 with the highest capacity. The fulvics and phenol were eluted with 0 1 N sodium hydroxide.

In a series of small column breakthrough studies at pH 8 and empty bed detention time (EBDT) of 2.1 min, McGuire (1977) compared the capacity of XE-340, XAD-2, and XAD-7 resins to that of Filtrasorb-400 for the constituents of a four-mixture solution: nitromethane, *n*-butanol, methyl ethyl ketone (MEK), and 1,4-dioxane. Extremely small adsorptive capacities were exhibited by the noncarbonaceous resins XAD-2 and XAD-7 in comparison with GAC and XE-340. This is in agreement with results from pilot plant studies (Suffet *et al.*, 1978a,b). While the adsorption capacities were similar, distinct differences were observed in adsorption kinetics in column studies. Breakthrough of each of the four components in the mixture began simultaneously in the XE-340 resin column. The breakthrough curves were also similar in shape. These results are in sharp contrast to those observed in the GAC column. There was evidence of displacement of dioxane by the other compounds, i.e., breakthrough of all components did not occur simultaneously, nor were the shapes of the breakthrough curves similar. The difference in breakthrough behavior between XE-340 and GAC suggests that adsorption on XE-340 may not involve competition to the same extent as on GAC.

Neely (1980) used a 10.2-cm-long, 15-ml bed volume of XE-340 and XAD-4 in columns to follow the breakthrough of 1 ppm of chloroform in drinking water with 2 ppm TOC. The flow rate was 4 gpm/ft^3. On the XAD-4 column, 10% breakthrough was observed at 12 hr, whereas on the XE-340 column, 10% breakthrough did not occur until 180 hr.

To summarize, few studies applying resin for treatment of water supplies have been completed. Present data for chloroform adsorption indicate relative adsorption capacity on XE-340 versus GAC of 3:1 to 5:1 at high chloroform concentrations (Neely, 1980) and approximately

1:1 at low chloroform concentrations (Chudyk *et al.*, 1979). Data on other low-molecular-weight organics are not available. The degree of competition between organic compounds with potential health effects on polymeric adsorbants has not been studied.

COLUMN STUDIES—PILOT SCALE

Studies on a pilot scale column have been performed to determine the efficiency of carbonaceous and neutral SDVB resins to remove the chemical species found in municipal water supplies. Suffet *et al.* (1978a,b) studied Filtrasorb-400, XAD-2, and XE-340 in pilot columns as a posttreatment of chlorinated Philadelphia drinking water from the Delaware River. They used computer-reconstructed gas-chromatographic weekly profiles of 1- and 3-day composite samples and GC/MS to assess 27 identified compounds (BP 60°C to 280°C). In one study, XAD-2 was found to have a much lower capacity than Filtrasorb-400 for the removal of the species that were present. They observed very early breakthrough for most compounds on XAD-2. A further series of tests involving XE-340 showed that XE-340 possessed adsorptive capacities that were generally much like those of Filtrasorb-400 for nonpolar low-molecular-weight organic compounds.

Suffet *et al.* (1978a,b) also observed that GAC removed both high- and low-molecular-weight organics, whereas XE-340 removed the lower-molecular-weight organics. They cautioned that the data are largely qualitative and that interpretation of results are complicated by the highly variable nature of the organic content of the influent to the adsorption column.

Wood and DeMarco (1980) compared the ability of XE-340, IRA-904, an anion exchanger, and Filtrasorb-400 GAC to remove purgeable organics, as defined by the technique of Bellar *et al.* (1974), and THMFP as defined by Stevens *et al.* (1976). Determinations were made on raw groundwater, lime-softened water, and finished water from Hialeah, Florida. Breakpoint chlorination was practiced to produce a 3-ppm free chlorine residual. They determined that GAC offered the best promise for the removal of TOC, THMFP, and purgeable halogenated organic compounds in the finished water. The XE-340 did not remove any THMFP whereas GAC removed 20% from finished water.

Table IV-10 shows that XE-340 always has a greater adsorption capacity than GAC for individual volatile halogenated organics in raw and finished water in 6.4-cm deep beds with 6.2 min EBDT. A value for XE-340 3 times greater than for GAC was generally observed despite a reduction of 30% TOC in finished water. These results were also

TABLE IV-10   Comparative Removal of Volatile Chlorinated Organic Compounds by XE-340 and GAC in Pilot Columns After Different Stages of Water Treatment at Hialeah, Florida[a]

Compound	Stage of Treatment	Average Concentration, μg/liter	Ratio of average capacity of XE-340 to GAC	
			By Volume	By Weight
Chloroform	Finished	67.3 (Range 45-90)[b]	4.9	4
cis-1,2-Dichloro-ethane	Raw	21-29 ($\geq$85% of Vol. TOX)[c]	3.6	3
	Lime-softened	20-25	3.1	2.5
	Finished	11-19 (10% of Vol. TOX)[c]		
Bromodi-chloro-methane	Finished	37-47	3.4	2.8
Dibromo-chloro-methane	Finished	12-34	3	2.5

[a] Wood and DeMarco, 1980.
[b] High points of 110 and 130 μg/liter at day 14 and 112, respectively, are the only points outside the range shown.
[c] Vol. TOX = Volatile total organic halogens.

observed for other purgeable halogenated organics and agree with isotherm data.

A review of specialized studies of the use of XAD resins has been completed by Kennedy (1973). He reported that the XAD-4 resin was particularly advantageous for the removal of chlorinated pesticides and phenols from industrial wastewater. He determined that the XAD-8 resin was the best for removal of color from Kraft mill wastes.

Symons (1980) evaluated the efficiency of XE-340 in removing THM's. With an empty bed contact time of 10 min, the column removed all THM compounds for 10 weeks from an influent that had a THM concentration of approximately 125 μg/liter. The effluent concentration rose to 25 μg/liter in the next 20 weeks as the influent concentration dropped steadily to 50 μg/liter.

Humic material did not interfere with adsorption of chloroform on XE-340 during isotherm studies (Chudyk *et al.*, 1979). This was confirmed in part in pilot plant studies for adsorption on XE-340. Wood and DeMarco (1980) did not observe the removal of THMFP from finished water. However, XE-340 did remove 24% of the THMFP from raw water. Competition between organics with potential health effects is not known at present.

Regeneration of Polymeric Adsorbents

The removal of adsorbed species from polymeric resins may be accomplished by various means. Kennedy (1973) found that XAD-4, when loaded with chlorinated pesticides, was readily regenerated by either acetone or isopropyl alcohol and that the regenerant could be readily reclaimed for further use. Kennedy also reported that XAD-8, when loaded with Kraft mill color bodies, could be regenerated with a weak base. Crook *et al.* (1975) regenerated XAD-4 with 4% sodium hydroxide when loaded with phenolic wastes.

Gustafson and Lirio (1968) regenerated XAD-1 and XAD-2 with 1% sodium hydroxide when columns were saturated with phenol. Ninety-nine percent of the phenol was eluted at a flow rate of 1 gal/ft³/min. Regeneration of XAD-1 and XAD-2 by low-polarity solvents or solutions of acid or base for the opposite material was also suggested. They recommended a dilute base for regeneration of organic color bodies in industrial wastes.

Slejko and Meigs (1980) stated that XE-340 may be regenerated efficiently by steam. XE-340 may be used for shorter periods between regenerations than GAC materials and that after 3 to 4 days in an adsorption mode an *in-situ* regeneration using 37 lb of 110°C steam per cubic foot of resin is adequate to clean the bed of all steam–purgeable species. Over an extended period of operation, possible buildup of organics that are not steam-purgeable caused the investigators to suggest a periodic washing with ethyl alcohol.

The Rohm and Haas Co. (1977) reported that carbonaceous resins (XE-340, 347, 348) may be regenerated by water-miscible solvents, such as acetone or methanol, or by water-immiscible solvents, such as toluene and xylene, both followed by a flow of steam to clear the bed of regenerant. For compounds with low boiling points that are not accompanied by heavier adsorbates, or for those compounds that form low-boiling azeotropes with water, steam is an effective primary regenerant. The investigators also suggested that acid or base regenerants should be effective for the removal of certain ionic organics, but presented no data to support this.

Chudyk *et al.* (1979) investigated the regeneration of an SDVB resin and a XE-340 resin, which had been loaded with MIB or chloroform. Atmospheric steam and/or ethyl alcohol were used as the regenerants. Slejko and Meigs (1980) described how this carbonaceous resin could be purged of chloroform with steam. Steam removed only 5% of the adsorbed MIB while ethanol removed only 20%. However, there were no successive saturation regenerations to determine if MIB applied in subsequent cycles could be recovered.

The SDVB resin proved to be easier to regenerate by these means. The MIB recovery with steam was 23%. This was followed by a further 53% recovery by ethyl alcohol, yielding a total of 76%. A replicate determination yielded recoveries of 34% by steam and a further 34% for the alcohol, for a total of 68%.

Summary, Conclusions, and Recommendations

ANION EXCHANGE RESINS

Much of the limited experience with the use of anion exchange resins to remove humic material has been gained from processing water for electronics and power utilities. In these cases, the anion exchange resins have effectively removed humic material. Resins have been preferred over GAC or PAC by these industries (Kunin 1972, 1976). Laboratory and pilot plant studies have shown that strong base anion exchange resins can remove humic materials as well as or better than GAC. The adsorption capacity is a function of the composition of the aqueous solution.

Present studies indicate that nitrosamines may be generated by passage of water over a strongly basic resin. The exact mechanism has yet to be demonstrated. Since the resins concentrate the potential reactants for forming nitrosamines and also accumulate potential catalysts (iron and copper), the published data on the formation of nitrosamines on anion exchange resins suggest that the use of such resins for potable water should be reconsidered. It may be possible to use anion exchange resins in conjunction with GAC. The resin would remove the bulk of the humic material and the GAC would remove the remainder of the humic material as well as any nitrosamines that had been generated, if any. However, there are no data for such possible systems.

The data on the use of anion exchange resins have been based primarily upon resins that either have been regenerated only a few times or have been in their virgin states. Such data are highly unrealistic for the water treatment industry. For example, the question of acceptable loss of capacity upon regeneration can be addressed only after regenerations are completed. Since regeneration is completed with either brine or caustic, the disposal of waste regenerant can also present serious environmental problems.

POLYMERIC ADSORBENTS

Experience with synthetic resins and polymeric adsorbents to remove organic compounds from drinking water is limited in comparison with the use of GAC or PAC. Laboratory studies and the few recent pilot plant studies indicate that the synthetic carbonaceous adsorbents of the XE-340 type do not have the broad-spectrum adsorption properties of GAC and that they selectively adsorb lower-molecular-weight organics but apparently do not readily adsorb humic material. However, the data indicate some promise for special situations such as the removal of toxic organics from sources contaminated with low-molecular-weight organics (Wood and DeMarco, 1980). The synthetic carbonaceous adsorbents are still in their experimental and developmental stages. Some published data show their greater efficiency with chloroform and related low-molecular-weight organics.

There is a lack of information on the effect of chlorine disinfectant before the use of resins under conditions at water treatment plants. Combined chlorine residuals were observed in the effluent during pilot column studies with XE-340 (Suffet et al., 1978b). Since attrition of the resin by chlorine is possible (Kunin, 1976), subsequent studies should consider dechlorination before the adsorption step. Under these conditions, microbial growth should also be monitored.

There is a lack of regeneration information for XE-340. Questions remain concerning the effectiveness of steam for regeneration, the use of solvents for regeneration and their potential health effects, and the number of times resins must be recycled in order to compete economically. These adsorbents may have excellent possibilities for small plants or well waters that are plagued only with haloforms or other low-molecular-weight compounds, but regeneration studies must be completed to evaluate their utility. The subcommittee recommends that:

1. A survey of several plants using anion exchange resins should be conducted to determine their performance for removal of humic

material. Most of these plants are industrial plants operating in the United States, Great Britain, and the Federal Republic of Germany.

2. The possible formation of nitrosamines on anion exchange resins must be studied.

3. Studies should be made on synthetic carbonaceous adsorbents for systems that use them in conjunction with anion exchange resins or following GAC. Dechlorination before the resin bed treatment should be considered.

4. Studies on the use of the synthetic carbonaceous resins for treating contaminated well waters should be expanded to include regeneration systems. The effect of chlorine on the adsorption process and resin attrition should also be studied.

5. Pilot column tests on different waters along with appropriate laboratory studies are needed to answer the following crucial questions concerning the regeneration of all resins. What is the rate of loss of capacity due to fouling? What type of regenerant will work best? How will the disposal of regenerant be handled?

ANALYTICAL METHODS TO MONITOR ADSORBENT UNIT PROCESSES IN WATER TREATMENT

This chapter has focused on individual compounds of potential harm to health. Thus, the primary purpose of this section is to evaluate the availability of analytical methods to monitor the operation of adsorbent processes for these compounds at a water treatment plant. The following questions are addressed:

1. Can the monitoring for individual compounds of potential harm to health be completed in other than a research laboratory?

2. Can nonspecific parameters be substituted for monitoring of individual compounds?

The chemical compounds entering an adsorption treatment process are both high- and low-molecular-weight organic compounds with a wide range in polarity. The Committee on Safe Drinking Water (National Academy of Sciences, 1977) estimated that 90% by weight of the total organic matter in drinking water is composed of high-molecular-weight organics. This would correspond to natural organic compounds of little-known toxicological importance (Class V; U.S. Environmental Protection Agency, 1978c), but these compounds may affect the process by competitive adsorption or support of microbial growth. A fraction of these high-molecular-weight organic compounds are precursors that react with disinfectants to produce "disinfectant by-products" (Class III; U.S. Environmental Protection Agency, 1978c). The remaining 10% of the total organic matter includes, but is not limited to, volatile synthetic organic chemicals that are present in source water and organic chemicals that are disinfection by-products (Classes II and IV; U.S. Environmental Protection Agency, 1978c). A subgroup of the chemicals in the last group are the potentially harmful chemicals (Interagency Regulatory Liaison Group, 1978; National Academy of Sciences, 1977; National Cancer Institute, 1978).

The primary goal of influent analysis is to monitor specific potentially harmful chemicals so that removal efficiencies can be established. The optimum monitoring method is to measure quantitatively the compounds of concern over the entire period of operation. Because concentrations in the influent may vary greatly over time (see section on competition), infrequent grab sampling might not be sufficient for an adequate evaluation of material entering the column. Since minute-to-minute sampling is presently impractical, the variability of these organics in the influent can best be followed by on-line composite sample collection. The variability of the load of humic substances, which include the precursors to compounds that might affect human health, should also be measured. Also, the general load of total organic matter as DOC can be used to follow mass loading of the carbon filter.

Chemical compounds in the effluent may be the same as those that entered the carbon bed, or they may have been changed by chemical or microbial action within the bed. The variability of species type and concentration in the column influent are also reflected in variable effluent concentrations. Competitive effects occur when a strongly adsorbed compound enters the bed and displaces a more weakly adsorbed compound. In this case, the concentration of the displaced compound may be higher in the effluent than in the influent until a new equilibrium is reached. A reequilibration effect is observed when the concentration of a compound in the influent decreases. This compound then desorbs from the carbon. Again, the concentration in the effluent could be higher than in the influent until a new equilibrium is established. This discussion indicates that effluent concentrations are dependent on influent concentrations, in addition to the adsorption dynamics on the column, and would therefore tend to vary.

In addition to monitoring influent and effluent, it may be desirable to monitor the contents of the GAC bed itself to determine when breakthrough will occur. By determining the location in the bed of the different compounds with potential health effects, one can evaluate column performance as well as the remaining capacity of the column. Indications of pending breakthrough may be easier to evaluate by determining the location of the specific organics.

Monitoring Specific Pollutants of Potential Harm to Health

Since 1975, a massive effort to identify organic compounds in drinking water by gas chromatography/mass spectrometry (GC/MS) has resulted in an inventory of volatile, relatively nonpolar, soluble organics that are isolated from water by volatilization, solvent extraction, or solid phase adsorption (Keith, 1976). More than 700 compounds have been isolated by these methods and by methods utilizing reverse osmosis as the concentration and isolation tool (U.S. Environmental Protection Agency, 1978b). In the United States, the concentration and frequency of occurrence of THM's are the highest of the volatile organics in drinking water due to the use of chlorination for disinfection (Symons *et al.*, 1975).

Two different analytical approaches can be used to determine specific organic compounds of potential harm to health. In one approach individual compounds that have been selected because of health implications are analyzed. In the second, a general "screening" procedure for the isolation of organic compounds is used and the compounds of interest are selectively determined from the same sample matrix.

ANALYSES OF INDIVIDUAL COMPOUNDS WITH A POTENTIAL TO AFFECT HEALTH

Table IV-2 lists specific pollutants of potential harm to health that should be monitored. Specific analytical methods for each of these or groups of these are being developed (Keith and Telliard, 1979). The analysis of THM's is reviewed below to point out general principles of analysis for specific pollutants.

THM's consist of chloroform, dichlorobromomethane, dibromochloromethane, and bromoform. The existing techniques for THM analysis have been reviewed (National Academy of Sciences, 1978). Routine monitoring methods are batch analyses, the purge and trap procedure (Bellar *et al.*, 1974), and liquid–liquid extraction (Henderson *et al.*, 1976; Mieure, 1977; Richard and Junk, 1977). Some investigators used other methods such as headspace analysis (Kaiser and Oliver, 1976) and direct water injection (Nicholson *et al.*, 1977). The limitations of direct water injection have been documented by Pfaender *et al.* (1978).

THM's are now routinely measured in many laboratories, primarily by the purge and trap method (Bellar *et al.*, 1974). Keith (1978) reported ± 20% of the true value for 90% of the individual THM's (≥ 10 ppb) by this method. He judged that the lowest concentration at which an accurate analysis can be obtained during routine monitoring was no less than 1.5 μg/liter, and he reported background levels of 0.5 μg/liter. Dressman *et al.* (1979) and Reding *et al.* (in press) obtained comparable results regarding the overall precision of the purge and trap analysis and the three liquid–liquid extraction methods for routine monitoring of drinking water.

THM monitoring as well as THMFP data for evaluation of GAC columns has been based upon a 15-min daily composite (U.S. Environmental Protection Agency, 1978b), but it is not known if this composite accurately represents the load on an adsorbent. Studies are needed to determine if a 15-min composite is justified. Recently, Westrick and Cummins (1978) have developed THM data for sewage treatment using an outline composite sampler that can collect a sample without headspace. Composite sample collection for evaluation of the control of THM's may give a more representative picture of the THM load on a column.

Appropriate blanks and quality control check samples must be completed to ensure accuracy and reproducibility. Sample transport, pretreatments (e.g., addition of a dechlorination agent), and storage are of concern because of THM volatility and precursor reactivity (Brass *et al.*, 1977). Primary calibration standards are needed, as are control samples. Interlaboratory studies to determine the accuracy of analysis are useful as part of the overall quality control program. Thus, quality assurance programs should be instituted to maintain the reliability of monitoring data. Quality assurance, as described by Miller (1979), minimizes errors resulting from sample site selection, sampling frequency, reference materials, and data acquisition systems, as well as from the analytical method itself.

SCREENING PROCEDURES

The screening procedure consists of a qualitative identification of individual compounds and their subsequent quantitative analysis. A general sequence followed for screening of trace organics is: Sample → Isolation Method → Concentration → Chromatographic Separation → Qualitative Identification → Quantification.

One key to the screening procedure is the isolation method that defines the type of compound to be studied and can simultaneously analyze for compounds that are potentially harmful to health. Each method will

TABLE IV-11   Methods of Isolation of Organic Chemicals from Aqueous Samples for General Screening Procedures and Specific Analysis[a]

Sample State	Isolation Techniques	Collection Phase
Vapor		
	Headspace analysis	Gas
	Purge and trap	Solid
Solution		
	Liquid-liquid extraction (LLE)	Liquid
	Adsorption by solids	Solid
	Carbon adsorption method (CAM)	
	Macroreticular resins (MRR)	
	Chromatographic liquid phases	
	Porous polyurethane foam	
	Freeze concentration	Solid
	Reverse osmosis	Aqueous-Concentrate

[a] Update of Suffet and Radzuil, 1976

isolate material selectively. Suffet and Radziul (1976) have described the methods that can isolate chemicals with health implications (see Table IV-11). For example, the less-polar-volatile organics of potential harm to health are isolated by methods such as the purge and trap volatile organic analysis (b.p. $\leq 150°C$) (Grob and Zurcher, 1976), liquid–liquid extraction (Yohe *et al.*, in press), and macroreticular resin accumulators (Chriswell *et al.*, 1977). These methods must be supplemented by specific analyses for compounds that are not isolated by the specific extraction method.

The complex group of trace organics in the extracted sample is chromatographed, and a sample profile or fingerprint is obtained. This constitutes an information pattern in each chromatographic analysis. When the profile is compared to a profile of a set of standards of the known compounds, a tentative identification of the sample components can be made. If standard curves are made for each of the components, an estimate of the amount of the tentatively identified compound can be made. When many profiles of influents and effluents are plotted in the same manner, chromatographic profiles can be compared and differences noted. GC/MS analyses must be used to confirm the identification of the compounds tentatively identified by the isolation method. Examples of the screening of the organic compounds in the influent and effluent of adsorption processes have been reported for purge and trap analyses (Steiglitz *et al.*, 1976; Wood and DeMarco,

1980), resin accumulators (Suffet *et al.*, 1978), and liquid–liquid extraction (Yohe *et al.*, in press). To monitor an adsorption process for pollutants of potential harm to health concern that are volatile or can be detected by GC techniques, only selected GC/MS analyses may be necessary. GC analysis can be used for monitoring purposes if concentration limits for pollutants are defined.

Nonspecific Organic Analysis

Nonspecific organic analyses lumps together a large number of organic compounds under one collective measurement umbrella. All of the nonspecific analyses should be evaluated on the basis of specific organic compounds identified in Table IV-2.

General organic analyses have been tested extensively by several investigators in an attempt to replace or supplement the complex GC or GC/MS analysis in water treatment monitoring. Correlation among general organic analyses and organic compounds with possible health effects has been attempted in order to develop an economical and rapid monitor for the use of GAC processes.

Stevens and Symons (1973) concluded that no current tests completely measure the total concentration of organic compounds in water. The primary analyses that have been routinely substituted for measurement of the total concentration are elemental, e.g., TOC, DOC, purgeable organic carbon (POC), or nonvolatile TOC (NVTOC), and general organic analyses, e.g., COD and the carbon chloroform extracts (CCE). UV absorbance and fluorescence have also been used to follow the efficiency with which organics are removed by GAC. Organic carbon analyses and UV absorbance have been used for process control of GAC plants in the Federal Republic of Germany. The ratio of DOC to UV absorbance was found to change after different water treatment processes.

Symons *et al.* (1975) indicated that NVTOC is a dominant factor influencing the creation of THM's. These workers describe NVTOC as a "reasonable indicator" of THM precursors in drinking water in an 80-city survey. They reported that some correlation existed between NVTOC and CCE data but these data were rather scattered. For drinking water, the NVTOC method did not correlate well with the UV absorbance method of Dobbs *et al.* (1972), the fluorescence method of Sylvia (1973), or an emission fluorescence scanning (EMFS) method. The two fluorescence methods correlated well with each other.

Sylvia and Donlan (1980) demonstrated a correlation between TOC and fluorescence from numerous water sources. This is comparable with data of Snoeyink *et al.* (1977), who reported that fluorescence could be used to monitor adsorption of the lower-molecular-weight fraction of humic material. The EPA (U.S. Environmental Protection Agency, 1978c) has stated that TOC tends to give excessive weight to naturally occurring high-molecular-weight compounds, which are not believed to be hazardous, and that TOC is not a suitable criterion for the design of GAC systems.

Brodtmann *et al.* (1980) used TOC, UV absorbance, fluorescence, and EMFS during two full-scale water treatment studies with GAC adsorption at the Jefferson Parish Water Plant on the Mississippi River in Louisiana. Samples were collected three times a week from five plant locations during the study. Brodtmann *et al.* (1980) were unable to correlate any nonspecific organic analyses with each other or with organic compounds having health implications during this study. Wood and DeMarco (1980) and Cairo *et al.* (1980) also indicated that TOC and THMFP did not correlate well in pilot plant studies in Miami, Florida, and Philadelphia, Pennsylvania, respectively. There have been no successful correlations between breakthrough of specific organic compounds on a GAC column and the breakthrough of those components as measured by general organic parameters.

Table IV-2 shows that the halogenated organics as THM's and low-molecular-weight organics comprise many of the organics that are potentially harmful to health. Higher-molecular-weight organics containing halogens from partially chlorinated humic material are suspected of having implications for health (Sontheimer, 1974). The measurement of total organic halogen (TOX) by the pyrohydrolysis method has been developed in the Federal Republic of Germany by Kuhn and Sontheimer (1973a,b) and evaluated by Dressman *et al.* (1977). Other methods of TOX analysis exist, e.g., the use of UV oxidation after resin adsorption (Glaze *et al.*, 1977).

The objective of water treatment in the Federal Republic of Germany is to attain a finished water quality equal in all respects to that of high-quality groundwater (Kuhn *et al.*, 1978a,b). Since chlorinated organics are not naturally found in groundwater, they have been singled out for intensive study.

In the Federal Republic of Germany, TOX has been used to monitor breakthrough behavior of activated carbon filters and to determine the necessity of reactivation in drinking water treatment plants (Kuhn *et al.*, 1978a,b). Dissolved organic halogen (DOX) in water and the adsorbed organic chlorine on the GAC have also been studied in that country.

Steiglitz *et al.* (1977) reported that single substance analysis of Rhine River water by GC and GC/MS and elemental analysis by TOX indicates that only approximately 10% by weight of the DOX was identified by GC/MS analysis. There was no recognizable correlation between the concentration of DOX and the amounts of specific organics. Kuhn and Fuchs (1975), Sander et al. (1977), and Oliver (1978) showed that DOX increases after chlorination of natural water as do the THM's. The THM's do not account for all of the increase.

Dressman et al. (1977) modified the original pyrohydrolysis method (DOX and TOX) and defined it more properly as a semiquantitative measurement of carbon-absorbable organohalides (CAOX as Cl). They suggested that a reliable lower limit of sensitivity is no less than 10 μg/liter over background values of 10 μg/liter. These authors reported critical problems in accounting for the efficiency of the adsorption step on charcoal for all halogenated organic compounds and the contribution of other halides to the microcoulometric measurement of hydrochloric acid from the burning of charcoal in an oxygen steam environment at 1,000°C. An addition to the method to be used for disinfected waters individually analyzes the nonpurgeable CAOX as Cl and purgeable OX by the purge and trap method to determine the approximate CAOX as Cl. In drinking water the purgeable organic halogen can be 25% of the approximate CAOX as Cl organic halogen.

A differentiation should be made between the TOX measurement of raw water and finished drinking water after chlorination. For example, the raw water measurement may be composed predominantly of low-molecular-weight synthetic organic compounds from industrial origin. The finished water measurement would also include higher-molecular-weight organic compounds that were formed by chlorination during treatment as well as haloforms and possibly others.

The elemental analyses indicate changes of influent concentration, process trends, and general adsorption capabilities. The CAOX as Cl measurement could be a nonspecific analysis of choice, as many organics of potential harm to health are halogenated.

GAC Surface Phase Analysis

The primary purpose of monitoring the adsorbed material is to follow compounds as they move down through the column so that a warning can be provided when harmful compounds are about to break through. While the aqueous phase must be approached by composite sampling, the sampling of the GAC surface phase is somewhat simplified, since the adsorption mechanism stores a composite record on the surface of the absorbent.

Carbon samples can be obtained either by taking samples directly from the operational bed (Kuhn and Fuchs, 1976) or by sacrificing small columns that are run parallel to the main bed (Fuchs, 1974). If practical, sampling of the main bed is preferable, since it directly samples the process under investigation and avoids problems of scaling down large operations, especially for long composite times when biological growth can occur.

Kolle *et al.* (1975) reported a screening method that avoided the solvent desorption step by vacuum desorption of the volatile compounds from heated samples for analysis by GC and GC/MS. However, there are no experimental details concerning the compounds for which it is useful or its reliability.

Kolle *et al.* (1975) also determined several different profiles of the adsorption pattern for several different chlorinated compounds throughout the GAC bed. Kuhn and Fuchs (1976) have used TOX along the length of a GAC column to monitor breakthrough, but the technique needs further development so TOX can be correlated with specific compounds with health implications.

Summary, Conclusions, and Recommendations

The variability of the complement of organic compounds in the influent to the GAC column affects the efficiency of the adsorptive process for the compounds. On-line composite sampling augmented by grab sampling of the influent and effluent of the GAC column is necessary because of the variability produced by competitive adsorption, reequilibrium, and desorption.

The analysis of specific organic compounds of health concern on a regular basis will be time-consuming, expensive, and difficult at most water treatment plants. One approach that may be useful is a set of screening protocols, e.g., collection of headspace free samples for purge and trap and resin accumulators using on-line composite samplers. These samples would be be compared by chromatographic profiles augmented by GC/MS analyses. This approach would monitor specific organics with health implications at each water treatment plant.

Analytical techniques for monitoring the performance of adsorbent beds need further development. Correlations between nonspecific measurements and compounds of concern should be completed on a site-specific basis, since the specific organic compounds that must be controlled will probably vary among water supplies. The correlation of such measurements as UV absorbance, fluorescence, or analyses of organic carbon (e.g., TOC) with GAC breakthrough of specific organic compounds of concern has not been observed (Brodtmann *et al.*, 1980;

Symons *et al.*, 1975; Wood and Demarco, 1980). However, TOC remains an important measure of the mass loading of an adsorption column.

The correlation of TOX in the aqueous or absorbed phases with organic compounds of concern has not been sufficiently studied. TOX would indicate the mass loading for halogenated compounds and the total amount of chlorination products produced during a water treatment process. This should be developed for routine use, since many compounds with health implications are chlorinated.

THM precursors that participate in the haloform reaction have not been shown to correlate with nonspecific organic analysis. Although fluorescence has been used to monitor humic material (Snoeyink *et al.*, 1977; Sylvia and Donlon, 1980), it has not been shown to correlate with THMFP. TOC and THMFP did not correlate well in pilot column studies (Cairo *et al.*, 1980; Wood and Demarco, 1980). Organic carbon is a collective measure of all organic constitutents, only a few of which are haloform precursors.

On a weight basis, only approximately 10% of all the organic compounds in drinking water have been identified (National Academy of Sciences, 1977). The low-molecular-weight polar organics and the nonvolatile high-molecular-weight organics cannot be analyzed by the above-mentioned methods. The screening of these compounds is now becoming possible with the use of high-pressure liquid chromatography (HPLC) analysis. The coupling of HPLC and MS, which is under development, will further expand the analytical possibilities. Research on these techniques is needed to expand our understanding of the more polar organics in water supplies. There is only a minimum of knowledge concerning the health implications of these compounds.

The calibration standards for specific pollutant analysis and reference compounds for the comparison of analytical recovery between methods should be standardized to ensure that analytical methods are accurate and reproducible. Strict quality control and interlaboratory comparisons are integral parts of the validation program.

REFERENCES

Abrams, I.M. 1975. Macroporus condensate resins as adsorbants. Ind. Eng. Chem. Prod. Res. Dev. 12(2):108–112.

Alexander, M. 1973. Biotechnology report: nonbiodegradable and other recalcitrant molecules. Biotechnol. Bioeng. 15:611–647.

Alexander, M. 1974. Microbial formation of environmental pollutants. Adv. Appl. Microbiol. 18:1–73.

Aly, O.M., and S.D. Faust. 1965. Removal of 2,4-dichlorophenoxyacetic acid derivatives from natural waters. J. Am. Water Works Assoc. 57:221–230.

Andelman, J.B. 1973. World Health Organization, European standards for organic matter in drinking water. Pp. 55– 61 in V.L. Snoeyink, ed. Organic Matter in Water Supplies: Occurrence, Significance, and Control. Proceedings of the 15th Water Quality Conference, University of Illinois at Urbana-Champaign.

Andelman, J.B., and M.J. Suess. 1970. Polynuclear aromatic hydrocarbons in the water environment. Bull. WHO 43:479–508.

Anderson, R.B., and P.H. Emmett. 1947. Surface complexes on charcoal. Gas evolution as a function of vapor adsorption and of high-temperature evacuation. J. Phys. Colloid Chem. 51:1308–1329.

Andrews, G.F., and C. Tien. 1975. The interaction of bacterial growth, adsorption and filtration in carbon column treating liquid wastes. Am. Ind. Chem. Eng. Symp. Ser. 71(152):164–175.

Angeles, R.M., L.K. Keefer, P.P. Roller, and S.J. Uhm. 1978. Chemical models for possible nitrosamine artifact formation in environmental analysis. Pp. 109–115 in E.A. Walker, L. Griciute, M. Casteguaro, and R.E. Lyle, eds. Environmental Aspects of N-Nitroso Compounds. World Health Organization, International Agency for Research on Cancer, Lyon. IARC Scientific Publications No. 19.

Anonymous. 1977. Proceedings, Fifth United States/Japan Conference on Sewage Treatment Technology, Tokyo, Japan.

Applebaum, S.B. 1968. Demineralization by ion exchange in water treatment and chemical processing of other liquids. Pp. 7–22 in Chapter 2. Survey of the Impurities in Water, Their Harmful Effects in Industry, and Methods of Removing Them. Academic Press, New York.

Atkins, P.F., Jr., D.A. Scherger, R.A. Barnes, and F.L. Evans III. 1973. Ammonia removal by physical–chemical treatment. J. Water Pollut. Control Fed. 45:2372–2388.

AWWA Committee Report. 1977. Measurement and control of organic contaminants by utilities. J. Am. Water Works Assoc. 69:267–271.

Ayanaba, A., and M. Alexander. 1973. Microbial formation of nitrosamines *in vitro*. Appl. Microbiol. 25:862-868.

Ayanaba, A., and M. Alexander. 1974. Transformations of methylamines and formation of a hazardous product, dimethylnitrosamine, in samples of treated sewage and lake water. J. Environ. Qual. 3:83–89.

Babcock, D.B., and P.C. Singer. 1977. Chlorination and coagulation of humic and fulvic acids. Proceedings of the 97th Annual American Water Works Association Conference, Anaheim, Calif. Paper No. 16-6, 16 pp.

Baldauf, G. 1978. Untersuchungen ueber die konkurrierende Adsorption von zwei Stoffgemischen an Aktivkohle. Ph.D. dissertation. University of Karlsruhe, Department of Chemical Engineering, Federal Republic of Germany.

Balzli, M.W., A.I. Liapis, and D.W.T. Rippin. 1978. Applications of mathematical modelling to the simulation of multi-component adsorption in activated carbon columns. Trans. Inst. Chem. Eng. 56:145–156.

Bauer, R.C., and V.L. Snoeyink. 1973. Reactions of chloramines with active carbon. J. Water Pollut. Control Fed. 435:2290–2301.

Behrman, A.S., and H. Gustafson. 1935. Behavior of oxidizing agents with activated carbon. Ind. Eng. Chem. 27:426–429.

Bellar, T.A., J.J. Lichtenberg, and R.C. Kroner. 1974. The occurrence of organohalides in chlorinated drinking water. J. Am. Water Works Assoc. 66:703–706.

Benedek, A. 1977. The effect of ozone on activated carbon adsorption—a mechanistic analysis of water treatment data. Presented at IOI Symposium on Advanced Ozone Technology. International Ozone Institute, Toronto, Ontario. 26 pp.

Besik, F. 1973. High rate adsorption-bio-oxidation of domestic sewage. Water Sewage Works 120:68–72.

Blackburn, A., and J.J. Kipling. 1955. Adsorption from binary liquid mixtures. Some effects of ash in commercial charcoal. J. Chem. Soc. Pt. IV:4103–4106.

Blanck, C.A. 1978. Taste and odor control utilizing granular activated carbon in the Plains region of the American Water Works System. Exhibit II of response to proposed regulations under the Safe Drinking Water Act as published in the *Federal Register* of Feb. 9, 1978. Submitted by Calgon Corp., Aug. 31, 1978.

Boening, P.H., D.D. Beckmann, and V.L. Snoeyink. 1980. Activated carbon vs. resin adsorption of humic substances. J. Am. Water Works Assoc. 72(1):54–59.

Boethling, R.S., and M. Alexander. 1979. Effect of concentration of organic chemicals on their biodegradation by natural microbial communities. Appl. Environ. Microbiol. 37(6):1211–1216.

Bohnsack, G. 1962. Behavior of anion-exchange resins toward humic acids. Mitt. Ver. Grosskesselbesitzer No. 76:53-58. 1979. (Chem. Abstr. 57:2884f, 1962)

Borneff, J. 1980. Elimination of carcinogens (excluding haloforms) by active carbon. In I.H. Suffet and M.J. McGuire, eds. Activated Carbon Adsorption of Organics from the Aqueous Phase. Proceedings of the 1978 ACS Symposium in Miami Beach, Fla. Ann Arbor Science Publishers, Inc., Ann Arbor, Mich.

Brass, H.J., M.A. Feige, T. Halloran, J.W. Mello, D. Munch, and R.F. Thomas. 1977. The national organic monitoring survey: sampling and analysis of purgeable organic compounds. Pp. 393–416 in R.B. Pojasek, ed. Drinking Water Quality Enhancement Through Source Protection. Ann Arbor Science Publishers, Inc., Ann Arbor, Mich.

Brodtmann, N., J. DeMarco, and D. Greenberg. 1980. Critical study of large-scale granular activated carbon filter units for the removal of organic substances from drinking water. In I.H. Suffet and M.J. McGuire, eds. Activated Carbon Adsorption of Organics from the Aqueous Phase. Proceedings of the 1978 ACS Symposium in Miami Beach, Fla. Ann Arbor Science Publishers, Inc., Ann Arbor, Mich.

Broitman, S.A., L.S. Gottlieb, and N. Zamcheck. 1964. Influence of neomycin and ingested endotoxin in the pathogenesis of choline deficiency cirrhosis in the adult rat. J. Exp. Med. 119:633–641.

Cairo, P.R., J.V. Radziul, I.H. Suffet, and M.J. McGuire. 1980. The application of bench-scale and pilot-scale studies for control of organic chemical contaminants in drinking water. In I.H. Suffet and M.J. McGuire, eds. Activated Carbon Adsorption of Organics from the Aqueous Phase. Proceedings of the 1978 ACS Symposium in Miami Beach, Fla. Ann Arbor Science Publishers, Inc., Ann Arbor, Mich.

Chambers, C.W, H.H. Tabak, and P.W. Kabler. 1963. Degradation of aromatic compounds by phenol adapted bacteria. J. Water Pollut. Control Fed. 35:1517–1528.

Choi, W.W., and K.Y. Chen. 1976. Associations of chlorinated hydrocarbons with fine particles and humic substances in nearshore surficial sediments. Environ. Sci. Technol. 8:782.

Chriswell, C.D., R.L. Ericson, G.A. Junk, K.W. Lee, J.S. Fritz, and H.J. Svec. 1977. Comparison of macroreticular resin and activated carbon as sorbents. J. Am. Water Works Assoc. 69:669–674.

Chudyk, W.A., V.L. Snoeyink, D.D. Beckman, and T.J. Temperly. 1979. Activated carbon vs. resin adsorption of 2-methylisoborneol and chloroform. J. Am. Water Works Assoc. 71(9):529–538.

Clifford, D.A., and W.J. Weber. 1978. Nitrate removal from water supplies by ion exchange. U.S. Environmental Protection Agency, Municipal Environmental Research

Laboratory, Water Supply Research Division, Cincinnati, Ohio. Report No. EPA/600-2-78-052. 311 pp.

Cohen, J.B., and J.D. Bachman. 1978. Measurement of environmental nitrosamines. Pp. 357–372 in E.A. Walker, L. Griciute, M. Casteguaro, and R.E. Lyle, eds. Environmental Aspects of N-Nitroso Compounds. World Health Organization, International Agency for Research on Cancer, Lyon. IARC Scientific Publications No. 19.

Cookson, J.T., Jr. 1978. Adsorption mechanisms: the chemistry of organic adsorption on activated carbon. Pp. 241–279 in P. N. Cheremisinoff and F. Ellerbusch, eds. Carbon Adsorption Handbook. Ann Arbor Science Publishers, Inc., Ann Arbor, Mich.

Crittenden, J.C. 1976. Mathematic modeling of fixed-bed adsorber dynamics—single components and multi-components. Ph.D. dissertation. Department of Civil Engineering, University of Michigan. 234 pp.

Crittenden, J.C., and W.J. Weber, Jr. 1978a. Predictive model for design of fixed-bed adsorbers: parameter estimation and model development. J. Environ. Eng. Div. Am. Soc. Civ. Eng. 104:185–197.

Crittenden, J.C., and W.J. Weber, Jr. 1978b. Predictive model for design of fixed-bed adsorbers: single-component model verification. J. Environ. Eng. Div. Am. Soc. Civ. Eng. 104:433–443.

Crittenden, J.C., and W.J. Weber, Jr. 1978c. Model for design of multicomponent adsorption systems. J. Environ. Eng. Div. Am. Soc. Civ. Eng. 109:1175–1195.

Crook, E.H., R.P. McDonnell, and J.T. McNutly. 1975. Removal and recovery of phenols from industrial waste effluents with Amberlite XAD polymeric adsorbents. Ind. Eng. Chem. Prod. Res. Dev. 14(2):113–118.

Culp, R.L., and S.P. Hansen. 1978. Carbon adsorption enhancement with ozone. Presented at the 50th Annual Water Pollution Control Federation Meeting, Anaheim, Calif.

Dahm, D.B., R.J. Pilie, and J.P. Lafornara. 1974. Technology for managing spills on land and water. Environ. Sci. Technol. 8:1076–1079.

Daniels, S.L. 1972. The adsorption of microorganisms onto solid surfaces: a review. Pp. 211–253 in Chapter 19. Developments in Industrial Microbiology, Proceedings of the 28th General Meeting of the Society for Industrial Microbiology. Published by American Institute of Biological Sciences, Washington, D.C.

Davis, T.A. 1977. Electro-regenerated ion-exchange deionization of drinking water. Final report. U.S. Environmental Protection Agency, Health Effects Research Laboratory, Cincinnati, Ohio. Report No. EPA/600/1-77-035. 83 pp.

Dietz, V.R., and J.L. Bitner. 1972. The reaction of ozone with adsorbent charcoal. Carbon 10:145–154.

DiGiano, F.A., G. Galdauf, B. Frick and H. Sontheimer. 1978. A simplified competitive equilibrium adsorption model. Chem. Eng. Sci. 33:1667–1673.

DiLuzio, N.R., and T.J. Friedmann. 1973. Bacterial endotoxins in the environment. Nature 244:49–51.

Directo, L.S., C.-L. Chen, and R.P. Miele. 1977. Independent Physical-Chemical Treatment of Raw Sewage. Final Report. U.S. Environmental Protection Agency, Municipal Environmental Research Laboratory, Cincinnati, Ohio. Report No. EPA/600/2-77/137. 119 pp.

Dobbs, R.A., R.H. Wise, and R.B. Dean. 1972. The use of ultra-violet absorbance for monitoring the total organic carbon content of water and wastewater. Water Res. 6:1173–1180.

Dobbs, R.A., R.J. Middendorf, and J.M. Cohen. 1978. Carbon adsorption isotherms for toxic organics. U.S. Environmental Protection Agency, Office of Research and

Development, Municipal Environmental Research Laboratory, Cincinnati, Ohio. 131 pp.

Donnet, J.B., L. Geldreich, D. Ferry, and F. Hueber. 1961. Effect of oxidation on the structure of amorphous carbon. Compt. Rend. 252:1146–1148. (Chem. Abstr. 55:13979b, 1961)

Donnet, J.B., J.C. Bouland, and J.Jaeger. 1963. The internal structure of carbon black particles. Compt. Rend. 256(25):5340-5343. (Chem. Abstr. 59:8208g, 1963)

Dressman, R.C., E.F. McFarren, and J.M. Symons. 1977. An evaluation of the determination of total organic chlorine (TOCl) in water by adsorption on ground granular activated carbon by pyrohydrolysis and chloride ion measurement. In The Proceedings of the 5th Annual American Water Works Association Water Quality Technology Conference, Water Quality in the Distribution System, Kansas City, Mo., 1977. Paper 3A-5. 14 pp.

Dressman, R.G., A.A. Stevens, J. Fair, and B. Smith. 1979. Comparison of methods for determination of trihalomethanes in drinking water. J. Am. Water Works Assoc. 71(7):392–396.

Dubinin, M. M. 1966. Porous structure and adsorption properties of active carbons. Pp. 51–120 in P.L. Walker, Jr., ed. Chemistry and Physics of Carbon, Vol. 2. Marcel Dekker, New York.

Eberhardt, M. 1976. Experience with the use of biologically effective activated carbon. Pp. 331–347 in H. Sontheimer, ed. Translation of Reports on Special Problems of Water Technology. Volume 9—Adsorption. Conference held in Karlsruhe, Federal Republic of Germany, 1975. U.S. Environmental Protection Agency, Municipal Environmental Research Laboratory, Cincinnati, Ohio. Report No. EPA-600/9-76-030.

Eberhardt, M., S. Madsen, and H. Sontheimer. 1974. Untersuchungen zur Verwendung biologisch arbeitender Acktivkohlefilter bei der Trinkwasseraufbereitung. Heft 7, Engler-Bunte-Instit, der Universitaet Karlsruhe, Federal Republic of Germany. EPA translation TR-77-503 (Investigations of the use of biologically effective activated carbon filters in the processing of drinking water.) 48 pp.

Fiddler, W., and W.I. Kimoto. 1979. Role of adsorbant (activated carbon and ion exchange resins) use in municipal water treatment in nitrosamine formation in drinking water. EPA-570/9-78-008, April 18, 1979, IAG # EPA-D7-01130.

Fiddler, W., J.W. Pensabene, R.C. Doerr, and C.J. Dooley. 1977. The presence of dimethyl- and diethylnitrosamines in deionized water. Food Cosmet. Toxicol. 15:441–443.

Fochtman, E.G., and R.A. Dobbs. 1980. Adsorption of carcinogenic compounds by activated carbon. In I.H. Suffet and M.J. McGuire, eds. Activated Carbon Adsorption of Organics from the Aqueous Phase. Proceedings of the 1978 ACS Symposium in Miami Beach, Fla. Ann Arbor Science Publishers, Inc., Ann Arbor, Mich.

Ford, C.T., and Boyer, J.F. 1973. Treatment of ferrous acid mine drainage with activated carbon. U.S. Environmental Protection Agency. Environmental Protection Technology Series. Report No. EPA-R2-73-150. 127 pp.

Freer, J.H., and M.R.J. Salton. 1971. The anatomy and chemistry of gram-negative cell envelopes. Pp. 67–126 in G. Weinbaum, S. Kadis, and S.J. Ajl, eds. Microbial Toxins, Vol. 4. Academic Press, New York.

Frick, B., R. Bartz, H. Sontheimer, and F.A. DiGiano. 1980. Predicting competitive adsorption effects in granular activated carbon filters. In I.H. Suffet and M.J. McGuire, eds. Activated Carbon Adsorption of Organics from the Aqueous Phase. Proceedings of the 1978 ACS Symposium in Miami Beach, Fla. Ann Arbor Science Publishers, Inc., Ann Arbor, Mich.

Fritz, W. 1978. Konkurrierende Adsorption verschiedener organischer Wasserinhaltstoffe in Aktivkohlefiltern. Ph.D. dissertation. Department of Chemical Engineerng, University of Karlsruhe, Federal Republic of Germany.

Fuchs, F. 1974. Direction for the determination of activated carbon charges. Engler-Bunte Institute of the University of Karlsruhe, Federal Republic of Germany. 15 pp.

Gans, H., and K. Matsumoto. 1974. Are enteric endotoxins able to escape from the intestine? Proc. Soc. Exp. Biol. Med. 147:736–739.

Garten, V.A., and D.E. Weiss. 1959. Functional groups in activated carbon and carbon black with ion- and electron-exchange properties. Pp. 295–313 in Proceedings of the Third Conference on Carbon held at the University of Buffalo, Buffalo, N.Y. Pergamon Press, New York.

Gauntlett, R. 1975. A comparison between ion-exchange resins and activated carbon for the removal of organics from water. Water Research Technology Report TR10, Medmenham Laboratory, England.

George, A.D., and M. Chaudhuri. 1977. Removal of iron from groundwater by filtration through coal. J. Am. Water Works Assoc. 69:385–389.

Giusti, D.M., R.A. Conway, and C.T. Lawson. 1974. Activated carbon adsorption of petrochemials. J. Water Pollut. Control Fed. 46:947–965.

Glaze, W.H., G.R. Peyton, and R. Rawley. 1977. Total organic chlorine as water quality parameter: adsorption/microcoulometric method. Environ. Sci. Technol. 11:685–690.

Gough, T.A., K.S. Webb, and M.F. McPhail. 1977. Volatile nitrosamines from ion exchange resins. Food Cosmet. Toxicol. 15:437–440.

Greve, P.A., and S.L. Wit. 1971. Endosulfan in the Rhine River. J. Water Pollut. Control Fed. 43:2338–2348.

Grob, K., and F. Zurcher. 1976. Stripping of trace organic substances from water. Equipment and procedures. J. Chromatogr. 117:285–294.

Guirguis, W.A., J.S. Jain, Y.A. Hanna, and P.K. Sirvastava. 1976. Ozone application for disinfection in the Westerly Advanced Wastewater Treatment Facility. Pp. 363–381 in E.G. Fochtman, R.G. Rice, and M.E. Browning, eds. Forum on Ozone Disinfection. International Ozone Institute, Cleveland, Ohio.

Guirguis, W., T. Cooper, J. Harris, and A. Ungar. 1978. Improved performance of activated carbon by pre-ozonization. J. Water Pollut. Control. Fed. 50:308–320.

Gulbrandson, R., C.M. Janicek, H. Klusterman, and R.L. Witz. 1972. Treating colored water with macroreticular resins. Am. Soc. Agric. Eng. Pap. Paper 72–711. 19 pp.

Gustafson, R.L., and J.A. Lirio. 1968. Adsorption of organic ions by anion exchange resins. Ind. Eng. Chem. Prod. Res. Dev. 7(2):116–120.

Hager, D.G., and J.L. Rizzo. 1974. Removal of toxic organics from wastewater by adsorption with granular activated carbon. Presented at U.S. Environmental Protection Agency Technology Transfer Session on Treatment of Toxic Chemicals, Atlanta, Ga.

Haller, H.D. 1978. Degradation of mono-substituted benzoates and phenols by wastewater. J. Water Pollut. Control Fed. 50:2771–2777.

Hart, P.J., F.J. Vastola, and P.L. Walker, Jr. 1967. Oxygen chemisorption on well cleaned carbon surfaces. Carbon 5:363–371.

Helfgott, T.B., F.L. Hart, and R.G. Bedard. 1977. An index of refractory organics. Office of Research and Development, U.S. Environmental Protection Agency Report No. EPA-600/2-77-174. Robert S. Kerr Environmental Research Laboratory, Ada, Okla.

Henderson, J.E., G.R. Peyton, and W.H. Glaze. 1976. A convenient liquid–liquid extraction method for the determination of halomethanes in water at the parts-per-billion level. Pp. 105–133 in L.H. Keith, ed. Identification and Analysis of Organic Pollutants in Water. Ann Arbor Science Publishers, Inc., Ann Arbor, Mich.

Herzing, D.R., V.L. Snoeyink, and N.F. Wood. 1977. Activated carbon adsorption of the odorous comopunds 2-methylisoborneol and geosmin. J. Am. Water Works Assoc. 69:223–228.

Hinrichs, R.L., and V.L. Snoeyink. 1976. Sorption of benzenesulfonates by weak base anion exhange resins. Water Res. 10:79–87.

Hofstad, T., and T. Kristoffersen. 1970. Chemical characteristics of endotoxin from *Bacteroides fragilis* NCTC 9343. J. Gen. Microbiol. 61:15–19.

Hsieh, J. 1974. Liquid phase multicomponent adsorption in fixed bed. Ph.D. dissertation Department of Chemical Engineering, Syracuse University, N.Y.

Hsieh, J.S.C., R.M. Turian, and C. Tien. 1977. Multicomponent liquid phase adsorption in fixed bed. Am. Ind. Chem. J. 23:263–275.

Huang, C.-P. 1978. Chemical interactions between inorganics and activated carbon. Pp. 281–329 in P.N. Cheremisinoff and F. Ellerbusch, eds. Carbon Adsorption Handbook. Ann Arbor Science Publishers, Inc., Ann Arbor, Mich.

Huang, C.-P., and M.-H. Wu. 1975. Chromium removal by carbon adsorption. J. Water Pollut. Control. Fed. 47:2437–2446.

Hutchinson, M., and J.W. Ridgway. 1977. Microbiological aspects of drinking water supplies. Pp. 179–218 in F.A. Skinner and J.M. Shewan, eds. Aquatic Microbiology. Society for Applied Bacteriology Symposium Series No. 6. Academic Press, London.

Inhoffer, W.R. 1978. Sorptive properties of granular activated carbon and infrared regeneration at Little Falls, New Jersey. Presented at the 98th Annual Conference of the American Water Works Association, Atlantic City, N.J. Paper No. 10-5. 18 pp.

Interagency Regulatory Liaison Group. 1978. Regulators release chemical hit list. Chem. Eng. News 56:50.

Ishizaki, C., and J.T. Cookson, Jr. 1974. Influence of surface oxides on adsorption and catalysis with activated carbon. Pp. 201–231 in A.J. Rubin, ed. Chemistry of Water Supply, Treatment, and Distribution. Ann Arbor Science Publishers, Inc., Ann Arbor, Mich.

Jain, S.J., and V.L. Snoeyink. 1973. Competitive adsorption from bisolute systems on active carbon. J. Water Pollut. Control Fed. 45:2463–2479.

Jayes, D.A., and I.M. Abrams. 1968. A new method of color removal: development report. N. Engl. Water Works Assoc. 82:15–25.

Jekel, M. 1977. Biological treatment of surface waters in activated carbon filters. Presented at the meeting of the Water Research Center (England), KIWA (Netherlands) and EBI (Federal Republic of Germany), Engler-Bunte Institute, Karlsruhe University, Federal Republic of Germany.

Jeris, J.S., and R.W. Owens. 1975. Pilot-scale, high rate biological denitrification. J. Water Pollut. Control Fed. 47:2043–2057.

Jeris, J.S., C. Beer, and J.A. Mueller. 1974. High rate biological denitrification using a granular fluidized bed. J. Water Pollut. Control Fed. 46:2118–2128.

Jeris, J.S., R.W. Owens, R. Hickey, and F. Flood. 1977. Biological fluidized-bed treatment for BOD and nitrogen removal. J. Water Pollut. Control Fed. 49:816–831.

Jorgensen, J.H., J.C. Lee, and H.R. Pahren. 1976. Rapid detection of bacterial endotoxins in drinking water and renovated wastewater. Appl. Environ. Microbiol. 32:347–351.

Jossens, L., J.M. Prausnitz, W. Fritz, E.U. Schlunder, and A.L. Myers. 1978. Thermodynamics of multi-solute adsorption from dilute aqueous solutions. Chem. Eng. Sci. 33:1097–1106.

Kaiser, K.L.E., and B.G. Oliver. 1976. Determination of volatile halogenated hydrocarbons in water by gas chromatography. Anal. Chem. 48:2207–2209.

Kavanaugh, M.C. 1978. Coagulation for removal of trihalomethane precursors at the Ralph D. Bollman Treatment Plant. Presented at the 98th Annual Conference of the American Water Works Association, Atlantic City, N.J. Paper No. 15-3. 21 pp.

Keinath, T.M., and R.P. Carnahan. 1973. Mathematical modeling of heterogeneous sorption in continuous contractors for wastewater decontamination. Final Report. Contract No. DADA-17-72-C-2034, Clemson University, S.C. 173 pp. Available from NTIS as AD-777 530.

Keith, L.H., ed. 1976. Identification and Analysis of Organic Pollutants in Water. Ann Arbor Science Publishers, Inc., Ann Arbor, Mich. 718 pp.

Keith, L.H. 1978. Comment of L.H. Keith re: Proposed amendment to National Interim Primary Drinking Water Regulations. June 1978.

Keith, L.H., and W.A. Telliard. 1979. Priority pollutants. I. A perspective view. Environ. Sci. Technol. 13(4):416–423.

Kennedy, D.C. 1973. Macroreticular polymeric adsorbents. Ind. Eng. Chem. Prod. Res. Dev. 12(1):56–61.

Kipling, J.J. 1965. Adsorption from Solutions of Non-Electrolytes. Academic Press, New York. 328 pp.

Klotz, M., P. Werner, and R. Schweisfurth. 1976. Investigations concerning the microbiology of activated carbon filters. Pp. 312–330 in H. Sontheimer, ed. Translation of Reports on Special Problems of Water Technology. Volume 9—Adsorption. Conference held in Karlsruhe, Federal Republic of Germany, 1975. U.S. Environmental Protection Agency, Municipal Environmental Research Laboratory, Cincinnati, Ohio. Report No. EPA-600/9-76-030.

Knorr, M., and D. Schenk. 1968. Synthesis of polycyclic aromatic compounds by bacteria. Arch. Hyg. Bakteriol. 152:282–285.

Kolle, W. 1976. Use of macroporous ion exchangers for drinking water purification. Pp. 405–413 in H. Sontheimer, ed. Translation of Reports on Special Problems of Water Technology. Volume 9—Adsorption. Conference held in Karlsruhe, Federal Republic of Germany, 1975. U.S. Environmental Protection Agency, Municipal Environmental Research Laboratory, Cincinnati, Ohio. Report No. EPA-600/9-76-030.

Kolle, W., H. Sontheimer, and L. Steiglitz. 1975. Quantification tests of activated carbon for water works based on adsorption properties for organic chlorine. Vom Wasser 44:203–217.

Kuhn, W., and F. Fuchs. 1975. Investigations on the significance of organic chlorine compounds and their adsorbability. Vom Wasser 45:217–232.

Kuhn, W., and H. Sontheimer. 1973a. Several investigations on activated charcoal for the determination of organic chloro compounds. Vom Wasser 41:65–79.

Kuhn, W., and H. Sontheimer. 1973b. Analytic determination of chlorinated organic compounds with temperature programmed pyrohydrolysis. Vom. Wasser 41:1. (Translated TR 169-75 by EPA)

Kuhn, W., H. Sontheimer, L. Steiglitz, D. Maier, and R. Kurz. 1978a. Use of ozone and chlorine in water utilities in the Federal Republic of Germany. J. Am. Water Works Assoc. 70:326–331.

Kuhn, W., H. Sontheimer, and R. Kurz. 1978b. Use of ozone and chlorine in water works in Federal Republic of Germany. Pp. 426–442 in R.G. Rice and J.A. Cortruvo, eds. Ozone/Chlorine Dioxide Oxidation Products of Organic Materials. International Ozone Institute, Inc., Cleveland, Ohio.

Kunin, R. 1972. Ion Exchange Resins. Krieger Publ. Co., Huntington, N.Y. 504 pp.

Kunin, R. 1973. Helpful hints in ion exchange technology (conclusion). Amber-Hi-Lites No. 132. Rohm and Haas Co., Philadelphia. 5 pp.

Kunin, R. 1974a. Ion exchange technology in medicine and the pharmaceutical industry. Part I. Amber-Hi-Lites No. 142. Rohm and Haas Co., Philadelphia. 7 pp.

Kunin, R. 1974b. Ion exchange technology in medicine and the pharmaceutical industry. Part II. Amber-Hi-Lites No. 143. Rohm and Haas Co., Philadelphia. 4 pp.

Kunin, R. 1976. Use of macroreticular polymeric adsorbents for treatment of waste effluents. Soc. Plast. Eng. Tech. Pap. 22:248–250.

Kunin, R., and D.G. Downing. 1971. New ion exchange systems for treating municipal and domestic waste effluents. Chem. Eng. Prog. Symp. Ser. 67(107):575–580. (Chem. Abstr. 74:102799n, 1971)

Larsen, E.C., and J.H. Walton. 1940. Activated carbon as a catalyst in certain oxidation-reduction reactions. J. Phys. Chem. 44:70–85.

Lawrence, J., and H.M. Tosine. 1976. Adsorption of polychlorinated biphenyls from aqueous solutions and sewage. Environ. Sci. Technol. 10:381–383.

Levin, J., and F.B. Bang. 1964. The role of endotoxin in the extracellular coagulation of *Limulus* blood. Bull. Johns Hopkins Hosp. 115:265–274.

Lombana, L.A., and D. Halaby. 1978. Carbon regeneration systems. Pp. 905–922 in P.N. Cheremisinoff and F. Ellerbusch, eds. Carbon Adsorption Handbook. Ann Arbor Science Publishers, Inc., Ann Arbor, Mich.

Love, T.O. and J.M. Symons. 1978. Operational aspects of granular activated carbon adsorption treatment. Unpublished paper of U.S. Environmental Protection Agency, Drinking Water Research Division.

Love, O.T., Jr., J.K. Carswell, R.J. Miltner, and J.M. Symons. 1976. Treatment for the prevention or removal of trihalomethanes in drinking water. Appendix 3 in J. Symons, ed. Interim Guide for the Control of Chloroform and Other Trihalomethanes. U.S. Environmental Protection Agency, Water Supply Research Division, Municipal Environmental Research Laboratory, Cincinnati, Ohio. 54 pp.

Ludzack, F.J., and M.B. Ettinger. 1960. Chemical structures resistant to aerobic biochemical stabilization. J. Water Pollut. Control Fed. 32:1173–1200.

McCarty, P.C., D. Argo, and M. Reinhard. 1979. Operational experiences with activated carbon adsorbers at Water Factory 21. Presented at Practical Applications of Adsorption Techniques in Drinking Water by NATO/CCMS, on May 1–2, 1979, Reston, Va. U.S. Environmental Protection Agency, Office of Drinking Water.

McCreary, J.J., and V.L. Snoeyink. 1977. Granular activated carbon in water treatment. J. Am. Water Works Assoc. 69:437–444.

McElhaney, J., and W.R. McKeon. 1978. Enumeration and identification of bacteria in granular activated carbon columns. In Proceedings of the 6th Annual American Water Works Association. Water Quality Technical Conference, Louisville, Ky. (Dec. 1978).

McGuire, M.J. 1977. The optimization of water treatment unit processes for the removal of trace organic compounds with an emphasis on the adsorption mechanism. Ph.D. thesis. Drexel University, Philadelphia, Pa.

McGuire, M.J., and I.H. Suffet. 1978. Adsorption of organics from domestic water supplies. J. Am. Water Works Assoc. 70:621–636.

McGuire, M.J., and I.H. Suffett. 1980. The calculated net adsorption energy concept. In I.H. Suffet and M.J. McGuire, eds. Activated Carbon Adsorption of Organics from the Aqueous Phase. Proceedings of the 1978 ACS Symposium in Miami Beach, Fla. Ann Arbor Science Publishers, Inc., Ann Arbor, Mich.

McGuire, M.J., I.H. Suffet, and J.V. Radziul. 1978. Assessment of unit processes for the removal of trace organic compounds from drinking water. J. Am. Water Works Assoc. 70:565–572.

Magee, V. 1956. The application of granular active carbon for dechlorination of water supplies. Proc. Soc. Water Treat. Exam. 5:17–40. (Chem. Abstr. 54:11342f, 1960)

Mahon, J.H. 1979. Selected carbon isotherms conducted on single organic compounds. Calgon Corp., Pittsburgh, Pa.

Maimonides, M.B. 1185. The Book of Cleanness, The Code of Maimonides Book X. Treatise II, pp. 97–146. Yale University Press, New Haven, Conn., 1954.

Maqsood, R., and A. Benedek. 1977. Low-temperature organic removal and denitrification in activated carbon columns. J. Water Pollut. Control Fed. 49:2107–2117.

Marshall, K.C. 1976. Interfaces in Microbial Ecology. Harvard University Press, Cambridge, Mass. 156 pp.

Martin, R.J., and K.S. Al-Bahrani. 1977. Adsorption studies using gas–liquid chromatography. II. Competitive adsorption. Water Res. 11:991–999.

Mathews, A.P. 1975. Mathematical modeling of multi-component adsorption in batch reactors. Ph.D. dissertation. Department of Civil Engineering, University of Michigan. 207 pp.

Merk, W. 1978. Konkurrierende Adsorption verschiedener organischer Wasserinhaltstoffe in Aktivkohlefiltern. Ph.D. dissertation. Department of Chemical Engineering, University of Karlsruhe, Federal Republic of Germany.

Middleton, F.M., and A.A. Rosen. 1956. Organic contaminants affecting the quality of water. Public Health Rep. 71:1125–1133.

Mieure, J.P. 1977. A rapid and sensitive method for determining volatile organohalides in water. J. Am. Water Works Assoc. 69:60–62.

Miller, S. 1979. Federal environmental monitoring: will the bubble burst? Environ. Sci. Technol. 12:1264–1269.

Miller, G.W., R.G. Rice, C.M. Robson, R.L. Scullin, and W. Kuhn. 1978. An assessment of ozone and chlorine dioxide technologies for treatment of municipal water supplies. U.S. Environmental Protection Agency, Municipal Environmental Research Laboratory, Water Supply Research Division, Cincinnati, Ohio. Report No. EPA-600/2-78-147. 588 pp.

Mills, A.L., and M. Alexander. 1976. Factors affecting dimethylnitrosamine formation in samples of soil and water. J. Environ. Qual. 5:437–440.

Morikawa, K., T. Shirasaki, and M. Ikada. 1969. Correlation among methods of preparation of solid catalysts, their structures, and catalytic activities. Pp. 97–133 in D.D. Eley, H. Pines, and P.B. Weisz, eds. Advances in Catalysis, Vol. 20. Academic Press, New York.

Mueller, G., and H. Bernhardt. 1976. Comparative bacteriological examinations on activated charcoal filter using chlorinated and ozonized ground and reservoir water. Forum Umwelt Hyg. 2(27):393–396. Translated TR-77-311 by EPA.

Murin, C.J., and V.L. Snoeyink. 1979. Competitive adsorption of 2,4 dichlorophenol and 2,4,6 trichlorophenol in the nanomolar to micromolar concentration range. Environ. Sci. Technol. 13:305.

National Academy of Sciences. 1977. Drinking Water and Health. Safe Drinking Water Committee, National Research Council. Washington, D.C. 939 pp.

National Academy of Sciences. 1978. Chloroform, Carbon Tetrachloride, and Other Halomethanes: An Environmental Assessment. Washington, D.C. 294 pp.

National Academy of Sciences. 1979. Toxicity of Selected Drinking Water Contaminants. Safe Drinking Water Committee. National Research Council. Washington, D.C. 421 pp.

National Cancer Institute. 1978. Human health considerations of carcinogenic organic chemical contaminants in drinking water. Fed. Reg. 43:29148–29150.

Neely, J.W. 1980. A model for the removal of trihalomethanes from water by Ambersorb XE-340. In I.H. Suffet and M.J. McGuire, eds. Activated Carbon Adsorption of Organics from the Aqueous Phase. Proceedings of the 1978 ACS Symposium in Miami Beach, Fla. Ann Arbor Science Publishers, Inc., Ann Arbor, Mich.

Nicholson, A.A., O. Meresz, and B. Lemyk. 1977. Determination of free and total potential haloforms in drinking water. Anal. Chem. 49:814–819.

Nolan, J.P. 1975. The role of endotoxin in liver injury. Gastroenterology 69:1346–1356.

Nolan, J.P., and M.V. Ali. 1968. Endotoxin and the liver. I. Toxicity in rats with choline deficient fatty livers. Proc. Soc. Exp. Biol. Med. 129:29–31.

Oliver, B.G. 1978. Chlorinated non-volatile organics produced by the reaction of chlorine with humic material. Can. Res. 11:21.

Parkhurst, J.D., F.D. Dryden, G.N. McDermott, and J. English. 1967. Pomona activated carbon pilot plant. J. Water Pollut. Control Fed. 39:R70–R81.

Peel, R., and A. Benedek. 1975. The modeling of activated carbon adsorbers in the presence of bio-oxidation. Presented at the American Institute of Chemical Engineers 68th Annual Meeting, The Design of Carbon Adsorption Systems Session, Los Angeles, Calif., Nov. 16–20. Paper 85-D. 12 pp.

Pfaender, F.K., A.A. Stevens, L. Moore, and J.R. Hass. 1978. Evaluation of direct aqueous injection method for analysis of chloroform in drinking water. Environ. Sci. Technol. 12:438–441.

Pitter, P. 1976. Determination of biological degradability of organic substances. Water Res. 10:231–235.

Pitter, P., P. Kucharova-Rosolova, L. Richtrova, R. Palyza, K. Hubnerova-Hajkova, and H. Radkova. 1974. Relation between the structure and biological degradability of organic compounds. Pts. III–VI. Sb. Vys. Sk. Chem. Technol. Praze. Technol. Vody F19:43–109.

Poggenburg, W., C. Engels, F.J. Weissenhorn, F. Fushs, and H. Sontheimer. 1974. Investigations on the application of activated carbon to the processing of Rhine riverbank filtrate. Sonderdruck aus der DVGW-Schroftenreihe Wasser Nr. 7. DVGW Publication Series No. 7.

Prober, R., J.J. Pyeha, and W.E. Kidon. 1975. Interaction of activated carbon with dissolved oxygen. Am. Ind. Chem. Eng. J. 21:1200–1204.

Puri, B.R. 1970. Surface complexes on carbons. Pp. 191–282 in P.L. Walker, Jr., ed. Chemistry and Physics of Carbon, Vol. 6. Marcel Dekker, New York.

Radke, C.J., and J.M. Prausnitz. 1972a. Thermodynamics of multi-solute adsorption from dilute liquid solutions. Am. Ind. Chem. Eng. J. 18:761–768.

Radke, C.J., and J.M. Prausnitz. 1972b. Adsorption of organic solutes from dilute aqueous solution on activated carbon. Ind. Eng. Chem. Fund. 11:445–451.

Randtke, S.J. 1978. Discussion [of]: Improved performance of activated carbon by pre-ozonization, by W. Guirguis, T. Cooper, J. Harris, and A. Ungar. J. Water Pollut. Control Fed. 50:2602–2603.

Reding, R., W.B. Kollman, M.J. Weisner, and H.J. Brass. In press. The Analysis of Trihalomethanes in Drinking Water by Liquid–Liquid Extraction. ASTM Special Technical Publication No. STP 686. Symposium on Organic Pollutants, Denver, Colo., June 19–20, 1978.

Rhead, T.F.E., and R.V. Wheeler. 1912. The combustion of carbon. J. Chem. Soc. Trans. 101:846–856.

Rhead, T.F.E., and R.V. Wheeler. 1913. The mode of combustion of carbon. J. Chem. Soc. Trans. 103:461–489.

Rice, R.G., G.W. Miller, C.M. Robson, and W. Kuhn. 1978. A review of the status of preozonization of granular activated carbon for removal of dissolved organics and ammonia from water and wastewater. Pp. 485–537 in P.N. Cheremisinoff and F. Ellerbusch, eds. Carbon Adsorption Handbook. Ann Arbor Science Publishers, Inc., Ann Arbor, Mich.

Richard, J.J., and G.A. Junk. 1977. Liquid extraction for the rapid determination of halomethanes in water. J. Am. Water Works Assoc. 69:62–64.

Rideal, E.K., and W.M. Wright. 1925. Low temperature oxidation at charcoal surfaces. Part I. The behaviour of charcoal in the absence of promoters. J. Chem. Soc. 127:1347–1357.

Rideal, E.K., and W.M. Wright. 1926. Low temperature oxidation at charcoal surfaces. Part II. The behaviour of charcoal in the presence of promoters. J. Chem. Soc. 128:1813–1821.

Robeck, G.G., K.A. Dostal, J.M. Cohen, and J.F. Kreissl. 1965. Effectiveness of water treatment processes in pesticide removal. J. Am. Water Works Assoc. 57:181–200. (Chem. Abstr. 62:11532e, 1965)

Rohm and Haas Co. 1977. Ambersorb carbonaceous adsorbents. Bulletin 1E-231. R&H Co., Philadelphia. 19 pp.

Rosene, M.R., and M. Manes. 1976. Application of the Polanyi adsorption potential theory to adsorption from solution on activated carbon. 6. Competitive adsorption of solids from water solution. J. Phys. Chem. 80:953–959.

Rosene, M.R., and M. Manes. 1977. Application of the Polanyi adsorption potential theory to adsorption from solution on activated carbon. 9. Competitive adsorption of ternary solid solutes from water solution. J. Phys. Chem. 81:1646–1650.

Rosene, M.R., M. Ozcan, and M. Manes. 1976. Application of Polanyi adsorption potential theory to adsorption from solution on activated carbon. 8. Ideal, non-ideal, and competitive adsorption of some solids from water solution. J. Phys. Chem. 80:2586–2589.

Sander, R., W. Kuhn, and H. Sontheimer. 1977. Study of the reaction of chlorine with humic substances. Z. Wasser Abwasser Forsch. 10(5):155–160.

Schalekamp, M. 1976. Use of activated carbon in the treatment of lake water. Pp. 128–159 in H. Sontheimer, ed. Translation of Reports on Special Problems of Water Technology. Volume 9—Adsorption. Conference held in Karlsruhe, Federal Republic of Germany, 1975. U.S. Environmental Protection Agency, Municipal Environmental Research Laboratory, Cincinnati, Ohio. Report No. EPA-600/9-76-030.

Schmidt, K. 1974. Effectiveness of standard drinking water preparation for eliminating pesticides and other pollutants. Gas Wasserfach, Wasser-Abwasser 115:72–76.

Schweinberg, F.B., and J. Fine. 1960. Evidence for a lethal endotoxemia as the fundamental feature of irreversibility in three types of traumatic shock. J. Exp. Med. 112:793–800.

Semmens, M., J.K. Edzwald, M. Taylor, and R. Sanks. 1978. Organics removal by coagulation—a review and research needs. Presented at the 98th Annual AWWA Conference, Atlantic City, N.J. 35 pp.

Shands, J.W., Jr. 1975. Endotoxin as a pathogenetic mediator of gram-negative infection. Pp. 330–335 in D. Schlessinger, ed. Microbiology—1975. American Society for Microbiology, Washington, D.C.

Shevehenko, M.A., P.V. Marchenko, P.N. Taran, and E.V. Kravets. 1974. Removal of some pesticides from drinking water by adsorption methods. Vodosnabzh. Sanit. Tekh. (USSR) 10:31–32.

Slejko, F.L., and G. Meigs. 1980. Economic analysis of employing Ambersorb XE-340 carbonaceous adsorbent in trace organics removal from drinking water. In I.H. Suffet and M.J. McGuire, eds. Activated Carbon Adsorption of Organics from the Aqueous Phase Proceedings of the 1978 ACS Symposium in Miami Beach, Fla. Ann Arbor Science Publishers, Inc., Ann Arbor, Mich.

Smith, R.N. 1959. The chemistry of carbon–oxygen surface compounds. Q. Rev. (Lond.) 13:287–305. (Chem. Abstr. 54:9464c, 1960)

Snoeyink, V.L., and J.J. McCreary. 1978. Reaction of activated carbon with aqueous chlorine and other disinfection agents. Technical Progress Report, U.S. Environmental Protection Agency, Grant No. R 805-293-01, Department of Civil Engineering, University of Illinois at Urbana-Champaign, Urbana. 33 pp.

Snoeyink, V.L., W.J. Weber, Jr., and H.B. Mark. 1969. Sorption of phenol and nitrophenol by active carbon. Environ. Sci. Technol. 3:918.

Snoeyink, V.L., H.T. Lai, J.H. Johnson, and J.F. Young. 1974. Active carbon: dechlorination and the adsorption of organic compounds. Pp. 233–252 in A.J. Rubin, ed. Chemistry of Water Supply, Treatment, and Distribution. Ann Arbor Science Publishers, Inc., Ann Arbor, Mich.

Snoeyink, V.L., J.J. McCreary, and C.J. Murin. 1977. Activated carbon adsorption of trace organic compounds. Final report. U.S. Environmental Protection Agency, Municipal Environmental Research Laboratory, Cincinnati, Ohio. Water Supply Research Division. Report No. EPA/600/2-77/223. 129 pp.

Snoeyink, V.L., W.A. Chudyk, D.D. Beckman, P.H. Boening, and T.J. Temperly. 1978. Bench scale evaluation of resins and activated carbons for water purification. Project Report, Iowa State University Subcontract EPA-R-804433, U.S. Environmental Protection Agency, Cincinnati, Ohio.

Sontheimer, H. 1974. Use of activated carbon in water treatment practice and its regeneration. Report on the Water Research Conference at the University of Reading (England) 3–5 April 1973 on Activated Carbon in Water Treatment.

Sontheimer, H., E. Heilker, M.R. Jekel, H. Nolte, and F.H. Vollmer. 1978. The Muelheim process. J. Am. Water Works Assoc. 70:393–396.

Sridharan, N., and G.F. Lee. 1972. Coprecipitation of organic compounds from lake water by iron salts. Environ. Sci. Technol. 6:1031–1033.

Steiglitz, L., W. Roth, W. Kuhn, and W. Leger. 1976. Behavior of organic halogen compounds in the purification of drinking water. Vom Wasser 47:347–377.

Stevens, A.A., and J.M. Symons. 1973. Measurement of organics in drinking water. Proceedings of the American Water Works Association Technology Conference on Water Quality, 1973, Cincinnati, Ohio. Paper No. 23. 26 pp.

Stevens, A.A., C.J. Slocum, D.R. Seeger, and G.G. Robeck. 1976. Chlorination of organics in drinking water. J. Am. Water Works Assoc. 68:615–620.

Stumm, W., and G.F. Lee. 1961. Oxygenation of ferrous iron. Ind. Eng. Chem. 53:143.

Suffet, I.H., and J.V. Radziul. 1976. Guidelines for the quantitative and qualitative screening of organic pollutants in water supplies. J. Am. Water Works Assoc. 68:5230–5240, Addendum:69:174, 1977.

Suffet, I.H., L. Brenner, J.T. Coyle, and P.R. Cairo. 1978a. Evaluation of the capability of granular activated carbon and XAD-2 resin to remove trace organics from treated drinking water. Environ. Sci. Technol. 12:1315–1322.

Suffet, I.H., J.V. Radziul, P.R. Cairo, and J.T. Coyle. 1978b. Evaluation of the capability of granular activated carbon and resin to remove trace organics from treated drinking water. In R.L. Jolley, ed. Water Chlorination: Enviornmental Impact and Health Effects, Vol. II. Ann Arbor Science Publishers, Inc., Ann Arbor, Mich.

Suidan, M.T., V.L. Snoeyink, and R.A. Schmitz. 1977. Reduction of aqueous free chlorine with granular activated carbon—pH and temperature effects. Environ. Sci. Technol. 11:785–789.

Sylvia, A.E. 1973. Detection and measurements of microorganisms in drinking water. J.N. Engl. Water Works Assoc. 87(2):183–199.

Sylvia, A.E., and R.J. Donlan. 1980. The use of fluorescence in monitoring removal of organics in drinking water. In I.H. Suffet and M.J. McGuire, eds. Activated Carbon Adsorption of Organics from the Aqueous Phase. Proceedings of the 1978 ACS Symposium in Miami Beach, Fla. Ann Arbor Science Publishers, Inc., Ann Arbor, Mich.

Symons, J.M. 1980. Applications of activated carbon to drinking water treatment: pilot plant. In I.H. Suffet and M.J. McGuire, eds. Activated Carbon Adsorption of Organics from the Aqueous Phase. Proceedings of the 1978 ACS Symposium in Miami Beach, Fla. Ann Arbor Science Publishers, Inc., Ann Arbor, Mich.

Symons, J.M., T.A. Bellar, J.K. Carswell, J. DeMarco, K.L. Kropp, G.G. Robeck, D.R. Seeger, C.J. Slocum, B.L. Smith, and A.A. Stevens. 1975. National organics reconnaissance survey for halogenated organics. J. Am. Water Works Assoc. 67:634–648.

Thurman, E.M., G.R. Aiken, and R.C. Malcolm. 1978a. The use of macroreticular nonionic resins to preconcentrate trace organic acids from water. Proc. 4th Joint Conf. Environ. Pollut.

Thurman, E.M., R.C. Malcolm, and G.R. Aiken. 1978b. Prediction of capacity factors for aqueous organic solutes adsorbed on porous acrylic resins. Anal. Chem. 50:775.

Tien, C. 1980. Bacterial growth on adsorption interactions in granular activated carbon column. In I.H. Suffet and M.J. McGuire, eds. Activated Carbon Adsorption of Organics from the Aqueous Phase. Proceedings of the 1978 ACS Symposium in Miami Beach, Fla. Ann Arbor Science Publishers, Inc., Ann Arbor, Mich.

Tillsworth, T. 1974. Organic and color removal from water supplies by synthetic resinous adsorbents. Institute of Water Resources, U.S. Department of the Interior, Office of Water Resources Research. Report No. IRW-50. (NTIS # PB 233068). 56 pp.

U.S. Environmental Protection Agency. 1974. Recommended list of priority pollutants—revised. National Resources Defense Council vs Train, 510 F2d 692 (DC Cir 1974).

U.S. Environmental Protection Agency. 1975. National Interim Primary Drinking Water Regulations. Fed. Reg. 59566–59588, Dec. 24, 1975.

U.S. Environmental Protection Agency. 1976a. Interim treatment guide for the control of chloroform and other trihalomethanes. J.M. Symons, ed. Municipal Environmental Research Laboratory, Water Supply Research Division, Cincinnati, Ohio. 261 pp.

U.S. Environmental Protection Agency. 1976b. The Proceedings of the 4th United States/Japan Conference on Sewage Treatment Technology. 600/9-76-023, Oct. 1976.

U.S. Environmental Protection Agency. 1978a. Statement of basis and purpose for an amendment to the National Interim Primary Drinking Water Regulations on a Treatment Technique for Synthetic Organic Chemicals. Office of Water Supply, Criteria and Standards Division.

U.S. Environmental Protection Agency. 1978b. Interim primary drinking water regulations: control of organic chemical contaminants in drinking water. Fed. Reg. 43(28):5756–5780.

U.S. Environmental Protection Agency. 1978c. Interim treatment guide for controlling organic contaminants in drinking water using granular activated carbon. In J.M. Symons, ed. Support document for U.S. Environmental Protection Agency Interim Primary Drinking Water Regulations, Control of Organic Chemical Contaminants in

Drinking Water; Fed. Reg. 43(28):5756–5780, Feb. 9, 1978. Municipal Environmental Research Laboratory, Water Supply Research Division, Cincinnati, Ohio. 207 pp.

van der Kooij, D. 1976. Some investigations into the presence and behaviour of bacteria in activated carbon filters. Pp. 348–354 in H. Sontheimer, ed. Translation of Reports on Special Problems of Water Technology. Volume 9—Adsorption. Conference held in Karlsruhe, Federal Republic of Germany, 1975. U.S. Environmental Protection Agency, Municipal Environmental Research Laboratory, Cincinnati, Ohio. Report No. EPA-600/9-76-030.

van der Kooij, D. 1978. Investigations concerning the relation between microorganisms and adsorption processes in granular activated carbon filters. Presented at the Conference on Oxidation Techniques in Drinking Water Treatment, Karlsruhe, 11–15 Sept. 1978. 16 pp.

van Lier, W.C., A. Graveland, J.J. Rook, and L.J. Schultink. 1976. Experiences with pilot plant activated carbon filters in Dutch waterworks. Pp. 160–181 in H. Sontheimer, ed. Translation of Reports on Special Problems of Water Technology. Volume 9—Adsorption. Conference held in Karlsruhe, Federal Republic of Germany, 1975. U.S. Environmental Protection Agency, Municipal Environmental Research Laboratory, Cincinnati, Ohio. Report No. EPA-600/9-76-030.

Van Rossum, P., and R.G. Webb. 1978. Isolation of organic water pollutants by XAD resins and carbon. J. Chromatogr. 150:381.

Verschuren, K. 1977. Handbook of Environmental Data on Organic Chemicals. Van Nostrand Reinhold Co., New York.

Verstraete, W., and M. Alexander. 1973. Heterotrophic nitrification in samples of natural ecosystems. Environ. Sci. Technol. 7:39–42.

von Dreusche, C., Jr. 1978. Process aspects of regeneration in a multiple–hearth furnace. Pp. 923–953 in P.N. Cheremisinoff and F. Ellerbusch, eds. Carbon Adsorption Handbook. Ann Arbor Science Publishers, Inc., Ann Arbor, Mich.

Weber, W.J., Jr. 1966. Fluid-carbon columns for sorption of persistent organic pollutants. Proc. 3rd Int. Conf. Water Pollut. Res. Water Pollut. Control Fed. Pap. No. 12, Sec. 1, Munich, Federal Republic of Germany.

Weber, W.J., Jr. 1972. Adsorption. Pp. 199–259 in W.J. Weber, Jr., ed. Physicochemical Processes for Water Quality Control. Wiley-Interscience, New York.

Weber, W.J., Jr. 1977. Integrated biological and physico-chemical treatment for reclamation of wastewater. Ind. Water Eng. 14(7):20–27.

Weber, W.J., Jr. 1978. Discussion [of]: Improved performance of activated carbon by pre-ozonization, by W. Guirguis, T. Cooper, J. Harris, and A. Ungar. J. Water Pollut. Control Fed. 50:2781–2783.

Weber, W.J., Jr., and J.P. Gould. 1966. Sorption of organic pesticides from aqueous solution. In Organic Pesticides in the Environment. Advances in Chemistry Series 60. American Chemical Society, Washington, D.C.

Weber, W.J., Jr., and T.M. Keinath. 1967. Mass transfer of perdurable pollutants from dilute aqueous solution in fluidized adsorbers. Chem. Eng. Prog. Symp. 63(74):79–89.

Weber, W.J., Jr., and J.C. Morris. 1963. Kinetics of adsorption of carbon from solution. J. Sanit. Eng. Div. Am. Soc. Civ. Eng. 89(SA2):31–59.

Weber, W.J., Jr., and J.C. Morris. 1964a. Equilibria and capacities for adsorption on carbon. J. Sanit. Eng. Div. Am. Soc. Civ. Eng. 90(SA3):79–107.

Weber, W.J., Jr., and J.C. Morris. 1964b. Adsorption in heterogeneous aqueous systems. J. Am. Water Works Assoc. 56:447–456.

Weber, W.J., Jr., C.B. Hopkins, and J. Bloom. 1970. Physicochemical treatment of municipal wastewater. J. Water Pollut. Control Fed. 42:83–99.

Weber, W.J., Jr., L. D. Friedman, and R. Bloom. 1972. Biologically extended physico-chemical treatment. In S. H. Jenkins, ed. Proceedings of the 6th International Conference on Water Pollution Research (Jerusalem). Advances in Water Pollution Research, pp. 641–656.

Weber, W.J., Jr., M. Pirbazari, M. Herbert, and R. Thompson. 1977. Effectiveness of activated carbon for removal of volatile halogenated hydrocarbons from drinking water. Pp. 125–141 in J.A. Borchardt, J.K. Cleland, W.J. Redman, and G. Olivier, eds. Viruses and Trace Contaminants in Water and Wastewater. Ann Arbor Science Publishers, Inc., Ann Arbor, Mich.

Weber, W.J., Jr., M. Pirbazari, and G.L. Melson. 1978a. Biological growth on activated carbon: An investigation by scanning electron microscopy. Environ. Sci. Technol. 12:817–819.

Weber, W.J., Jr., M. Pirbazari, and M.D. Herbert. 1978b. Removal of halogenated organic and THM precursor compounds from water by activated carbon. Proceedings of the 98th American Works Association Conference. Paper No. 15–1, Atlantic City, N.J.

Weiss, D.E. 1962. The catalytic properties of amorphous carbons. Pp. 65–72 in Proc. Conf. Carbon, 5th, University Park, Pa. 1961. Volume 1. Macmillan Co., New York. (Chem. Abstr. 58:13182b, 1963)

Westrick, J.J., and M.D. Cummins. 1978. Collection of automatic composite samples without atmospheric exposure. Draft Report EPA, March 1978.

Wolff, W. F. 1959. A model of active carbon. J. Phys. Chem. 63:653.

Wood, P., and J. DeMarco. 1980. Effectiveness of various adsorbents in removing organic compounds from water. In I.H. Suffet and M.J. McGuire, eds. Activated Carbon Absorption of Organics from the Aqueous Phase. Proceedings of the 1978 ACS Symposium in Miami Beach, Fla. Ann Arbor Science Publishers, Inc., Ann Arbor, Mich.

Yin, E.T., C. Galanos, S. Kinsky, R.A. Bradshaw, S. Wessler, O. Luderitz, and M.E. Surmiento. 1972. Picogram-sensitive assay for endotoxin: Gelatin of *Limulus polyphemus* blood cell lysate induced by purified lipopolysaccharides lipid A from Gram-negative bacteria. Biochem. Biophys. Acta 261:284–289.

Ying, W.C., and W.J. Weber, Jr. 1978. Bio-physiochemical adsorption systems for wastewater treatment: predictive modeling for design and operation. Presented at the 33rd Annual Purdue Industrial Waste Conference, Purdue University, West Lafayette, Ind.

Yohe, T.L., I.H. Suffet, and R.J. Grochowski. In press. Development of a teflon helix continuous liquid–liquid extraction apparatus and its application for the analysis of organic pollutants in drinking water. ASTM Special Technical Publications. STP 686. Symposium on Organic Pollutants, Denver, Colo., June 19–20, 1978.

Zogorski, J.S. 1975. The adsorption of phenols onto granular activated carbon from aqueous solution. Ph.D. thesis. Rutgers University, The State University of New Jersey, New Brunswick.

Appendix

1977 AMENDMENT TO SAFE DRINKING WATER ACT

Appendix A in the 1977 NAS publication *Drinking Water and Health* (p. 905) is entitled "Legislation and Terms of Reference of the Study." It describes the purpose of the legislation, gives an abridged summary of it, explains why it was needed, and describes what subjects are to be addressed in the National Academy of Sciences study mandated by the Safe Drinking Water Act of 1974 (PL93–523).

Section 1412(e)(2) of the 1974 act called for results of the NAS study to be reported to Congress no later than two (2) years after the date of enactment of the title.

The Safe Drinking Water amendments of 1977 authorized continuation of the agreement with the NAS to revise the study "reflecting new information which has become available since the most recent previous report [and which] shall be reported to Congress each two years thereafter."

Index

383

PAC (*see* powdered activated carbon)
PAH (*see* polynuclear aromatic hydrocarbons)
parasites, 35–36, 48, 67–71
particulates, disinfection effects, 9–11
pathogens, waterborne diseases, 5–6
pesticides, ozonization by-products, 220–
221
phenolic humic model compounds, 161
phenolic substances, reactions, 155
phenols
chlorine dioxide reactions, 196
in competition, 277
ozonization by-products, 210–213
Philadelphia, Pa., water treatment, 276,
287, 298
pilot plant studies, 288, 298, 300, 308–309,
343
Planctomyces, 309
poliovirus, 27, 30–35, 40–41, 46, 49–50,
58–59, 68, 71–72, 78, 80, 90, 93, 97
pollutants
monitoring, 358–361
potential health hazards, 358–359
screening procedures, 359–361
pollution control, carbon regeneration,
270–271, 332–336
polymeric adsorbents, 337–339, 347–353
polynuclear aromatic hydrocarbons,
206–208, 270
chlorination by-products, 163–164
leaching of chemicals, 332
Pomona, Calif., 304, 333
potable water, 186–187
potassium halide—effect on THM formation, 187
potassium permanganate, 297
analytical methods, 99
biocidal activity, 99–101
determination, 99
disinfection, 98–102
E. coli inactivation, 100
mechanism of action, 101
oxidizing agent, 98
production and application, 99
residual, 99
Potomac River, free chlorine–viruses reactions, 31
powdered activated carbon, 252, 255–256,
271, 273–275
prechlorination, 8–9, 303–304

precursors, 140–144
microbial activity, 311
THM, 344–345
preozonization, 298–302
presedimentation, raw water treatment, 8
pretreatment chemicals, organics—adsorption reaction, 270
protozoan parasites, 35
Pseudomonas aeruginosa, 16, 25, 27, 88
Pseudomonas alcaligenes, 15–16
Pseudomonas fluorescens, 45
Pseudomonas sp., 308–310
public water supplies
chlorination, 5
disinfectants, 184–186
disinfection, 5
residuals—disinfection effects, 10–11
pulp and paper industry, 191

Quebec Province, ozonization, 202

radiation, ionizing, disinfection, 94–98
raw water quality, 8–9
recalcitrant organic compounds, 294–295
residuals
disinfection effects, 10–11 (*see also* individual agents)
resinous adsorbents, 338–340
resorcinol, 160–161
Rhine River
bank filtration, 271
breakpoint chlorination, 159
Rotterdam, Netherlands, chlorinated
drinking water, 185
Rouen-la-Chapelle, France, ozonization,
203

Safe Drinking Water Act (PL 93-523), 144
Salmonella montevideo, 89
Salmonella typhi, 13, 25, 27, 30, 45, 75, 84,
88–89, 92–93, 96–97, 104
Schecter method, 48
Schuylkill River, Pa., treatment plant, 153
seawater ozonization, 205
sewage effluent, 155, 157–159, 187–189
Shigella dysenteriae, 25, 27, 88
Shigella flexneri, 45, 84, 96
silver disinfection, 102–106
silver–sulfhydryl complexes, 105
SNORT (*see* stabilized neutral orthotol-
idine method)